The Neuropsychology Casebook

D.L. Orsini W.G. Van Gorp K.B. Boone

The Neuropsychology Casebook

With 27 Illustrations

Springer-Verlag New York Berlin Heidelberg
London Paris Tokyo

DONNA L. ORSINI
Clinical Neuropsychologist, Daniel Freeman Memorial Hospital, Inglewood, California 90301, USA; Clinical Assistant Professor of Psychology, University of Southern California School of Medicine, Los Angeles, California 90033, USA

WILFRED G. VAN GORP
Chief, Neuropsychology Assessment Laboratory, West Los Angeles Veterans Administration Medical Center, Los Angeles, California 90073, USA; Assistant Professor in Residence, Departments of Psychiatry and Biobehavioral Sciences, UCLA School of Medicine, Los Angeles, California 90024, USA

KYLE BRAUER BOONE
Assistant Clinical Professor of Neuropsychology, Departments of Psychiatry and Biobehavioral Sciences, UCLA School of Medicine, Los Angeles, California 90024, USA; Research Associate and Clinical Supervisor (Neuropsychology), Department of Psychiatry, Harbor-UCLA Medical Center, Los Angeles, California 90509, USA

Library of Congress Cataloging-in-Publication Data
Orsini, Donna Lotstein.
The neuropsychology casebook.
Includes bibliographies.
1. Clinical neuropsychology—Case studies.
I. Van Grop, Wilfred G. II. Boone, Kyle Brauer.
III. Title. [DNLM: 1. Head Injuries—case studies.
2. Nervous System Diseases—case studies.
3. Neurologic Examination—case studies.
4. Neuropsychological Tests. WI 141 076n]
RC386.5.077 1988 616.8 87-32325

Softcover reprint of the hardcover 1st edition 1988

Typeset by Publishers Service, Bozeman, Montana.

9 8 7 6 5 4 3 2 1

ISBN-13: 978-1-4612-8371-3 e-ISBN-13: 978-1-4612-3836-2
DOI: 10.1007/978-1-4612-3836-2

Preface

The Neuropsychology Casebook was developed to fill the existing gap in the current body of literature on clinical neuropsychology. Although texts are available that describe neuropsychological tests and others provide information on syndromes, this volume provides descriptions of neuropsychological test performance for individuals with various syndromes. It was designed to illustrate the process of clinical interpretation of test findings and report writing for the individual case. Our aims are to provide both the student and practicing professional with a collection of actual neuropsychological case studies that typify many of the cardinal disorders or syndromes frequently seen by practicing clinical neuropsychologists. We have not provided an exhaustive survey of case studies representing many of the disorders commonly seen in neuropsychology; rather, we have focused on a few select cases that illustrate some of the more common disorders.

This book includes detailed case reports complete with referral questions, historical information, relevant neuroradiological findings, actual neuropsychological test data, and clinical interpretations that take into account all available information on the patient. The cases are discussed in the chapter commentaries with reference to how each compares and contrasts with the prototypic case for that disorder or syndrome. Such case studies help to highlight the various types of behavioral and cognitive sequelae associated with common clinical disorders. The case studies, which are examined through an hypothesis-testing approach, are also aimed at demonstrating how neuropsychological principles and methods are applied.

Case presentations are based on actual patients referred for neuropsychological evaluation. The majority of these cases were referred to the UCLA Neuropsychiatric Institute where each patient was evaluated by one of the authors while serving as post-doctoral fellows in the UCLA Neuropsychology Training Program. A number of cases were also selected from patients evaluated under the supervision of Dr. Van Gorp at the West Los Angeles Veterans Administration Center (Brentwood Division) and from the Harbor–UCLA Medical Center, Department of Psychiatry, where they were evaluated under the supervision of Dr. Boone.

We are deeply indebted to Dr. Paul Satz for his close guidance and support while we were his trainees as post-doctoral neuropsychology fellows at UCLA.

It is out of the tradition of case example, taught to us by Dr. Satz, that this book is written.

We also would like to acknowledge the support of the UCLA fellows, past and present, West Los Angeles Veterans Administration staff and interns, and Harbor-UCLA interns, including Allen Brandon, Louis D'Elia, Julianne Fishman, Patricia Gross, Robert Kern, Cheryl Lanktree, Alexander Piatka, and David Schretlen. We also acknowledge the helpful comments of Dean Delis in his review of an earlier stage of a section of our manuscript. Special thanks are also extended to individuals who have been supportive as well as inspirational to our work, Drs. Jeffrey Cummings and Frank Benson. Finally, we would like to thank our families—Enzo Orsini, Lauren Orsini, Rodney Boone, and Steve Buckingham—for their support and encouragement during the course of this project.

DONNA L. ORSINI
WILFRED G. VAN GORP
KYLE BRAUER BOONE

Contents

Introduction

Purpose of the Neuropsychological Evaluation

Neuropsychological assessment has gained increasing popularity over the past decade as its contributions have become widely recognized. Consequently, neuropsychologists are now more commonly employed in such settings as acute care and rehabilitation hospitals, clinics, and private offices. The overall benefits of a thorough neuropsychological evaluation are manifold—to determine the effects of a brain insult on cognitive and emotional functioning; to provide a description of the extent and quality of cognitive, emotional, and/or motor dysfunction; to provide a measure of the patient's potential and course of recovery following brain injury; to provide a calculated estimate of the baseline (or premorbid) level of functioning; to assist in the formulation of a differential diagnosis; to help determine localization of lesion; and to facilitate educational, vocational, and rehabilitation planning.

The neuropsychological evaluation can offer a measure of the patient's overall pattern of cognitive strengths and weaknesses. Moreover, repeated assessments over time provide an index of behavioral change that allows factors such as treatment interventions, progression or improvement of illness, aging, and developmental growth to be systematically evaluated. The differential diagnosis between a CNS-based disease and a process that is primarily "functional" in origin is an important aspect of the neuropsychological evaluation, particularly as it impacts on the method of treatment intervention.

Neuropsychological evaluations generally prove to be useful in a variety of contexts. Individuals who potentially could benefit from a neuropsychological evaluation include: 1) patients with known central nervous system (CNS) dysfunction such as stroke, head injury, tumor, or dementia for assessment of cognitive/emotional functioning aimed at providing information regarding degree of deficits and the extent of sparing of functioning; 2) individuals with suspected, but undocumented, CNS dysfunction to ascertain the presence of any cognitive dysfunction; or 3) individuals undergoing treatment (i.e., medication, surgery) that may effect a cognitive/behavioral change secondary to the intervention.

The Neuropsychological Evaluation

A thorough neuropsychological evaluation includes: 1) careful review of all available medical records; 2) a detailed interview with the patient and/or family member; and 3) the quantitative and qualitative assessment of cognitive, motor, and emotional functioning, and interpretation of these findings.

Interview

The interview process is an integral part of the neuropsychological examination as it provides an opportunity to gather data on the patient's background and presenting problems that will moderate interpretation of the test scores. It also offers an opportunity for the examiner to formulate hypotheses regarding the patient's underlying cognitive deficits, which can be tested during the evaluative process. For this reason, the interview should be conducted before the testing whenever possible. It is often useful to interview a family member or significant other in addition to the patient. This is particularly worthwhile when the patient's ability to supply historical information is in question, such as in the case of a demented individual. During collection of historical information and test administration, the examiner should note the patient's mental status, mood and affect, general response style, test-taking attitude, personality attributes, speech characteristics (prosody, fluency), and general physical appearance (grooming, physical anomalies). Also, it is helpful to determine the patient's degree of insight regarding his or her illness and reasons for the evaluation. All of these factors will prove useful in making a differential diagnosis.

Information regarding the patient's background is significant because it helps the examiner to formulate a working hypothesis of the patient's premorbid state of functioning. Data regarding occupational and educational attainments of the patient and immediate family members may provide an index of the patient's endowed intelligence and cognitive potential. Such information is valuable in the interpretation of test results and when making estimates related to extent and quality of cognitive loss following brain injury.

Specific aspects of the personal history to be queried include basic information regarding the patient's age, gender, cultural background, educational level and performance, and occupational status and history. Information regarding self-professed handedness and familial sinistrality may uncover subtle differences in brain organization that could underlie different methods of approaching cognitive tasks. A detailed account of past insults to the central nervous system should also be obtained, such as head injuries sustained in childhood or adulthood. It is important to determine whether the patient has had any past hospitalizations, surgeries, or treatment, or has been exposed to toxic substances (i.e., paint, asbestos, lead).

Indicators of the patient's premorbid strengths and weaknesses are important to consider as well. These kinds of data could be obtained by asking the patient which subjects he or she performed best and worst in school or by identifying hobbies. Information should be collected regarding birth and developmental history, such as language and motor milestones in particular, to provide data regarding possible developmental slowness or learning disabilities. It should be determined whether the patient has engaged in previous psychological or neuropsychological testing, and if so, those results should be obtained for comparative purposes. Also, information regarding intake of alcohol and recreational and prescribed drugs should be obtained. It is important to ascertain whether the patient has had any chronic illnesses or is currently taking any medications. Information regarding whether the patient has incurred injury to his upper extremities is important for interpretation of the results of the motor examination. Furthermore, the examiner is advised to question whether the patient has had any past psychiatric hospitalizations or treatment, any unusual perceptual experiences such as auditory or visual hallucinations, strange sensations, depression, or suicidal ideation or plans. It is also important to ascertain whether there is a family history of psychiatric and/or neurologic illnesses.

A description of the patient's presenting cognitive, physical, and psychological complaints and symptoms should be obtained. This should include information regarding whether the symptoms developed insidiously or acutely, data that could bear importance in the differential diagnosis, for example, of a vascular disorder. Accordingly, the examiner should investigate whether the patient has had any recent changes in either sleeping or eating habits, hand preference or strength, cognitive state, or mood.

Testing Approach

The evaluative process provides a measure of the patient's cognitive and emotional strengths and weaknesses, helps in formulating a diagnosis of the illness, and leads to recommendations to help improve the patient's quality of life. Often recommendations are most useful when they provide strategies (i.e., mnemonic) to help the person adapt to or cope with cognitive problems. Toward this aim, it is necessary to first understand the pattern of neuropsychological performance; that is, the specific nature of the patient's deficits and preserved abilities. A flexible approach that tests hypotheses in a systematic fashion is quite helpful toward this goal.

The hypothesis-testing approach, based on the teaching of A.R. Luria (1966; 1973), provides an exemplary framework for neuropsychological assessment. Essentially, this approach entails testing patient-specific hypotheses regarding locus, quality, and extent of brain impairment. These hypotheses can be generated based on the information obtained from medical records, the interview, and from the referring source. Specific tests are then administered to help determine the degree of impairment or preservation of various cognitive functions. After a deficit is identified on screening, additional tasks can be administered to more carefully delineate the nature of the dysfunction. For example, a gross memory impairment may be uncovered upon brief examination, which then may be followed by careful verbal versus nonverbal, free recall versus recognition memory testing to ascertain the quality and extent of memory impairment. In the final analysis, each patient is administered a battery of tests unique to his/her symptomatology. Luria strongly advocated focusing on the manner in which a person solves a task and not only on the quantitative score derived from the test. This emphasis on the process in which a task is solved is also advocated by Edith Kaplan (1983). For example, a patient eventually might be able to copy a complex line drawing, but the strategy may be quite haphazard and inefficient, suggesting some compromise although the final product may be within normal limits. Moreover, test interpretation is never based on a single test score but on the overall profile of test performance as a whole.

The hypothesis-testing approach differs from a predesignated or standard battery approach, such as the Halstead-Reitan Battery (Reitan & Davison, 1974) or Luria-Nebraska Battery (Golden, Hammeke, & Purisch, 1978), in several ways. The standard battery approach generally entails administration of a fixed set of tasks to each patient regardless of presenting symptomatology. Because of its rigid nature, the battery approach confers less flexibility and is often less proficient at determining the individual profile of abilities and weaknesses. Generally, it also focuses less on the quality or manner in which the patient performs a task and more on the test score, and may thereby tend to overlook important subtleties. This is particularly true if the battery is administered by a technician not trained in neuropsychology, who may miss methods of the patient's task solving approach that represent characteristic types of dysfunction. Another problem with the battery approach, particularly by the Halstead-Reitan Battery, is length of test administration. Tests are administered that may not be pertinent to the individual patient. A long battery may not only be costly for the patient, but can also be very arduous and tiresome for the impaired patient. Another significant concern with fixed batteries such as the Halstead is that they are not able to sufficiently measure memory, language, or "frontal lobe" functioning. Recently, our knowledge regarding these areas of cognition has vastly increased, and new and more sophisticated tests have been devised. The hypothesis-testing approach allows ready incorporation of such new tasks; batteries, by their fixed nature, remain locked to the knowledge available at the time of the battery development.

Another problem with the battery approach is misuse by untrained individuals. For example, the Luria-Nebraska Battery (Golden et al., 1978) has a high probability for diagnostic errors by individuals who have had no formal training in brain behavior relationships. The Luria-Nebraska Battery carries the illusion of straightforward locus-function determinations. The presence of 14 scales that purport to link structure with function invite misuse of this battery by individuals who are not fully knowledgeable regarding neuropsychological theory. Adding to this problem is the fact that questions have been raised regarding the development and validity of the batteries. For example, users of the Luria-Nebraska Battery are at a disadvantage because the samples used in standardizing it have not been well controlled for age, education, and medication, among other factors

(Adams, 1980). There are additional problems concerning the validity of the scoring system as well (Adams, 1979; Spiers, 1981).

Although each predesignated battery may be too rigid by itself, it is often useful to incorporate some of the tasks from the batteries when they are warranted. In this regard, some of the tasks from the Halstead-Reitan Battery can be used very effectively without requiring the administration of the entire battery.

We utilize various tasks in an effort to survey a functional area (i.e., intelligence, attention and concentration, verbal and nonverbal memory, language, perception and sensation, motor skill). Table I lists some tasks that are often useful for adults when measuring cognitive, emotional, and motor functioning.

More detailed information regarding the tests, including descriptions, can be found for most of these tests in Lezak's (1976; 1983) texts on neuropsychological assessment. It should be noted that some of the functional categories overlap, hence some tasks can be included in more than one category (i.e., the Rey-Osterrieth Complex Figure can provide information regarding both memory and perceptual functioning).

The hypothesis-testing approach to assessment can be used with the measures listed in Table I. For example, if poor performance on the Block Design and Object Assembly subtests of the WAIS-R are uncovered, the examiner may hypothesize that the patient has problems in visual-motor integration. To test whether these problems are also found without a motor component, the Hooper Visual Organization Test may be administered. If the patient performs within the normal range on this measure, one tenable hypothesis is that visual perceptual processes are intact and that the deficit lies in constructional ability. Another example – the patient who presents with reduced ability to generate vocabulary definitions on the vocabulary subtest of the WAIS-R can be administered the PPVT-R to assess whether an actual loss of vocabulary is present or whether the deficit lies mainly in the expression of linguistic knowledge.

Test Interpretation

Interpretation of the neuropsychological test performance should consider factors related to individual variability, qualitative analysis, test-taking behavior, test conditions, test score conversions, and normative data. Each of these factors is discussed in the following sections.

Individual Variability

Results of the neuropsychological exam should be considered in light of the individual's unique background information. Such background variables, discussed earlier, include cultural background, native language, handedness, educational and occupational attainments, and endowed intelligence. An individual from a different culture and for whom English is a second language

TABLE I. Useful tests for measuring functional neuropsychological competence in adults.

Intelligence	
	Wechsler Adult Intelligence Scale–Revised (WAIS-R)
Attention/Concentration	
	Digit Span
	Trail Making
	Wechsler Memory Scale–Mental Control subtest
	Continuous Performance Test
	Serial 7s Subtraction
Language	
	Boston Diagnostic Aphasia Examination
	Boston Naming Test
	Controlled Word Association Test (FAS)
	Reitan-Indiana Aphasia Screening Exam
	Token Test
	Peabody Picture Vocabulary Test–Revised (PPVT-R)
Verbal Memory	
	California Verbal Learning Test
	Rey Auditory Verbal Learning Test
	Shopping List Test
	Wechsler Memory Scale
	Logical Memory subtest with delayed recall[a]
	Associate Learning subtest with delayed recall[a]
Nonverbal Memory	
	Wechsler Memory Scale–Visual Reproductions subtest with delayed recall[a]
	Rey-Osterrieth Complex Figure with 3 minute delayed recall
Perceptual/Organizational	
	Rey-Osterrieth Complex Figure–Copy format
	Hooper Visual Organization Test
	Beery Visual Motor Integration Test
	Draw-a-Clock
Sensory	
	Halstead-Reitan Sensory-Perceptual Exam
Motor	
	Finger Tapping
	Grooved Pegboard
	Grip Strength
	Lateral Dominance Exam
Frontal Systems	
	Wisconsin Card Sorting Test
	Rey Tangled Lines
	Auditory Consonant Trigrams
	Stroop Test
Personality	
	Minnesota Multiphasic Personality Inventory
	Sentence Completion
	Thematic Apperception Text
Academic Achievement	
	Wide Range Achievement Test–Revised (WRAT-R)
	Peabody Individual Achievement Test (PIAT)

[a] Delayed recall is typically assessed 20–60 minutes following the initial presentation (Lezak, 1983).

typically will be at a disadvantage on most standardized tests that have been normed on English-speaking Americans. Also, bilingual individuals for whom English is a second language often perform verbal tasks more poorly than nonverbal tasks. In addition, task performance may be influenced by the person's genetic manual laterality.

The individual's level of intellectual functioning should be considered when interpreting neuropsychological test scores. For example, verbal memory functioning should be interpreted within the context of one's verbal intellectual functioning as they are expected to be at comparable levels. The person's educational level and occupational role can provide a general means to estimate the premorbid intellectual level of the patient. This is most important in ascertaining the extent, if any, of the cognitive loss following brain injury. For example, a person with a law degree employed as an attorney presenting with low average intellectual functioning following a brain injury may be suspect for recent deterioration in cognitive processing abilities. In comparison, another person who scores in the low average range on intellectual testing, who has a considerably lower educational and occupational level, may be less likely to have presenting low intellectual level explained by a recent brain insult. Overall, most scores should be interpreted in light of IQ and educational and occupational attainments.

Qualitative Analysis

The process by which the patient solves a task may lend generous insights into the underlying deficit. Kaplan (1983) provides an excellent example of this in her description of the process approach to the Block Design task. She points out that brain-damaged individuals will frequently solve this task in a characteristic fashion depending on the laterality of the lesion. Individuals with damage to the right side of the brain generally fail to attend to the gestalt of the geometric pattern, whereas those with left-sided damage are able to preserve the configuration matrix but tend to display simplification and confusion.

Test-Taking Behavior

Test performance can be affected by a host of behavioral considerations. For example, factors such as low motivation, anxiety, fatigue, or the transient effects of medication may generate the appearance of a deficit or may exacerbate real deficits. Moreover, performance may be manipulated by a patient with attempts to feign a deficit, either consciously or unconsciously. Other times, a patient's impulsive style in task solving will denigrate test performance. Equally important in test score interpretation is the patient's familiarity with the test materials. If the patient has been exposed to a particular test before, practice effects may spuriously elevate test performance. However, depending on the type of brain injury, brain-injured individuals may not always manifest practice effects (Shatz, 1981).

Test Conditions

Test conditions that are less than optimal may generate apparent, but not real, deficits; other times they may enhance real deficits. Poor test conditions are caused by noise, inadequate lighting, and distractions, among other factors. Realistically, optimal test conditions are not always possible. This is particularly true for the hospital patient who may require bedside test administration. Testing under such conditions may be hampered by intrusions of hospital staff during task administration, particularly during attention testing. Also, a hospital roommate may induce distractions and noise factors. Moreover, it is not always possible to administer all tests that are considered important due to time constraints or limited patient cooperation.

Test Score Conversions

Raw test scores can be converted to standard scores to reflect how the individual's performance deviates from the average. The Z-score represents the amount of deviation of a score from the mean of the population from which it is drawn. It can be computed using the following formula:

$$Z = \frac{\text{raw score} - \text{mean score}}{\text{standard deviation}}$$

The normal curve has a mean of zero and a standard deviation of one. The distance in standard units that a score is from the mean of a comparison standard will determine test performance. It is generally accepted that differences of two standard deviations or more may be considered significant, whereas differences of one to two standard deviations suggest a trend (Payne & Jones, 1957).

Converting the raw score to a percentile is also helpful in describing how the individual's performance differs from an average score on that particular measure. Percentiles are also more readily understood by the general public than are Z-scores. Percentile equivalents can be calculated based on a table of normal curve functions (see Appendix, Table A), which presents percentile ranks from 1 to 99 and corresponding Z-score equivalents. To show how to use this table, we will take an example of a finger tapping normative score, which has a mean of 45.2 and a standard deviation of 6.0. An individual who obtains a score of 50.6 will be compared with the norm by converting his or her raw score into a score using the standard formula above:

$$\frac{50.6 - 45.2}{6.0} = .90$$

Using the table, one can see that the percentile equivalent to a Z-score of +.90 is 82. Therefore, this individual's ability level on the Finger Tapping Test is found to be at the 82nd percentile. To interpret this percentile in terms of ability level, refer to the commonly accepted classification of ability levels (see Appendix,

Table B). This table indicates that the finger tapping score of 50.6, with a corresponding Z-score of .90 and a percentile rank of 82, is within the high average range of ability.

Normative Data

Interpretation of test performance is based on how the individual's performance differs from a comparison standard and generally involves the way "normal," or non-brain-damaged, people perform on the particular measure. A major problem in neuropsychological assessment at this time is that few tests are properly normed. A well normed test involves administering the measure to a large sample of individuals with stratified sampling. Accordingly, one of the best normed measures is the Wechsler Adult Intelligence Scale–Revised (WAIS-R) (Wechsler, 1955; 1981), which has been normed on a large sample of individuals classified by age, sex, race, geographic region, occupation, education, and urban-rural residence. Unfortunately, few neuropsychological tests have been standardized in this manner. Moreover, normative information may differ for the same tests based on different researchers collecting normative data on small sample sizes. Variations in test scores may reflect sample differences including age, sex, cultural background, and educational level. This often renders differences in test interpretation depending on which norms were used to interpret the patient's test performance. Another problem is that it is often quite difficult to locate normative data on certain tests. In light of these problems, we present a list of references for normative data for the majority of tests discussed in the case presentations that appear in subsequent chapters (see Appendix, Table C). It should be noted that additional normative data are also available for many of these tests.

Report Writing

There are various ways to write an effective neuropsychological report, thereby precluding the idea of any one ideal approach. However, there are some key features that can enhance the usefulness of any neuropsychological report.

The effectiveness of a neuropsychological report can be augmented when the following factors are included:

1. Statement of the referral question–the referring professional's reason for requesting a neuropsychological examination
2. Presenting symptoms–behavioral, cognitive, and/or neurological
3. Background and historical information on the patient
4. Behavioral observations of the patient during the evaluation
5. List of neuropsychological and psychological tests administered
6. Test results and interpretation presented by functional system–intelligence, memory, language, and motor, for example
7. Summary impressions, conclusions, and recommendations

The above factors provide a general outline for basic report writing. It is often helpful to begin a report by stating the reason for the referral, the source of the referral, and what is expected to be accomplished by the neuropsychological evaluation. A thorough history of the patient's background is also critical, including presenting illness and/or symptoms, medical history, and educational and occupational levels. Background historical information should present an integrated summary of information obtained from the medical chart, referring source, and the interview. Behavioral observations of the patient during the evaluation are also useful information. This should include the person's test-taking attitude, mental status, mood and affect, general response style, personality attributes, speech characteristics, and general physical appearance. A list of the tests administered is also helpful, particularly to other psychologists whose familiarity with them will enhance their understanding of the report. It is our general practice to include in each report a list of the tests administered, with scores listed in the report text, rather than a data summary sheet. However, for the purposes of this book, we have provided a data summary sheet that also provides names of the tests administered. Finally, the report should conclude with a summary of findings with appropriate recommendations. In this section, the facts from the patient's background history, behavior during evaluation, and test results can be integrated to form impressions and conclusions regarding his or her problems, their underlying etiology, and ways in which to treat the patient. It is useful to include specific treatment intervention strategies, particularly to aid in plans for rehabilitation.

Accordingly, a report that uses subsections based on the above points can be very effective and straightforward. The following outline can be used:

Outline for a Neuropsychological Report

Name of Patient:
Patient's Birthdate:
Patient's Hospital Identification Number (if any):
Date of Evaluation:

Reason for Referral—specific referral questions.
Pertinent History—age, sex, handedness, education, occupation, medical and psychiatric history, description of symptoms.
Behavioral Observations—test-taking behavior, mood, affect, salient personality characteristics, attire, grooming.
Tests Administered—list of individual tests.
Test Results—listed by function, including scores converted to percentiles and descriptive statements of the manner in which tests were approached and attempted.

Function

Gross Cognitive
Intelligence

Attention/Concentration
Language
Perceptual/Organizational
Memory
  Verbal
  Nonverbal
Motor
Sensory
Frontal Systems
Academic Achievement
Personality

Summary Impression—integration of the results with statements as to possible diagnosis and treatment recommendations.

Our approach is to present the test results by functional systems (i.e., intelligence, memory, visual spatial, motor, language). This assists in making decisions regarding localization of dysfunction and helps to target behaviors for rehabilitation efforts. A thorough neuropsychological report should include not only test score equivalents but also descriptive statements regarding the manner in which the tasks were approached and/or solved. The latter type of information may lend insights into the nature of the underlying deficits.

Summary

The information presented in this introduction has been designed to assist in: 1) determining the circumstances under which a neuropsychological evaluation is useful, 2) understanding the essentials of the neuropsychological exam, 3) presenting some commonly used tasks, 4) providing a test interpretation guide, and 5) furnishing a format for report writing.

The chapters that follow should clarify some of these points by providing actual neuropsychological reports. Each chapter begins with a brief, general overview of the condition and presents some basic cognitive findings that may be revealed on neuropsychological exam. These brief chapter introductions are not intended as conclusive summaries or critiques of the literature. Rather, they may offer the student or trainee a synopsis of general neuropsychological correlates of the syndromes, thereby providing a framework for understanding the case presentations. Case reports are then presented to illustrate the process of clinical interpretation of test findings and report writing. We have not provided an exhaustive selection of cases to fit all the various types of syndromes or disorders seen in neuropsychology. Rather, a few cases were selected that are believed to typify the more common types of disorders referred to neuropsychologists in a clinic or acute care setting. The case presentations are based on actual patients who were referred for neuropsychological evaluation in a hospital or clinic and identifying factors have been obscured to protect confidentiality. Case presentations include historical information, reason for referral, test data (both quantitative and qualitative), a quantitative test data summary sheet, and summary interpretation and recommendations. The case presentations illustrate how to integrate historical information, test data, and qualitative indices to aid in patient diagnosis, care, and rehabilitation planning.

The case studies, which are examined through an hypothesis-testing approach, are also aimed at demonstrating how neuropsychological principles and methods are applied. Each chapter concludes with a brief commentary that helps to illuminate or highlight important features.

REFERENCES

Adams, K. (1979). Linear discriminant analysis in clinical neuropsychology research. *Journal of Clinical Neuropsychology, 1*, 259–272.

Adams, K. (1980). In search of Luria's battery: A false start. *Journal of Consulting and Clinical Psychology, 48*, 511–516.

Bornstein, R.A. (1985). Normative data on selected neuropsychological measures from a nonclinical sample. *Journal of Clinical Psychology, 41*, 651–659.

Butters, N., Wolfe, J., Granholm, E., & Martone, M. (1986). An assessment of verbal recall, recognition, and fluency abilities in patients with Huntington's disease. *Cortex, 22*, 11–32.

Comalli, P.E., Wapner, S., & Werner, H. (1962). Interference effects of Stroop color-word test in childhood, adulthood, and aging. *Journal of Genetic Psychology, 100*, 47–53.

Delaney, R.C., Rosen, A.J., Mattson, E.H., & Novelly, R.A. (1980). Memory function in focal epilepsy: A comparison of nonsurgical, unilateral temporal lobe and frontal lobe samples. *Cortex, 16*, 103–117.

Folstein, M.F., Folstein, S.E., & McHugh, P.R. (1975). Mini-mental state: A practical method for grading the cognitive state of patients for the clinician. *Journal of Psychiatric Research, 12*, 189–198.

Golden, C., Hammeke, T., & Purisch, A. (1978). Diagnostic validity of a standardized neuropsychological battery derived from Luria's neuropsychological tests. *Journal of Consulting and Clinical Psychology, 46*, 1258–1265.

Haaland, K.Y., Linn, R.T., Hunt, W.C., & Goodwin, J.S. (1983). A normative study of Russell's variant of the Wechsler Memory Scale in a healthy elderly population. *Journal of Consulting and Clinical Psychology, 51*, 878–881.

Hulicka, I.M. (1966). Age difference in Wechsler Memory Scale scores. *Journal of Genetic Psychology, 109*, 135–145.

Kaplan, E. (1983). Process and achievement revisited. In S. Wapner & B. Kaplan (Eds.), *Toward a holistic developmental psychology.* Hillsdale, NJ: Lawrence Erlbaum.

Lezak, M. (1976). *Neuropsychological assessment.* New York: Oxford University Press.

Lezak, M. (1983). *Neuropsychological assessment* (2nd ed.). New York: Oxford University Press.

Luria, A.R. (1966). *Higher cortical functions in man.* New York: Basic Books.

Luria, A.R. (1973). *The working brain: An introduction to neuropsychology.* New York: Basic Books.

McCarthy, M., Ferris, S.H., Clarke, E., & Crook, T. (1981). *Experimental Aging Research, 7*, 127–135.

Mungas, D. (1983). Differential clinical sensitivity of specific parameters of the Rey Auditory-Verbal Learning Test. *Journal of Consulting and Clinical Psychology, 51*, 848–855.

Payne, R.W., & Jones, H.G. (1957). Statistics for the investigation of individual cases. *Journal of Clinical Psychology, 13*, 115–121.

Reitan, R.M., & Davison, L.A. (1974). *Clinical neuropsychology: Current status and applications*. New York: Hemisphere.

Shatz, M.W. (1981). WAIS practice effects in clinical neuropsychology. *Journal of Clinical Neuropsychology, 3*, 171–179.

Spiers, P. (1981). Have they come to praise Luria or to bury him? The Luria-Nebraska Battery controversy. *Journal of Clinical and Consulting Psychology, 49*, 331–341.

Stuss, D.T., Ely, P., Hugenholtz, M.D., Richard, M.T., LaRochelle, S., Poirier, C.A., & Bell, I. (1985). Subtle neuropsychological deficits in patients with good recovery after closed head surgery. *Neurosurgery, 17*, 41–47.

Stuss, D.T., Kaplan, E.F., Benson, D.F., Weir, W.S., Chiulli, S., & Sarazin, F.F. (1982). Evidence for the involvement of orbitofrontal cortex in memory functions: An interference effect. *Journal of Comparative and Physiological Psychology, 96*, 913–925.

Wechsler, D. (1955). *Manual for the Wechsler Adult Intelligence Scale*. New York: The Psychological Corporation.

Wechsler, D. (1981). *Manual for the Wechsler Adult Intelligence Scale—Revised*. New York: The Psychological Corporation.

1 Head Injury

Clinical neuropsychologists are evaluating an increasing number of head injured patients, largely because of rapid gains that are being made in the emergency medical treatment of such patients, thus decreasing the mortality rate. Another reason for the increase in referrals is that it is becoming ever more recognized that even seemingly minor head injury, including those cases with good recovery, often present with quantifiable and clinically relevant neuropsychological deficits that may not be evident on gross neurologic exam or neurobehavioral interview (e.g., Barth, Macciocchi, Giordani, Rimel, Jane, & Boll, 1983; Stuss, Ely, Hugenholtz, Richard, LaRochelle, Poirier, & Bell, 1985). Because referrals of head injured patients are on the rise and the clinician is likely to see a fair number of these cases, it is advisable for him or her to be well informed in the basic neuropathology of head injury and the concomitant implications for planning a sensitive and thorough neuropsychological assessment of these patients.

Presented below are what we believe to be the essentials for the professional to understand when planning and conducting a neuropsychological evaluation of the head injured patient. As is true with all overviews in this book, this is intended only as a survey of the most important concepts, and the reader is strongly encouraged to consult additional sources for more comprehensive information, such as the excellent work on closed head injury by Levin, Benton and Grossman (1982), and the chapter on head trauma in Adams and Victor (1985). Though there is a large literature regarding specific test findings on various measures in head injured patients, we will deemphasize presentation of a specific pattern of test findings in this overview because head injured patients are a heterogeneous group, precluding the illusion of "uniform deficits." However, we will provide principles that will allow the clinician to understand and develop an adequate neuropsychological test battery in order to carefully assess the head injured patient.

Types of Head Injury

Traditionally, classification of head injury has been divided into cases of open and closed injury, and because the two categories have different implications for evaluation, we will follow such division here.

Open Head Injury

In cases of open head injury, the scalp is lacerated, the skull is penetrated by an intruding object or force (such as a bullet, missile projectile, or fragments from exploding objects as are often seen during wartime), and a portion of the brain is directly damaged by the intruding object and/or fragments of the skull that may be depressed into brain tissue. In these cases, the point of penetration is usually clear, and neuroradiologic imaging such as CT or MRI scan will readily reveal the direct site of immediate damage. This localization of direct damage allows for the formulation of hypotheses regarding predictable deficits based on the area of the brain directly affected. For example, a bullet crossing through the lateral convexity of the left frontal lobe will usually prompt the neuropsychologist to assess frontal lobe functions and possible changes in attention abilities, executive problem-solving skills, motor dexterity and strength, and/or personality since the accident.

Unfortunately, knowledge of the direct site of impact in cases of open head injury may lure the neuropsychologist into focusing on a specific area or functional system at the cost of neglecting other functional areas that also may have been affected by the more diffuse effects found in head trauma. This latter component will be discussed more fully below.

Closed Head Injury

Closed head injury is produced by rapid acceleration followed by deceleration of the head, resulting in rapid linear and/or rotational movement of the brain against the hard, bony inner surface of the skull. As will be discussed below, predictions of impaired functioning based upon the "site" of this type of damage are not as easily made as no clear site of damage is often known. Unlike cases of open head injury, CT scan and other indices will likely reflect only the swelling or edema of the brain as a result of the injury, but generally no focal areas are seen on neuroimaging studies. The neuropsychologist should consider other factors affecting neuropsychological status following closed head injury, such as the point of impact and coup and contrecoup effects, neurological complications (e.g., hematoma), length of coma and post-traumatic amnesia, and age of the patient in the evaluation and assessment of sequelae following head injury. As is true for open head injury as well, older patients often have more medical complications and a slower recovery rate than younger patients.

Coup and Contrecoup Effects in Closed Head Injury

As the brain, sitting in its liquid medium and resting on its stem, is thrust against the hard, unmoving skull during impact or rapid acceleration/deceleration, *coup contusion* (or bruising of the brain under the point of impact) results. However, as the brain is thrust either forward or backward, or is rotated on its axis, it is not only bruised at the direct point of impact, but it is often thrust against the opposite or contralateral side of the skull, producing a *contrecoup effect* (i.e., bruising of the brain on the side opposite to the initial point of impact). Coup and contrecoup effects are essential for the neuropsychologist to understand because "localizing" signs seen in the test results initially can seem confusing if they point to focal areas of deficit not consistent with the initial site of impact. This is especially important because contrecoup effects are very common and have been estimated to range as high as 50% to 80% (Lezak, 1983).

Another factor for the neuropsychologist to consider is that the skull is not a uniformly smooth surface covering and protecting the brain. Certain bony irregularities may make bruising in some areas more likely. For instance, common sites of cerebral contusions or bruising are in the *frontal* and *temporal* lobes because of the "curved" shape of the cranium cradling these areas (cf., Adams & Victor, 1985). Thus, frontal and temporal areas are particularly vulnerable to injury following all types of closed head injury. Therefore, it is especially important for the neuropsychologist to assess frontal and temporal lobe functions fully in any closed head injury evaluation.

Frontal lobe damage may not be readily apparent on standard, highly structured psychometric tests, and inclusion of specific tests for frontal and temporal lobe functions is essential. This is cogently illustrated in a study by Stuss and coworkers (1985) who compared neuropsychological test results on 20 head injured patients with results on 20 normals, matched for age, sex, handedness, native language, and IQ. The head injured group had sustained head injury of varying levels of severity, but most importantly, all had returned to work and had been judged to have made a "good recovery." No significant differences were found between the head injured group and normal controls on most of the neuropsychological tests used, though selected tests measuring divided attention did show differences. The Consonant Trigrams Test—a sensitive test of attention and memory under conditions of interference—was the most discriminating test in the battery, and group differences were also found on the Stroop Test (time), the Digit Symbol subtest of the WAIS, Trails A, and Wisconsin Card Sorting Test (number of perseverative errors). Stuss and colleagues note that lowered performance consistently appeared on tests involving divided attention, and they concluded that the head injured individual is limited "in information processing capacity, either in terms of speed of processing or in terms of the amount of information that can be simultaneously handled." They noted that most neuropsychological tests would not disclose these deficits, and urged that tests specifically sensitive to frontal lobe functioning and divided attention be included in assessment of all head injured patients.

Language and memory functioning may also be differentially affected because of the vulnerability of the temporal lobes to damage in head trauma. Heilman, Safran, and Geschwind (1971), in a detailed study of closed head injured patients, found anomic aphasia to be the most frequent language abnormality in their group of patients. A similar finding was reported by Levin, Grossman, and Kelly (1976) who studied closed head injured patients of varying levels of injury with a variety of language tests. One of the most notable findings from their study was that nearly half showed deficits in naming or verbal fluency. Thus, deficits in confrontational naming and verbal fluency appear to be frequent sequelae of closed head injury in a wide array of patients sustaining varying degrees of injury.

Several studies have examined effects of head injury on memory functioning. In one such study, van Zomeren and van den Berg (1985) found that 84% of a sample of patients with severe closed head injury reported "forgetfulness" as their most common cognitive symptom. They also found that complaints including forgetfulness, slowness to respond or process information, and poor ability to concentrate and to divide attention between two competing activities correlated significantly with severity of injury.

It should also be noted that frontal lobe damage (and damage to other brain structures, particularly involving the limbic system) may cause changes in personality that may be misdiagnosed as strictly psychiatric in origin. Such characteristics include disinhibition, rage outbursts, inappropriate sexual gestures, pressured and rambling speech, and behavior resembling a manic episode.

Shearing/Tearing Effects

Quite apart from any coup or contrecoup effects are the microscopic white matter lesions resulting from the shearing and tearing of neuronal fibers of the brain not evident on CT scanning. Ommaya and Gennarelli (1974) documented the shearing effect that results as the brain rapidly rotates from the acceleration/deceleration forces and, not surprisingly, found the frontal and temporal lobes to be particularly affected by the shearing/tearing effects of closed head injury. In fact, these effects have been found on autopsy in patients sustaining even seemingly minor head injury and may well result in quantifiable deficits on neuropsychological tests (e.g., Stuss et al., 1985). This diffuse damage may well contribute to the "post-concussion syndrome," which is characterized by a compromise in attention, fatiguability, nervousness, low tolerance for noise, and generally lowered cognitive efficiency (Binder, 1986). Diffuse injury may also result from hypoxia or edema occurring after injury.

Medical Complications Producing Focal Damage in Closed Head Injury: Hematomas

In a subset of cases of head injury (estimated to range from 15% to 40%, depending on severity [Levin et al., 1982]), a hemorrhage will occur, resulting in a collection of blood over an area of the brain that eventually forms a clot. These are called *intracranial hematomas* and are serious in that they displace the rest of the brain and ventricles within the skull, exerting pressure on neighboring brain areas. Hematomas are most common in the frontal and temporal areas (Levin et al., 1982), again largely because of the bony irregularities of the skull in those regions. They are usually treated surgically, with evacuation procedures to reduce the clot and the concomitant pressure and displacement on adjacent brain tissue. Hematomas are classified according to the layer of brain covering in which they occur.

Extradural Hematoma

These hematomas occur between the skull and the dura covering of the brain. Though serious, they often do not result in as severe deficits as those associated with subdural hematomas.

Subdural Hematoma

This indicates a collection of blood in the subdural space. These hematomas tend to be more serious in terms of lasting neuropsychological sequelae.

In planning for a test battery to adequately assess a patient who has a history of hematoma(s), the neuropsychologist should take into account the anatomic location of the hematoma(s) and whether they were acute or chronic so that hypotheses may be formulated and tested and that appropriate functional areas may be assessed completely.

Prognostic Factors: Coma and Post-Traumatic Amnesia

It is often estimated that the greatest recovery takes place during the first year after injury, but some deficits may persist years following the injury, even in cases of mild injury (Binder, 1986).

It is useful for the clinician to understand certain features of the injury and subsequent recovery processes because of the important prognostic implications. Among these, probably the two most commonly used and relevant prognostic indicators are coma and duration of post-traumatic amnesia.

Coma

Depth and duration of coma, until the last decade or so, have been hard to quantify reliably because it was often uncertain exactly when coma ended and when a confusional state (or delirium) began. This has changed since the development of the Glasgow Coma Scale (Teasdale & Jennett, 1974), a standardized, objective rating scale on which the patient is assigned points for varying levels of behavior such as eye opening and motor and verbal responses. A cumulative score is obtained that can be plotted over several days (or compared with other patients) to reliably monitor depth and duration of coma. Coma has often been used to classify minor and severe head injury in research studies, which have sometimes correlated severity of coma with rate and degree of recovery. For instance, Glasgow Coma Scale (GCS) scores were found to be good predictors of survival rate from head injury and mortality (Jane & Rimel, 1982; Dye, Saxon, & Milby, 1981). Though many studies have used coma and GCS as indices of severity of injury, others have used post-traumatic amnesia and have found it to correlate even more highly with the rate of and degree of recovery.

Post-Traumatic Amnesia (PTA)

The extent of post-traumatic amnesia (i.e., the loss of memory or ability to acquire new information for events after the traumatic injury) is an important datum for the clinical neuropsychologist to measure because of its prognostic implications.

Russell (1932) first proposed the use of length of PTA as an index of the severity of head injury and found it predictive of discharge from the service because of disability. Various others (e.g., Von Wowern, 1966; Norman & Svahn 1961; Brooks and Aughton, 1979; Gronwall & Wrightson, 1981) found PTA to correlate with later cognitive problems. Brooks, Aughton, Bond, Jones, and Rizvi (1980) studied a group of 89 severely head injured patients two years post-injury, comparing both GCS score and length of PTA with various measures of cognitive performance. They found that GCS score did *not* correlate with later cognitive outcome although duration of PTA was an accurate predictor of subsequent cognitive performance. Bennett-Levy (1984), in a particularly well-designed study, examined long-term cognitive functioning in a consecutive series of 39 young adults with severe closed head injuries, two to five years post injury. He found significantly more impairment in his follow-up with patients whose PTA was greater than three weeks (particularly on tasks requiring long-term retention of complex materials or in which time constraints are important), whereas patients whose PTA was less than three weeks were generally unimpaired on the cognitive tests that were used at follow-up. Bennett-Levy concluded that at least in young adults, a threshold of lasting impairments may occur near the three week marker of PTA duration.

Caution should be exercised in formulating final conclusions regarding the prognostic value and limitations of various measures of injury, such as coma or PTA. The studies are not entirely consistent on this issue, perhaps because of the heterogeneous nature of the various samples with different ages, different types of head injury, different severity levels, different post-traumatic medical complications within the samples, the different schedules of cognitive assessment, practice effects, and appropriate comparison groups (Brooks et al., 1984).

Conclusions

It is quite difficult to make broad generalizations about head injured patients because the group is not homogeneous. However, existing commonalities permit certain conclusions regarding proper neuropsychologic assessment of these individuals.

1. Most studies indicate that greatest recovery from head injury occurs within the first year following the injury, though measurable recovery also has been shown to continue well beyond the one-year marker. In addition to actual brain recovery, improvements in functioning may result from rehabilitation and learned coping and compensatory strategies.
2. Many have challenged the widely held contention that greatest recovery occurs within the first year following the injury, and recent evidence suggests that specific cognitive deficits may persist years after the injury. Such impairment has been documented in "divided" attentional abilities and complaints of "forgetfulness."
3. The residual effects of head injury are usually referred to as the "post-traumatic or concussional syndrome," consisting of nervousness, irritability, fatigue, distractibility, lowered attention span, poor memory, emotional lability, and headache.
4. Because of the bony irregularities of the skull cavity, the frontal and temporal lobes are particularly susceptible to injury after head trauma. Thus, language, memory (both verbal and nonverbal), and "frontal systems" tasks should be an essential component in any evaluation of the head injured patient. Because a patient with frontal lobe damage will often perform normally on many structured psychometric tests, tests known to be more sensitive to frontal lobe dysfunction should be included in the battery, such as the Consonant Trigram Test, Wisconsin Card Sorting Test, Porteus Maze Test, Stroop Test, Trail Making Test A and B, Verbal Fluency, and Finger Tapping.
5. Focal deficits may arise from coup and contrecoup effects, as well as direct tissue damage by open injury. Medical complications, such as hematomas, may also produce focal neuropsychological findings. The clinician should not be confused by areas of focal deficit that may not correspond to the initial site of impact as they may result from contrecoup effects.
6. One of the most useful prognostic indicators may well be length of post-traumatic amnesia, with the general conclusion that the longer the amnesia (particularly over three weeks), the more serious the injury and expected neuropsychological sequelae. Although generally not as reliable in predicting future functioning, GCS ratings are often useful.
7. Certain psychiatric disorders may result from head trauma (Benson & Blumer, 1975; Binder, 1986). Behavioral changes or deficits following injury should be carefully evaluated as they are frequently misdiagnosed as functional in origin (e.g., Weinstein & Wells, 1981) rather than as resulting from direct neurologic injury with different implications for treatment. Common behavioral traits often seen include disinhibition, tactlessness, jocularity, anxiety, and aggression.
8. Finally, mention should be made of the importance, not only of thorough and comprehensive assessments in these patients, but also of serial assessments over time. Retesting of the same head injured patient (for instance, at six-month or yearly intervals) allows an estimation of the rate and degree of recovery over time. This information may also be quite important in providing

the patient and his/her family with realistic expectations regarding anticipated level of functioning and possible return to work or school.

References

Adams, R.D., & Victor, M. (1985). *Principles of neurology* (3rd ed.). New York: McGraw-Hill.

Barth, J.T., Macciocchi, S.N., Giordani, B., Rimel, R., Jane, J.A., & Boll, T.J. (1983). Neuropsychological sequelae of minor head injury. *Neurosurgery, 13,* 529–533.

Benson, D.F., & Blumer, D. (1975). *Psychiatric aspects of neurologic disease.* New York: Grune and Stratton, Inc.

Bennett-Levy, J.M. (1984). Long-term effects of severe closed head injury on memory: Evidence from a consecutive series of young adults. *Acta Neurol Scand, 70,* 285–298.

Binder, L.M. (1986). Persisting symptoms after mild head injury: A review of the post-concussive syndrome. *Journal of Clinical and Experimental Neuropsychology, 8,* 323–346.

Brooks, D.N., & Aughton, M.E. (1979). Psychological consequences of blunt head injury. *International Rehabilitation Medicine, 1,* 160–165.

Brooks, D.N., Aughton, M.E., Bond, M.R., Jones, P., & Rizvi, S. (1980). Cognitive sequelae in relationship to early indices of severity of brain damage after severe blunt head injury. *Journal of Neurology, Neurosurgery and Psychiatry, 43,* 529–534.

Brooks, D.N., Deelman, B.G., van Zomeran, A.H., van Dongen, H., van Harskamp, F., & Aughton, M.E. (1984). Problems in measuring cognitive recovery after acute brain injury. *Journal of Clinical Neuropsychology, 6,* 71–85.

Dye, O.A., Saxon, S.A., & Milby, J.B. (1981). Long-term neuropsychological deficits after traumatic head injury with comatosis. *Journal of Clinical Psychology, 37,* 472–477.

Heilman, K.M., Safran, A., & Geschwind, N. (1971). Closed head trauma and aphasia. *Journal of Neurology, Neurosurgery and Psychiatry, 34,* 265–269.

Gronwall, D. & Wrightson, P. (1981). Memory and information processing capacity after closed head injury. *Journal of Neurology, Neurosurgery and Psychiatry, 44,* 382–386.

Jane, J.A., & Rimel, R.W. (1982). Prognosis in head injury. *Clinical Neurosurgery, 29,* 346–352.

Levin, H.S., Benton, A.L., & Grossman, R.G. (1982). *Neurobehavioral consequences of closed head injury.* New York: Oxford University Press.

Levin, H.S., Grossman, R.G., & Kelly, P.J. (1976). Aphasic disorder in patients with closed head injury. *Journal of Neurology, Neurosurgery and Psychiatry, 39,* 1062–1070.

Lezak, M.B. (1983). *Neuropsychological assessment.* New York: Oxford University Press.

Norman, B., & Svahn, K. (1961). A follow-up study of severe brain injuries. *Acta Psychiat Scand, 37,* 236–264.

Ommaya, A.K., & Gennarelli, R.A. (1974). Cerebral concussion and traumatic unconsciousness: Correlation of experimental and clinical observations on blunt head injuries. *Brain, 97,* 633–654.

Russell, W.R. (1932). Cerebral involvement in head injury. *Brain, 55,* 549–603.

Stuss, D.T., Ely, P., Hugenholtz, H., Richard, M.T., LaRochelle, S., Poirier, C., & Bell, I. (1985). Subtle neuropsychological deficits in patients with good recovery after closed head injury. *Neurosurgery, 17,* 41–47.

Teasdale, G., & Jennett, B. (1974). Assessment of coma and impaired consciousness: A practical scale. *Lancet, 2,* 81–84.

Von Wowern, F. (1966). Posttraumatic amnesia and confusion as an index of severity in head injury. *Acta Neurol Scand, 42,* 373–378.

Van Zomeren, A.H., & Van den Berg, W. (1985). Residual complaints of patients two years after severe head injury. *Journal of Neurology, Neurosurgery and Psychiatry, 48,* 21–28.

Weinstein, G.S., & Wells, C.E. (1981). Case studies in neuropsychiatry: Post-traumatic psychiatric dysfunction– diagnosis and treatment. *Journal of Clinical Psychiatry, 42,* 120–122.

Case 1: Closed Head Injury Implicating Frontal Dysfunction[1]

Presenting Situation and Reason for Referral

Ms. H.B. is a 45-year-old, right-handed, Caucasian female who was initially referred by her neurologist for neuropsychological evaluation of cognitive changes associated with a closed head trauma. Approximately three weeks before the initial referral and testing, Ms. B. was involved in a motor vehicle accident and struck the right side of her forehead. She lost consciousness for an undetermined period of time. Although the length of post-traumatic amnesia is not known, she reports amnesia for the collision and for events during her subsequent two-and-one-half-week hospitalization. Since the injury, Ms. B. has been reported to indulge in inappropriate jocularity and seductive behavior, to exhibit poor insight, and to display difficulty in new learning and memory skills that represent changes in her functioning. She was evaluated initially three weeks post-injury and again six months post-injury. Ms. B. presented with complaints of memory problems–both in recalling information people have told her and material she has read, as well as difficulty recalling directions which leads her to become lost and disoriented when driving. In addition, she reports difficulty with mathematical computations and states that before her injury, she engaged in accounting and bookkeeping for others as a hobby, but is no longer able to perform these tasks. Finally, the patient also reports symptoms of depression and anxiety; she cries easily, which she has difficulty controlling, and experiences sleep and appetite disturbance.

Although Ms. B. has completed 14 years of schooling and worked in sales for a large company, she has not been able to return to work since the accident because of her cognitive complaints described above.

There is no history of prior head injury, significant medical illness, or drug or alcohol abuse, and no prior history of psychiatric treatment for her or her family members. The patient is currently on no medications.

Behavioral Observations

Ms. B. appeared for the initial testing session well groomed except for having nail polish on only some of her fingernails. She was quite vague when discussing her

[1] We usually list the names of tests administered here in lieu of a data summary sheet. However, for the purposes of this book, we are presenting the data summary sheet, which contains information regarding tests used in the evaluation.

cognitive difficulties, and even attempted to minimize them, saying she had difficulty remembering things before the accident as well. Initially, Ms. B. appeared very defensive and guarded, attempting to demean the assessment process, saying, "This is the most boring thing I have ever done." She also evidenced little overt anxiety over poor performance. On the second assessment, she appeared much more pleasant and cooperative, and although this defensive, caustic demeanor was not evident, she arrived 30 minutes late for the appointment. At this point, she was found waiting at the door of the examination room instead of in the waiting room as instructed earlier. Ms. B. reported no recollection of having been instructed where to go for the evaluation despite explicit instructions from the appointment secretary.

Tests Administered

See data summary sheet.

Test Results

Intelligence

Results of intellectual assessment from both evaluations place Ms. B. in the average range of intellectual ability. Overall, her intellectual scores were not significantly different across the two assessments some six months apart. Her individual subtest scores were also highly similar on both assessments, except for significant improvement on a task requiring her to sequentially order a set of pictures to tell a meaningful story (Picture Arrangement) from the first to the second assessment. Within the verbal domain, the patient's best performance was on tasks assessing her ability to think abstractly (Similarities), arithmetic computation skills requiring auditory concentration (Arithmetic), and on a task assessing her knowledge of the world about her (Information). Within the nonverbal domain, more variability was evident, with improvement noted on a nonverbal task requiring her to sequentially arrange pictures to tell meaningful stories (Picture Arrangement), whereas all other subtests were in the average range.

Attention and Concentration Processes

Performance on tests of attention and concentration was essentially within normal limits on both assessments although slightly lowered relative to overall intellectual skills. Mrs. B.'s performance on the two subtests of the WAIS-R most sensitive to disturbances in attention and concentration (Digit Span and Arithmetic) was essentially intact, though marginally but not significantly lower on the second assessment compared to the first. This is in contrast with her improved performance on a task requiring her to perform such tasks as reciting the letters of the alphabet, counting backwards from 20, and counting by 3s to 40, from the first to second assessment (Wechsler Memory Scale-Mental Control, up from the 20th percentile to the 58th percentile).

Language Functioning

Ms. B.'s spontaneous speech was unremarkable although she reports talking "more slowly" than prior to the injury. No language comprehension errors were noted on the comprehension section of the BDAE administered during the second evaluation.

The patient performed in the average range for her age on a formal confrontational naming test (Boston Naming Test) on both assessments. Conversely, Ms. B.'s word list generation skills (FAS) were in the low average/borderline range, being slightly poorer on the second examination than the first, indicating compromise on the second examination in list generation. Thus, though essential language mechanisms appear intact (comprehension, word finding), verbal fluency appears to have declined slightly over at least a six-month interval.

Sensory-Perceptual and Motor Exam

Ms. B. reported a preference for the use of her right hand, and she denies any history of peripheral injury to arms, hands, or shoulders. No finger agnosia was observed on either assessment. On initial exam, Mrs. B. exhibited several errors on her right hand on a sensory task involving identification of numbers traced on fingertips, though on the second testing six months later, no errors were evident. Thus, any sensory deficits (possibly associated with attentional deficits noted above) that may have existed on initial exam had resolved by the second examination.

On a motor test of finger tapping speed (Finger Tapping Test), performance was intact for her right (dominant) hand, but Ms. B. performed slightly more poorly than expected with her left hand (76th percentile, 1st assessment; 45th percentile, 2nd assessment). While a 10% dominant-hand advantage is expected, this patient showed a 19% dominant-hand advantage, evident during both testing sessions. Scores on a task involving the placing of pegs in slots (Grooved Pegboard) administered during the second testing session revealed normal performance with both hands. Interestingly, evaluation of grip strength (Hand Dynamometer) revealed essentially equal performance across hands, although performance for each hand was extremely depressed on the second assessment and much lower than that on initial testing. Thus, tests of motor performance were variable, with some evidence of decreased strength bilaterally, and possible declines in dexterity in the left hand.

Perceptual Organizational Skills

Visual perceptual skills were consistently within the average range across the two assessments (Hooper Visual Organization Test, Picture Completion).

Scores on visual-sequencing and visual-tracking tasks were variable. The patient performed within the average range on Trails A on the first assessment but within the borderline range on the second assessment. She performed in the low average range on Trails B on both assessments, suggesting some difficulty on more complex conceptual-tracking tasks. Of note, dramatic improvement was evidenced on a task requiring the sequencing of visual material (Picture Arrangement) on the second assessment relative to her performance on initial examination. In addition, improvement in maze performance was found on retesting: six months earlier, the patient was unable to complete the last two mazes on the WISC-R Mazes subtest, but on the second testing, she was able to complete all of the mazes accurately. Performance on the Digit Symbol subtest declined slightly on retesting.

Performance on constructional tasks was within the normal range and generally consistent across both testing sessions. Her copy of a complex two-dimensional figure was in the average range on both assessments (Rey-Osterrieth). Of note, however, was her performance on the second examination on a design fluency test (Design Fluency), a nonverbal analogue to the word generation task that requires the patient to generate novel, nonnameable paper and pencil designs. Ms. B. was unable to generate any designs within four minutes. She appeared to be attempting to comply with the task and after several seconds spontaneously commented, "You mean people can really put something down that has no name?" This is in sharp contrast to her performance six months earlier when she generated nine designs, though still below expected levels (mean score for normals is 16 designs in five minutes).

Learning and Memory

Results of tests of learning and memory were variable. Somewhat surprisingly, Ms. B.'s performance on tasks involving immediate recall of paragraph information reflected a substantial decline from the first to second assessment. Though she performed in the superior range (98th percentile) on the Wechsler Memory Scale-Logical Memory immediate recall subtest on initial exam, she performed in the low average range six months later (11th percentile). Following a 30-minute delay, she was able to recall 61% of the information originally learned on the initial assessment but, six months later, recalled 80% of the information learned on the immediate recall portion of the task. Thus, though she seems to have learned less material on the second assessment, her recall following an extended delay seems improved from that six months earlier, though this could be a statistical artifact of her lowered initial recall on the second assessment.

On a task involving learning of simple and more difficult word pairs (WMS-Associate Learning), Ms. B.'s intact performance on the easier word pairs was consistent across the two assessments, though her learning of the more difficult word pairs was slightly better on the initial assessment. Because of this decline in performance in learning the more difficult word pairs, Ms. B.'s overall performance score has declined from the high average to the low average range from the first to the second assessment.

The patient's word list learning (AVLT) indicated slight but consistent improvement on every learning trial from the first to second assessments, though her performance is still slightly below average. Her excellent recognition of the items compared with her difficulty in recall of the items following a 15-minute delay would implicate dysfunction in storage and/or retrieval mechanisms rather than in the original encoding of the information, which seems intact.

Ms. B. also evidenced a decline in her performance on a task involving the immediate recall of relatively simple geometric figures over the two assessments. Initially, she performed within the average range (WMS-Visual Reproduction, 58th percentile). However, six months later when given the same task, she performed in the low average range (23rd percentile). Though she could not recall any of the designs following a 30-minute delay on either assessment, she could correctly recognize them on both assessments when presented in multiple choice format. Finally, Ms. B.'s recall of a complex two-dimensional figure following a three-minute delay was below the 10th percentile on both examinations (Rey-Osterrieth).

Overall, memory scores reveal unusual variability across the two testing sessions. A marked and consistent impairment in delayed recall of nonverbal visual material is documented on the two testing sessions. In contrast, retention of verbal material over a delay appeared to improve. However, declines in the initial acquisition of novel verbal and nonverbal material was noted from first to second testing.

Tasks of Conceptual Shifting and Response Inhibition

Ms. B.'s performance on tasks in this domain reflects a significant improvement from scores obtained on initial testing. At that time, she was only able to complete two categories on the Wisconsin Card Sorting Test and exhibited excessive perseverative responses. Six months later, performance well within the normal range for her age was observed on this test; she was able to complete six categories, and the number of errors and perseverative responses was well within normal limits. The patient's performance was within normal limits on the Stroop Test on both initial and follow-up assessment six months later.

Summary and Impressions

Intellectual assessment was essentially consistent between the two testing sessions, indicating that Ms. B. is functioning within the average range of general intellectual ability.

The most striking findings on initial testing had been the consistently poor performance on various tasks traditionally associated with frontal lobe function, such as difficulty in word and novel-design generation, visual sequencing and alternation, maze solving, categorization, and mental flexibility (ability to shift set). On the second testing, the patient showed generally normal performance on tasks involving categorization and conceptual shifting, response inhibition, and planning (maze solving), but she continued to show relatively poor performance on tasks involving generation of material (word and novel-design generation) and alternation between tasks. Her scores on the word-fluency and design-fluency tasks were in fact poorer than on initial testing. Results from motor testing were inconclusive, but some of the data suggest that left-hand performance continued to be excessively depressed relative to right-hand performance, raising the question of right-frontal dysfunction. Also of note, upper limb motor strength deteriorated significantly from first to second testing.

Scores on memory testing continued to reflect deficiencies in delayed recall consistent with findings on initial exam. However, Ms. B. surprisingly performed much more poorly on the second testing in the initial learning of information (both verbal and nonverbal). This type of deterioration is not common in head injury, and the most probable explanation for the decreased learning ability would be interference associated with attentional difficulties, as performance on attentional tasks was variable and overall slightly depressed relative to intellectual scores.

Language skills and visual perceptual and constructional abilities were judged to be generally intact on both assessments.

Personality assessment was not completed, but we are concerned about the presence of numerous depressive symptoms including loss of interest in activities, sleep disturbance, appetite loss, loss of sex drive, and anxiety. Depression can interfere with such cognitive activities as learning of novel information through the disruption of attention and motivation. We suspect that the poorer scores on immediate recall noted on second evaluation, as well as the poorer performance on generation tasks, might be related to the apparent current depression. We believe that it might be beneficial for the patient to receive supportive psychotherapeutic treatment to treat her depression, and also to participate in support groups for head injury victims. If, following adequate treatment for depression, Ms. B.'s memory functioning does not improve, it may be beneficial for her to receive cognitive rehabilitation aimed toward improving her memory abilities.

Could some of the improvement noted in her performance between the initial and second testing sessions be the result of practice effects? This hypothesis must be entertained, though interestingly, Ms. B. declined on some measures (specifically, memory tasks). She did show improvement on some tasks that could be influenced by practice on multiple testings (i.e., Wisconsin Card Sorting Test and Mazes), and this influence cannot be ruled out as a factor contributing to her improved performance on these selected measures. That she did not improve on other measures and declined on some is a curious finding and not consistent with an hypothesis of generalized practice effects influencing overall performance.

The patient's initial complaint of difficulty in math skills is interesting in light of her intact performance on simple arithmetic calculations in this examination. It may be that in more complex, multi-step tasks, she has difficulty with the sequential calculating necessary in her everyday work environment.

The results presented above are somewhat encouraging because they show some possible recovery patterns in selected domains, consistent with mild recovery in individuals following brain injury. We must, however, offer the caveat that Ms. B. continues to show dysfunction on selected tests sensitive to frontal systems functioning and memory. It will be important to reexamine this patient in approximately six months to continue monitoring her course. It is also recommended that Ms. B. be encouraged to rely on memory aids, such as note pads and reminders, to cue her recall of learned information. A work environment with structure and routine will also facilitate her functioning.

Time 1 NEUROPSYCHOLOGY TEST SCORE SUMMARY SHEET

Patient: H.B. Age: 45 Sex: F Handedness: R

I. Intelligence WAIS-R Age-Corrected Scores

VERBAL			PERFORMANCE		
Information	13	(84 %ile)	Picture Completion	10	(50 %ile)
Digit Span	8	(25 %ile)	Picture Arrangement	7	(16 %ile)
Vocabulary	8	(25 %ile)	Block Design	8	(25 %ile)
Arithmetic	12	(75 %ile)	Object Assembly	10	(50 %ile)
Comprehension	8	(25 %ile)	Digit Symbol	10	(50 %ile)
Similarities	14	(91 %ile)			
VERBAL IQ =	99	(48 %ile)	PERFORMANCE IQ =	92	(30 %ile)

FULL SCALE IQ = 96 (39 %ile)

II. Attention/Concentration
Digit Span: 5 forward + 4 backwards = 9 Total (25 %ile)
Mental Control, WMS: 5 (20 %ile)
Trails A: 24" (64 %ile), Trails B: 97" (14 %ile)

III. Language
Boston Naming Test: 56 /60
Controlled Word Association: F (8) + A (7) + S (8) + Age Corr.= 27 (15-19 %ile)

IV. Perceptual/Organizational
Rey-Osterrieth Complex Figure Copy: 34 /36 (70-80 %ile)
Hooper Visual Organization Test: 23.5/30

V. Memory

VERBAL		NONVERBAL	
WMS Logical Memory	13.5 (98%ile)	WMS Visual Repro.:	9 (58%ile)
30 min. delay:	8.2	30 min. delay:	0
Percent retention:	61	Percent retention:	0

WMS Associate Learning	Easy 5 , 6 , 6	Rey-Osterrieth Fig:	34 (70-80 %ile)
	Hard 2 , 3 , 3	3 min. delay:	14 (<10 %ile)
	Score: 16.5 (80 %ile)		

Rey Auditory Verbal Learning Test (15 items):
T1:5 T2:6 T3:9 T4:10 T5:10 Recall after Interference: 7
15-min. Delayed Recall 5
Recognition: 12 Hits, 0 False Identifications

VI. Motor Exam	Dominant Hand	%ile	Nondom. Hand	%ile
Finger Tapping:	50.8	93	42	76
Grip Strength:	32.2	66	22.5	21

VII. Sensory	Dominant Hand	Nondominant Hand
Finger Gnosis:	0 errors	0 errors
Fingertip Number Writing:	several errors	0 errors

VIII. Frontal Systems
Stroop A: 42", Stroop B: 60", Stroop C: 133"
Wisconsin Card Sort: Categories: 2
WISC-R Mazes: 6
Design Fluency: 9

Time 2 NEUROPSYCHOLOGY TEST SCORE SUMMARY SHEET

Patient: H.B. Age: 45 Sex: F Handedness: R

I. Intelligence WAIS-R Age-Corrected Scores

VERBAL			PERFORMANCE		
Information	11	(63 %ile)	Picture Completion	10	(50 %ile)
Digit Span	7	(16 %ile)	Picture Arrangement	13	(84 %ile)
Vocabulary	10	(50 %ile)	Block Design	8	(25 %ile)
Arithmetic	11	(63 %ile)	Object Assembly	11	(63 %ile)
Comprehension	8	(25 %ile)	Digit Symbol	8	(25 %ile)
Similarities	15	(95 %ile)			
VERBAL IQ =	101	(52 %ile)	PERFORMANCE IQ =	99	(48 %ile)

FULL SCALE IQ = 100 (50 %ile)

II. Attention/Concentration
Digit Span: 4 forward + 4 backwards = 8 Total (16 %ile)
Mental Control, WMS: 7 (58 %ile)
Trails A: 41" (7 %ile), Trails B: 97" (14 %ile)

III. Language
Boston Naming Test: 57 /60
Controlled Word Association: F (6) + A (5) + S (9) + Age Corr.= 24 (5-9 %ile)

IV. Perceptual/Organizational
Rey-Osterrieth Complex Figure Copy: 33 /36 (60 %ile)
Hooper Visual Organization Test: 26/30

V. Memory

VERBAL		NONVERBAL	
WMS Logical Memory	5 (11%ile)	WMS Visual Repro.:	6 (23%ile)
30 min. delay:	4	30 min. delay:	0
Percent retention:	80	Percent retention:	0

WMS I	Easy	5 , 6 , 6	Rey-Osterrieth Fig:	33 (60 %ile)
Associate I	Hard	0 , 1 , 2	3 min. delay:	14 (<10 %ile)
Learning I	Score:	11.5 (22 %ile)		

Rey Auditory Verbal Learning Test (15 items):
T1: 6 T2: 9 T3: 11 T4: 11 T5: 11 Recall after Interference: 8
15-min. Delayed Recall: 7
Recognition: 13 Hits, 0 False Identifications

VI. Motor Exam

	Dominant Hand	%ile	Nondom. Hand	%ile
Finger Tapping:	45.8	77	37	45
Grip Strength:	6	<1	6.3	<1
Grooved Pegboard:	73	10	75	32

VII. Sensory

	Dominant Hand	Nondominant Hand
Finger Gnosis:	0 errors	0 errors
Fingertip Number Writing:	0 errors	0 errors

VIII. Frontal Systems
Stroop A: 46", Stroop B: 68", Stroop C: 135"
Wisconsin Card Sort: Categories: 6
WISC-R Mazes: 20
Design Fluency: 0

Case 2: Open Head Injury Associated with Frontal Lobe Dysfunction

Presenting Situation and Background Information

Mr. N. A. is a 61-year-old, right-handed, Caucasian male with a college education who was referred for neuropsychological assessment to clarify the extent of memory and general cognitive impairment following his severe head trauma some 20 years ago. Consultation was also requested to help clarify the role of the injury in producing the psychiatric condition described below.

The patient presents with a history of a severe head trauma from an automobile accident in which most of the right side of his face was crushed, producing a coma lasting three days. Length of post-traumatic amnesia and other details of the injury are not known. Before the accident, Mr. A. served in the Army Air Corps during World War II. Following the service, he went to college, where he majored in music, and from there pursued advanced study in music at an internationally renowned conservatory under musicians of great repute. After his tutorial, he began a career as a composer and sold some of his work for which he now receives royalties. About this time, Mr. A. received the severe closed head injury from an automobile accident described above. Following extensive medical and surgical treatment, he left the hospital with a notable right-sided facial dysplagia and later underwent corrective bone surgery for this. The patient also had left-sided motor weakness requiring him to use a cane for ambulation. He made a poor psychiatric recovery and was never able to work after the accident, living in various nursing homes over the past 20 years. The patient was admitted at this time because he exhibits constant intrusive verbalizations and obsessions that the "world is going to be destroyed by an atomic bomb," and that the FBI is hiding information about the Rosenbergs from the 1940s.

Mr. A. has no history of additional head injury, significant medical illness, or alcohol or other substance abuse. Of note, he was discharged from the military with a diagnosis of "nerves." However, he was never hospitalized for any psychiatric condition prior to his accident, and he reports no family psychiatric history. Neurologic examination revealed left-sided weakness, requiring the patient to walk with the assistance of a cane, and diminished reflexes on the left side. Currently, the patient is being treated with a low dosage of Haldol.

Behavioral Observations

Mr. A. appeared for the testing casually dressed and with a beard that partially hid his right facial disfigurement. He spoke in a dysarthric manner, largely because of his right-sided facial paralysis. He approached the testing situation in a cooperative manner, though he was unable to inhibit his obsessive and intrusive thoughts and every few seconds interrupted the examiner to ask or to repeat the date, and to state his concerns regarding the atomic bomb and the world coming to an end, the Rosenbergs, and the FBI or CIA. Mr. A. seemed to exert his best effort on all tasks and generally was able to focus on the tasks presented him except for his frequent but brief intrusions.

Tests Administered

See data summary sheet.

Test Results

Gross Cognitive Functioning

Mr. A. scored 28/30 on the Mini-Mental State Exam (MMSE), indicating grossly intact cognitive functioning. His only errors were in citing the day of the week and the name of the county. Otherwise, his performance was fully intact on this test.

Intelligence

Results of intellectual assessment indicate Mr. A. has a Verbal IQ of 104, a Performance IQ of 87, and a Full Scale IQ of 95 (37th percentile), placing him overall in the average range of intellectual ability. He evidenced a 17-point discrepancy in favor of his verbal abilities. Within the verbal domain, there was substantial intersubtest scatter, ranging from average performance on attentional tasks (Arithmetic, Digit Span), to high average to superior performance on tests of abstract thinking (Similarities), understanding of common social conventions (Comprehension), and knowledge of word usage (Vocabulary). Within the Performance tasks, Mr. A. performed in the low average to borderline range on several subtests involving visual perception (Picture Completion), grapho-motor tracking (Digit Symbol) and puzzle-solving (Object Assembly). He performed within the superior range on a task measuring his ability to sequentially arrange a series of pictures to tell a meaningful story (Picture Arrangement) and within the average range on a task measuring his ability to arrange a set of blocks to match a design (Block Design). Examination of those subtests most predictive of premorbid level of functioning together with his remarkable education and social/occupational achievements suggest that Mr. A. likely functioned at least in the superior range of intellectual ability at an earlier time.

Attention and Concentration

Variable performance was noted in this domain. As already noted, Mr. A. was easily distracted by his own intrusive ruminations about the FBI, the atomic bomb, and the Rosenbergs. Formal tests of attention revealed that he could repeat five digits forward and five backward (Digit Span), and on simple rote tasks he was able to rapidly and errorlessly count backwards from 20 to 1 and recite the alphabet, though he did make one error on a task requiring him to count forward by serial 3s (WMS-Mental Control). He was able to correctly spell "World" backwards. The patient performed in the borderline to impaired range on a speeded test of visual scanning, tracking, and alternation (Trail Making Test). Finally, on a sustained-attention task involving a response-inhibition component, Mr. A. performed in the average range on all three components of the test (Stroop Test). Thus, though simple selective attention abilities appear intact, some decrements were noted in higher level attention abilities and on tasks of visual scanning and tracking.

Language Functioning

Mr. A.'s spontaneous speech was noteworthy for his dysarthria resulting from his facial paralysis and for his many verbal intrusions. Formal language screening revealed a mild impairment in confrontational naming (Boston Naming Test = 43/60) with phonemic cues helpful on many words, and word list generation was profoundly impaired (FAS = 7, < 1st percentile). His comprehension, repetition, writing to dictation, and reading written material were grossly intact.

Perceptual Organizational Abilities

Lowered performance was noted on many of the tests in this domain despite normal vision in both eyes. Mr. A. performed below the 10th percentile on his copy of a complex two-dimensional figure (Rey-Osterrieth Complex Figure, see Figure 1.1), and his strategy in copying it was poor. On a task requiring him to either manually or mentally manipulate cut-up objects to form a whole, his performance was in the borderline range (Object Assembly = 5th percentile and Hooper Visual Organization Test = 18.5/30). In sharp contrast, his ability to

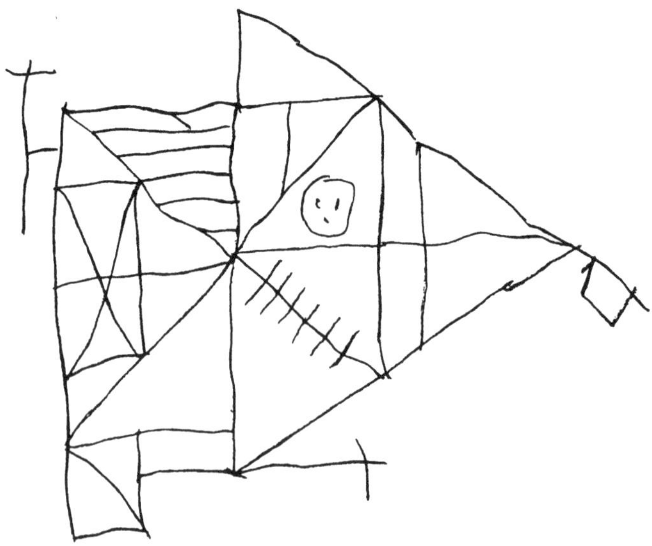

FIGURE 1.1. Case N.A. Rey-Osterrieth Complex Figure: copy. Reduced by 40%.

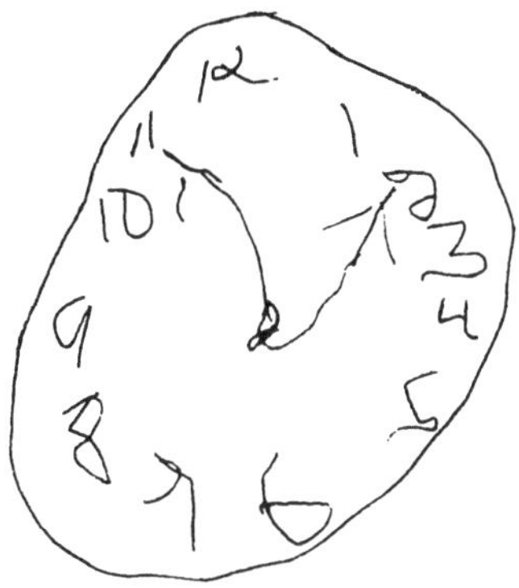

FIGURE 1.2. Case N.A. Draw-A-Clock. Reduced by 35%.

construct a set of blocks to match a design was within the average range (Block Design = 63rd percentile). His clock drawing was somewhat crude but contained all the numbers, and he set the hands correctly as requested at "10 past 11" (see Figure 1.2).

Verbal (Auditory) and Nonverbal (Visual) Learning and Memory

On a serial list-learning task of 10 related words (all shopping-list items), Mr. A. showed a modest learning curve; by the fifth learning trial he had learned seven of the 10 words. Following a 15-minute delay, he was able to recall six of the

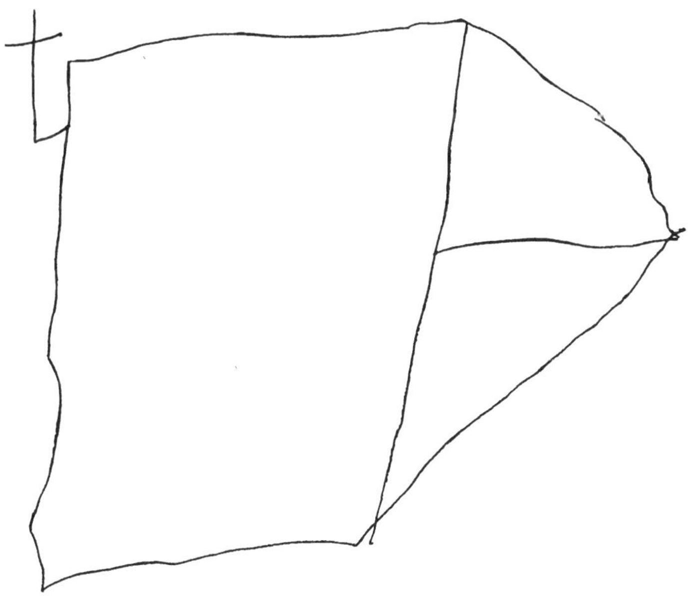

FIGURE 1.3. Case N.A. Rey-Osterrieth Complex Figure: delayed recall. Reduced by 40%.

words, indicating he could retain most of the originally learned information over a short delay. On a recognition portion of the test, the patient obtained nine correct identifications and two false-positive recognitions. On verbal paired-associate learning (WMS-Associate Learning), he readily learned the easy word pairs but could learn only one of the four more difficult word pairs by the third learning trial. His immediate recall of story passages (WMS-Logical Memory) was in the average range (45th percentile) for his age, and following a 30-minute delay, he recalled 79% of the originally learned information, a retention rate within normal limits.

Assessment of nonverbal memory was difficult because of the already noted impairment in visuo-construction skills. Mr. A. performed in the low average range (21st percentile) in his immediate recall of simple line drawings (WMS-Visual Reproduction), and following a 30-minute delay, he recalled 33% of the originally reproduced information, well below expected levels. Following a three-minute delay, Mr. A. could recall and reproduce only 25% of the originally reproduced complex figure (Rey-Osterrieth), again, well below expected levels (see Figure 1.3). To remove the constructional factor from assessment of nonverbal memory, the Benton Visual Form Discrimination Test-multiple-choice form was administered. (Before the delay was administered, the patient indicated evidence of adequate visual discrimination by matching all the sample items to the correct stimulus in match-to-sample multiple-choice paradigm.) In this task, the patient is shown the original stimulus for 10 seconds and, following a 15-second delay, is asked to choose from four choices the figure exactly matching the one shown earlier. On this test, Mr. A. correctly recognized eight of 14 designs, placing him in the low average range (13th percentile).

Thus, assessment of learning and memory skills revealed a decrement in learning and recall of both verbal and nonverbal memory, with greater decrement seen in the nonverbal domain. The use of a visual recognition format and percent of recall following a delay support the presence of decline in nonverbal memory over and above his visuo-spatial constructional impairment. It should be noted that his learning is aided by contextual cues, such as when information is presented in paragraph/story format versus merely a list of words.

Motor Exam

The patient denied any history of injury to his hands, arms, or shoulders. On a finger tapping test, Mr. A. exhibited a much greater than expected dominant-hand advantage (R=52, L=36). His dominant-hand finger tapping was superior (97th percentile), while his nondominant-hand performance was within the average range (30th percentile).

Tasks of Concept Learning, Set Shifting, and Response Inhibition

On the Wisconsin Card Sorting Test, Mr. A. showed notable impairment; he was unable to complete even one category and committed many perseverative errors. As already noted, he performed in the average range on a task of response inhibition (Stroop Test, Part C).

Summary and Impressions

Mr. A. presents with notable areas of compromise in higher cognitive functioning relative to estimated premorbid functioning. Simple attention abilities are within normal limits, but more complex attention tasks tapping sustained attention and visual scanning/tracking reveal impairment. Though the patient currently functions within the average range of intellectual ability, this most likely represents a serious decline in a man who once functioned in a high-level musical and intellectual environment. Although deficits appear in virtually every cognitive sphere, the most striking deficits appear in functions believed to be mediated by his nondominant hemisphere, including nonverbal memory, visuoconstructive abilities, visual tracking, and a notable decrement in finger tapping with his left hand relative to right-hand performance. In addition, there was some evidence of a mild anomia. Finally, many of the test results reflect significant compromise in functions traditionally associated with the frontal lobe (word list generation, motor asymmetries, categorization and ability to shift set, ability to inhibit intrusive or inappropriate thoughts). Behaviorally, quite significant is the patient's rather prominent preoccupation and inability to inhibit his statements concerning the Rosenbergs, the FBI, and the atomic bomb. It is likely that his inability to control his intrusive, perseverative, and obsessive thoughts and verbalizations of the Rosenbergs and the atomic bomb may well be the product of damage sustained to frontal systems structures, preventing him from screening out these distracting stimuli and inhibiting these repetitive thoughts.

Together, these results reflect the patient's overall cognitive/brain dysfunction, with the nondominant (right) hemisphere (both anterior and posterior) more severely affected. This is consistent with the history of right-sided skull damage in the accident and the resulting right-sided dysplagia.

Regarding the question of the etiology of the patient's obsessional preoccupation with the delusion of the Rosenbergs and the atomic bomb, much of the inappropriateness and disinhibition can no doubt be ascribed to the serious head injury the patient sustained some 20 years ago as described above. An additional factor that must also be entertained is that the patient was discharged from the military with a diagnoses of "nerves," suggesting a premorbid psychiatric condition in this individual. However, the fact that the patient was able to function quite successfully for several years following his military experience argues against any premorbid psychiatric disturbance accounting exclusively or even largely for the clinical picture we are currently seeing.

Because of the residual and serious impairment Mr. A. does have, it is recommended that the patient be evaluated by a cognitive rehabilitation/behavioral management service to determine if some degree of improvement can be obtained in his overall behavior so that it is somewhat more appropriate.

NEUROPSYCHOLOGY TEST SCORE SUMMARY SHEET

Patient: N.A. Age: 61 Sex: M Handedness: R

I. Gross Cognitive Functioning
Mini-Mental State Exam: 28/30

II. Intelligence WAIS-R Age-Corrected Scores

VERBAL			PERFORMANCE		
Information	9	(37 %ile)	Picture Completion	6	(9 %ile)
Digit Span	8	(25 %ile)	Picture Arrangement	14	(91 %ile)
Vocabulary	12	(75 %ile)	Block Design	11	(63 %ile)
Arithmetic	9	(37 %ile)	Object Assembly	5	(5 %ile)
Comprehension	12	(75 %ile)	Digit Symbol	6	(9 %ile)
Similarities	14	(91 %ile)			
VERBAL IQ =	104	(61 %ile)	PERFORMANCE IQ =	87	(19 %ile)

FULL SCALE IQ = 95 (37 %ile)

III. Attention/Concentration
Digit Span: 5 forward + 5 backwards = 10 Total (25 %ile)
Mental Control, WMS: 6 (46 %ile)
Trails A: 100" (<1 %ile), Trails B: 128" (3 %ile)

IV. Language
Boston Naming Test: 43/60
Controlled Word Association: F (3) + A (3) + S (1) + Age Corr.= 10 (1 %ile)

V. Perceptual/Organizational
Rey-Osterrieth Complex Figure Copy: 28/36 (<10 %ile)
Hooper Visual Organization Test: 18.5/30
Benton Visual Retention Test: 18/14

VI. Memory

VERBAL		NONVERBAL	
WMS Logical Memory	7 (45 %ile)	WMS Visual Repro.:	3 (21 %ile)
30 min. delay:	5.5	30 min. delay:	1
Percent retention:	79	Percent retention:	33

WMS Associate Learning	I Easy 6 , 5 , 6	Rey Osterrieth Fig:	28 (10 %ile)
	I Hard 0 , 0 , 1	3 min. delay:	7 (<10 %ile)
	I Score: 9.5 (29 %ile)		

Shopping List Test (10 items):
T1: 3 T2: 5 T3: 6 T4: 7 T5: 7 15 min. delay: 6
Recognition: 9 Hits, 2 False Identifications

VII. Motor Exam

	Dominant Hand	%ile	Nondom. Hand	%ile
Finger Tapping:	52	97	36	30

VIII. Frontal Systems
Stroop A: 65", Stroop B: 84", Stroop C: 153"
Wisconsin Card Sorting Test: 0 Categories

Case 3: Open Head Injury Associated with Frontal Lobe Dysfunction

Presenting Situation and Background Information

Ms. K.H. is a 30-year-old, right-handed, Caucasian female who was referred for neuropsychological assessment by her neurologist for evaluation of any residual cognitive impairment secondary to an open head trauma the patient sustained three years earlier.

Ms. H. was involved in a motor vehicle accident three years earlier, producing extensive facial disfigurement and a serious open head injury, and leaving her comatose for six weeks. Length of post-traumatic amnesia is not known. Associated with her injuries was the loss of her right eye and severe compression of the right frontal and zygomatic bones directly into right frontal cortical tissue. As a result, the patient was treated neurosurgically, and a portion of her right frontal lobe was removed. Upon recovery from coma, Ms. H. was unable to talk, walk, or eat, and she underwent extensive rehabilitation at a local rehabilitation hospital. Since that time, she has undergone numerous surgeries to rebuild the orbit of her right eye.

Prior to the accident, Ms. H. had been a successful college student in her sophomore year. Currently, however, she reports having difficulty in learning new information, "doing different things at once," and becoming "flustered and irritable" when encountering even minor setbacks. One year ago, Ms. H. attempted to complete two college courses but failed both despite considerable effort. Six months ago, she obtained employment as a receptionist but was soon fired because she had difficulty keeping track of more than one thing at once. She subsequently obtained two more jobs but left them because they required heavy bookkeeping and computer-programming skills, though she initially thought they would entail simple secretarial duties. She finally obtained a receptionist position with a local business but was again fired because she made "transpositions" in telephone numbers. Her past medical history is unremarkable, and there is no known history of other neurologic disease.

The patient is currently on no medications but had been on Dilantin on a prophylactic basis until three months ago. She occasionally drinks and uses marijuana but reports no serious past drug or alcohol abuse.

Behavioral Observations

Ms. H. appeared on time for the testing session, well groomed and appropriately attired. Her appearance was noteworthy for the scarring and disfigurement of her face and right orbit. Though she was generally pleasant and cooperative during most of the examination, she became irritable and mildly belligerent during two more demanding neuropsychological tests (Wisconsin Card Sorting Test and Auditory Consonant Trigrams Test).

Tests Administered

See data summary sheet.

Test Results

Intelligence

Intellectual assessment reveals a Verbal IQ of 94, a Performance IQ score of 89, and a Full Scale IQ of 91 (27th percentile), placing her in the average range of ability overall. No significant discrepancy was evident between Verbal and Performance scores, nor was there significant intersubtest variability among the various Verbal subtests. Some intersubtest scatter was evident, however, within the Performance domain, with Ms. H. performing best on tests of visuo-spatial constructional skills (Object Assembly, Block Design), and poorer on a task requiring her to sequentially arrange a series of pictures to tell a meaningful story (Picture Arrangement) and on a task measuring attention to visual details (Picture Completion).

Attention and Concentration

Ms. H.'s attention skills were intact on relatively simple, selective material but deteriorated rapidly when presented with more complex "divided-attention" tasks. She obtained a digit span forward of seven, and a backwards digit span of five (Digit Span). She could rapidly and accurately perform such rote tasks as counting backwards from 20, reciting the alphabet, and counting forward by serial 3s to 40 (WMS-Mental Control). Conversely, she scored below expected levels on the Auditory Consonant Trigrams Test, a divided-attention task that involves counting backwards aloud while keeping a string of three letters in mind. Notably poor performance was evident on a timed motor task requiring visual scanning and tracking (Trail Making).

Language Functioning

The patient's spontaneous speech was unremarkable except for a slight dysarthria. No difficulties were noted in her comprehension of task instructions. On an aphasia screening exam, she was able to name, spell, read aloud, repeat words and phrases, write to dictation, follow verbal commands, and discriminate right and left. No deficits were noted on a test of confrontational naming (Boston Naming Test-55/60) or on word list generation (age-corrected FAS=39, 55–59th percentile).

Perceptual Organizational Abilities

Scores on perceptual organization and constructional tasks were uniformly well within the normal range. Ms. H. scored at the 63rd percentile on the Block

Design and Object Assembly subtests of the WAIS-R, indicating average visuospatial construction skills. She also scored well within the normal range in her copy of a complex two-dimensional design (Rey-Osterrieth Complex Figure Test). In contrast, she scored at the 16th percentile on the Picture Completion subtest of the WAIS-R, measuring attention to visual details, and also in the low average range on the Hooper Visual Organization Test, a task requiring her to mentally manipulate cut-up objects to form a whole percept. Thus, variable performance was evident in this domain, though overall, most perceptual organization and construction abilities appear largely intact.

Motor/Sensory Perceptual Exam

The patient denied any history of injury to arms, hands, or shoulders. The patient reported to be right-hand dominant. On a brief sensory perceptual exam, Ms. H. was observed to make several errors with her left hand on an astereognosis test, whereas no errors were made with her right hand. No finger agnosia was observed. On a task of finger tapping speed (Finger Tapping Test), she scored well within the normal range with both hands, and a slight expected dominant-hand advantage was observed (74th percentile, dominant hand; 60th percentile, nondominant hand). Likewise, the patient's grip (Hand Dynamometer) strength revealed normal performance bilaterally with a slight (expected) dominant-hand advantage.

Verbal (Auditory) and Nonverbal (Visual) Learning and Memory

Ms. H.'s initial learning of novel verbal material appeared to be well within the normal range, although her delayed recall of the material was mildly depressed. When novel nonverbal material was presented, Ms. H. showed consistently depressed scores, both in her immediate and delayed recall of the material.

On a task involving the learning of rote word pairs (WMS-Associate Learning), the patient's performance was well within the normal range (67th percentile), although some variability was observed. This was likely related to attention factors (specifically, she recalled three of the four difficult word pairs on the first two trials, then recalled only two of the four on the third learning trial.) Following a 45-minute delay, she recalled only five of the six easy word pairs and one of the more difficult word pairs. Ms. H.'s learning of a 15-item list of unrelated words (AVLT) was well within the normal range, but again, some variability was observed across the five trials, again most likely due to attention factors. Following an interference task, she was able to recall 10 of the items but only recalled six of the 15 items on 30-minute delayed recall, although she correctly recognized 13 of the items in paragraph format with no false-positives. On a task involving the immediate recall of paragraph details (WMS-Logical Memory), the patient scored at the average range for her age. However, following a 30-minute delay, she was able to recall only 65% of the information originally learned, a retention rate slightly below the 80% usually expected in normal adults.

The patient's immediate recall reproduction of relatively simple geometric figures (WMS-Visual Reproduction) was within the low average range for her age (13th percentile), and following a 30-minute delay, she was only able to recall 12% of the information originally learned, well below expected levels. Additionally, her recall of a complex two-dimensional figure (Rey-Osterrieth) following a three-minute delay was well within the borderline to impaired range.

Conceptual Tracking and Response Inhibition

Ms. H. scored well within the normal range on a task involving categorization and shifting of set (she was able to complete six categories on the Wisconsin Card Sorting Test with 86 of the stimulus cards). In addition, normal performance was observed on the Stroop Test, which involves the screening out of distracting information and the inhibition of incorrect responses. Also of note, Ms. H. was able to generate 19 novel designs in five minutes on the Design Fluency Test, a performance well within expected limits. In contrast, she could not complete the last two mazes on the WISC-R. Finally, the patient made five errors on the Rey Tangled Lines Test, though this must be interpreted in light of the fact that she had use of only one eye. Thus, mild and selective deficits were noted on some tasks thought to assess frontal systems functioning, though most tasks in this domain were within normal limits.

Achievement Scores

The patient's scores on formal achievement testing (WRAT-R) were slightly below expectation in light of her current intellectual level. Specifically, she performed in the low average range on a sight reading task, in the low average range on a spelling task, and in the low average to borderline range on a mathematical task.

Summary and Impressions

Neuropsychological test scores reveal the presence of difficulties in learning and recall (particularly for nonverbal visual material), visual perception, sequencing and tracking, tactile perception with the left hand, and attention and concentration for complex material. These findings overall reflect a pattern of mild dysfunction lateralized to the right hemisphere. In addition, the patient scored lower than expected on formal academic achievement testing. Attenuation in achievement areas is not typically found in cases of open head injury, and raises the possibility of long-standing, subtle academic difficulties.

In contrast, intact performance was observed on basic language skills, motor functioning, conceptualization/abstraction, and general intellectual functioning.

We were pleased to observe that, in spite of the patient's partial right frontal lobectomy, only mild signs of frontal systems dysfunction were observed on formal testing. Specifically, she evidenced relatively poor performance on tasks of divided attention and on visual sequencing and tracking tasks, though her word list generation, novel design generation, sorting, set shifting, and response-inhibition skills were well within the normal range. Behavioral observations of difficulty at work on complex tasks might also be taken as an indicator of disruption in frontal systems functioning, and the patient's belligerence and irritability during the administration of difficult and/or ambiguous tasks also provide some indirect evidence of frontal lobe disruption. It is possible that her loss of an eye may well have impacted negatively her performance on the visual sequencing and tracking tasks, artificially lowering her scores in these areas.

Within an employment setting, the patient will require a position in which she will not be expected to learn and retain a lot of novel information and in which she will not have to continually or rapidly shift her attention from one task to another. She would function best in a very routinized job that changes little from day to day. Her intellectual abilities border on low average, and she should be placed in a job position that does not demand greater than low average intellectual capabilities. It should be noted that the patient's irritability and low frustration tolerance are probably more apt to cause her problems in the work place than any intellectual difficulties. She appears to become rather irritable in demanding situations in which there is a lack of structure and solutions to problems are not immediately obvious.

NEUROPSYCHOLOGY TEST SCORE SUMMARY SHEET

Patient: K.H. Age: 30 Sex: F Handedness: R

I. Intelligence WAIS-R Age-Corrected Scores

VERBAL			PERFORMANCE		
Information	9	(37 %ile)	Picture Completion	7	(16 %ile)
Digit Span	10	(50 %ile)	Picture Arrangement	6	(9 %ile)
Vocabulary	8	(25 %ile)	Block Design	11	(63 %ile)
Arithmetic	9	(37 %ile)	Object Assembly	11	(63 %ile)
Comprehension	9	(37 %ile)	Digit Symbol	9	(37 %ile)
Similarities	11	(63 %ile)			
VERBAL IQ =	94	(34 %ile)	PERFORMANCE IQ =	89	(23 %ile)

FULL SCALE IQ = 91 (27 %ile)

II. Attention/Concentration
Digit Span: 7 forward + 5 backwards = 12 Total (50 %ile)
Mental Control, WMS: 7 (55 %ile)
Trails A: 55" (<1 %ile), Trails B: 79" (11 %ile)

III. Language
Boston Naming Test: 55/60
Controlled Word Association: F (18) + A (9) + S (8) + Age Corr.= 39 (55-59 %ile)

IV. Perceptual/Organizational
Rey-Osterrieth Complex Figure Copy: 36/36 (100 %ile)
Hooper Visual Organization Test: 22.5/30

V. Memory

VERBAL		NONVERBAL	
WMS Logical Memory	9.25 (67 %ile)	WMS Visual Repro:	8 (13 %ile)
30 min. delay:	6	30 min. delay:	1
Percent retention:	65	Percent retention:	13

WMS Associate Learning I Easy 6 , 6 , 6 ; Hard 3 , 3 , 2 ; Score: 17 (67 %ile)

Rey Osterrieth Fig: 36 (100 %ile)
3 min. delay: 10 (<10 %ile)

Rey Auditory Learning Test (15 items):
T1: 7 T2: 13 T3: 10 T4: 11 T5: 11 Recall after Interference: 10
30-min. Delayed Recall: 6
Recognition: 13 Hits, 0 False Identifications

VI. Motor Exam

	Dominant Hand	%ile	Nondom. Hand	%ile
Finger Tapping:	48	74	42	60
Grip Strength:	29	36	28	44

VII. Sensory
Asterognosis: several errors with the nondominant hand
Finger Gnosis: intact
Fingertip Number Writing: intact

VIII. Frontal Systems
Stroop A: 50", Stroop B: 59", Stroop C: 112"
Wisconsin Card Sorting Test: 6 Categories
WISC-R Mazes: Could not solve last two
Aud. Consonant Trigrams: 41/60
Rey Tangled Lines: 5" average, 5 errors

IX. Achievement

	Percentile Rank
WRAT-R: Reading	11
Spelling	12
Arithmetic	9

Case 4: Closed Head Injury Associated with Multiple Cognitive Deficits

Reason for Referral and Presenting Situation

Mr. L.M. is a 43-year-old, right-handed, Caucasian male with a Master's degree in psychology who is seeking help in understanding the origins of his rage attacks. He is currently employed as an office worker for a small company. He was referred by the Neurobehavior Service for assistance in determining the extent of damage and sequelae from a closed head injury the patient received approximately 17 years ago while a soldier in the army. At that time, he was involved in a truck crash, resulting in a head injury with evidence of a skull fracture of the right zygoma. He was unconscious for 24 hours, after which confusion persisted, and the patient reports post-traumatic amnesia for eight weeks following the injury. Subdural hematomas were suspected but not found, and he underwent bifrontal and bitemporal burholes to evacuate the suspected hematomas. Since the injury, the patient has reported double vision, constant headache, and left-sided motor weakness in upper and lower extremities, and has had borderline hypertension. Most significant, however, is the persistence of "rage attacks" following his injury, along with forgetfulness and depression. Mr. M. has experienced episodes of rage in response to minor frustrations, during which he screams, breaks or smashes items (e.g., he has smashed a car windshield), or drives at speeds greatly in excess of the speed limit. Once he hit his wife after she yelled at him, and he described another incident at a restaurant in which he threw a chair through a window when the restaurant did not provide him with a highchair for his daughter. As he was throwing the chair through the window, he recalls thinking, "I don't want to do this," but still was unable to inhibit himself. Though his recall for details after the rage outbursts is poor, he does recall the incidents themselves. He also described an incident in which he recently exposed his genitals to a woman in a parking lot, though no other sexual disinhibition is reported.

Mr. M. has worked as a office worker for the past four years. He has a degree in psychology and is a licensed marriage counselor, though his current problems have prohibited him from practicing in this field. He reports having been an "A" student throughout school. Since the injury, however, he reports difficulty remembering dates, names, and faces. His inability to recall information relevant to cases at work is a source of frustration. He further states that he feels his memory problems do not increase with fatigue, but rather, as the number of environmental distractors increase. Mr. M. compensates for memory problems by writing notes to himself.

Mr. M. has been married for nine years. His wife is a post-graduate level professional. They have one child, a daughter. Though no incidents of child abuse have been noted, Mr. M.'s wife reports being at times fearful for the safety of herself and their daughter.

The patient's medical history prior to his accident is unremarkable, and there was no prior history of neurologic disorder. Family medical history is significant for the patient's father dying of emphysema and congestive heart failure at age 72. The patient's mother died from a cerebral vascular accident at the age of 69. One sister died at age 8 from complications associated with polio. Family history is also significant for alcoholism in a grandfather and several "nervous breakdowns" in his mother, though no additional details are known. The patient reports only occasional alcohol use, and he reports becoming "more mellow" after a drink.

Mr. M. had taken Valium and Librium to help with anger control approximately 10 years ago, though these medications were largely ineffective. He currently is prescribed no medications.

Behavioral Observations

The patient appeared as a friendly, pleasant, and cooperative individual who seemed eager to participate in the testing process. He was persistent and handled frustration well. He requested one short break during the testing and was quick to ask that testing resume. Mr. M. has some familiarity with the assessment instruments and states that he was trained with the older WAIS (not WAIS-R) some 10 years ago, though he had forgotten many of the items because he has not used the tests in the interim. Also, the patient states that he was administered various neuropsychological and personality tests at another hospital three years ago when he participated in a head injury study, though these findings are not currently available to us. He was very sensitive to embarrassment during the interview portion of the assessment, relying heavily on his wife to recall and verify details about his behavior and items pertaining to his personal history.

Mr. M.'s wife exhibited an aggressive, irritating style of communication, fielding questions for her husband and frequently correcting inaccuracies for him, forcefully influencing both the content and direction of the interview. It was often necessary to redirect the interview, though she would not allow the topic to change until she was certain she had made her point. Interestingly, Mrs. M. demonstrated some awareness of her interpersonal style, stating that she always has to have the last word in conflicts ("I have to be right.").

The results of the assessment are believed to be an accurate reflection of the patient's current level of cognitive and intellectual functioning.

Tests Administered

See data summary sheet.

Test Results

Gross Cognitive Functioning

Mr. M. obtained a score of 28/30 on the MMSE, indicating grossly intact cognitive functioning. He made two errors on recall of three words following a distractor.

Intelligence

On the WAIS-R, Mr. M. achieved a Verbal IQ of 120, a Performance IQ of 99, and a Full Scale IQ of 111. This places him in the high average range of functioning (77th percentile). There is a 21-point discrepancy between Verbal and Performance IQ scores, which is unlikely to be found in the normal population. Within the verbal domain, Mr. M. exhibited considerable variability, with scores ranging from the very superior to superior range on tasks assessing word knowledge (Vocabulary), ability to think abstractly (Similarities), and judgment (Comprehension), to the average range on a task assessing attention and concentration (Digit Span). Within the performance domain, there was less variability evident, with the patient performing in the high average range (84th percentile) on a task assessing attention to detail (Picture Completion) and in the average range on all other nonverbal intellectual tasks.

Attention and Concentration

Mr. M. obtained a digit span of seven forward and five backwards (Digit Span). He performed rapidly and accurately on an attention task requiring such rote skills as counting backwards from 20, reciting the alphabet, and counting forward by 3s to 40 (WMS-Mental Control). On a speeded graphomotor task of visual scanning and tracking (Trail Making Test A), Mr. M. performed in the low average range (12th percentile), whereas on a more complex graphomotor speeded task involving visual scanning, tracking, and set shifting, he performed within the average range (Trail Making Test B, 51st percentile). Thus, intact abilities were evident in attention tasks, with perhaps some variability evident in timed tasks involving visual scanning and tracking.

Language

The patient's spontaneous speech was fluent and meaningful. No deficits were noted on a test of confrontational naming abilities (Boston Naming Test). Word list generation, in which the patient was asked to generate as many words as possible beginning with "f," "a," and "s" (with one minute for each) was well above average (80–84th percentile). Gross assessment of comprehension, repetition, and spontaneous writing were all within normal limits. Thus, language abilities appeared grossly intact.

Perceptual Organizational Abilities

Mr. M. performed within the average range (60th percentile) on his copy of a complex two-dimensional figure (Rey-Osterrieth). Also, he performed within the average range (63rd percentile) on a visuo-spatial task requiring him to construct red and white blocks to match a design (Block Design) and on a visuo-spatial task requiring him to put together puzzle pieces to form a familiar object (Object Assembly, 37th percentile). Thus, no frank deficits were evident in perceptual organization tasks.

Learning and Memory

Variable performance was evident in this domain. Mr. M. performed at the 48th percentile (average range) in his immediate recall of story passages (WMS-Logical Memory). Following a 30-minute delay, he recalled 44% of the information originally learned, well below expected levels. On a serial list-learning task of 15 unrelated words (AVLT) presented over five trials, Mr. M. showed a modest learning curve; he was able to learn 11 of the words by the fifth trial, a performance below expectation for his verbal intellectual level. Following an interference trial, he was only able to recall seven of the originally learned words, again a performance below expected levels. Assessment of recognition of the words from a larger array indicated the patient was able to correctly recognize all 15 of the words with no false-positive identifications.

Mr. M. performed in the average range (70th percentile) in his immediate recall reproduction of simple line drawings (WMS-Visual Reproduction), but following a 30-minute delay, he recalled only 20% of the originally learned information, though he was able to correctly recognize all four designs. He performed well below the 10th percentile in his recall of a complex two-dimensional figure (Rey-Osterrieth) following a three-minute delay. Overall, performance on memory tasks suggests deficits in both verbal and nonverbal memory with recognition preserved, suggesting probable intact initial encoding of the inforation but deficits in retrieval and/or storage mechanisms.

Motor

On the Finger Tapping Test, the patient achieved a 30% dominant hand advantage, despite no peripheral injury or anomaly. Performance with the nondomiant right hand was within the borderline impaired range (7th percentile), whereas performance with the dominant left hand was within the high average range (83rd percentile).

Frontal Systems Measures

On the Wisconsin Card Sorting Test, Mr. M. demonstrated no performance difficulty. He was able to complete six categories with 78 cards, and few perseverative errors were noted. On the Auditory Consonant Trigrams task, involving recall of consonants following distractors of varying delays, the patient showed no performance deficit. However, Mr. M. performed in the impaired range on a response-inhibition task (Stroop Test, Part C). Thus, these measures revealed variable performance on tasks of divided attention and abstract concept learning.

Personality Assessment

Mr. M.'s responses to personality assessment indicate a significant amount of psychological distress. His responses to the MMPI indicate a self-critical style and possibly a cry for help. Testing does suggest at least moderate levels of depression with accompanying vegetative symptoms (sleep and appetite disturbance), anxiety, low self-esteem, and a preoccupation with somatic concerns. The patient is also acknowledging strange and peculiar thoughts, feelings of derealization, hearing strange things when alone, and smelling strange odors.

Personality testing indicates conflicts stemming from childhood experiences with family as well as current marital discord. The patient feels rejected and unloved; he is very frightened over abandonment and conflicted over dependency needs. Apparently, his wife does many things for him that he used to do for himself. Due to a fear of losing control, he responds with resentment and withdrawal, as opposed to asserting himself. As the resentment builds, his ability to inhibit aggressive and hostile impulses is even further reduced. In disagreements, his wife feels a need to "be right" that, in conjunction with her husband's poor impulse control, seems to predispose him to losing control of his aggressive impulses.

Summary and Conclusions

The pattern of deficits revealed spotty performance with many areas surprisingly preserved in light of the patient's remarkable head injury. Though Mr. M. is currently functioning overall in the high average range of intelligence, his significant 21-point superiority of Verbal over Performance scores suggests disproportionate compromise in the nonverbal domain. While this discrepancy is rare in the general population, these scores may indeed reflect the patient's endowed pattern of intellectual functioning. On the other hand, the lower Performance IQ, in conjunction with evidence of a left-sided weakness, would be consistent with disproportionate right-hemisphere involvement. Difficulties in both verbal and nonverbal memory currently displayed by Mr. M. are common in patients with closed head injury, given the vulnerability of the temporal lobes to such an injury. The noteworthy behavioral change following the injury characterized by severe difficulties inhibiting his immediate impulses suggests frontal systems disturbance; the patient performed normally on most "frontal" tests but scored poorly on one measure tapping ability to inhibit incorrect responses and maintain a course of action despite distractors. Finally, the presence of depression, anxiety, restlessness, and poor impulse control – in addition to the dysfunction noted above – are consistent with a post-concussion syndrome, although the positive family psychiatric history raises the possibility that the patient may have been predisposed to psychiatric disturbance even without the head injury.

Given the patient's poor impulse control, psychotherapeutic intervention is strongly recommended to reduce the risk of assaultiveness, especially to his wife and young daughter. The patient's wife would likely benefit from involvement in this therapy as her behavior appears to contribute to the increased risk of assaultiveness from Mr. M. The patient expressed a desire to improve the quality of his relationship with his daughter, and we recommend that she be evaluated and treated for any untoward effects from her father's condition. The family should be *closely monitored* to insure the safety of the daughter, given the potential for child abuse. Providing the family with much needed support may serve as an emotional safety valve for the patient and his family, and we strongly recommend the patient and his family receive ongoing therapeutic contact to monitor and reassess his potential for acting out.

NEUROPSYCHOLOGY TEST SCORE SUMMARY SHEET

Patient: L.M. Age: 43 Sex: M Handedness: R

I. Gross Cognitive Functioning
Mini-Mental State Exam: 28 /30

II. Intelligence WAIS-R Age-Corrected Scores

VERBAL			PERFORMANCE		
Information	12	(75 %ile)	Picture Completion	13	(84 %ile)
Digit Span	8	(25 %ile)	Picture Arrangement	10	(50 %ile)
Vocabulary	16	(98 %ile)	Block Design	11	(63 %ile)
Arithmetic	10	(50 %ile)	Object Assembly	9	(37 %ile)
Comprehension	16	(98 %ile)	Digit Symbol	10	(50 %ile)
Similarities	15	(95 %ile)			
VERBAL IQ =	120	(91 %ile)	PERFORMANCE IQ =	99	(47 %ile)

FULL SCALE IQ = 111 (77 %ile)

III. Attention/Concentration
Digit Span: 7 forward + 5 backwards = 12 Total (25 %ile)
Mental Control, WMS: 9 (89 %ile)
Trails A: 40" (12 %ile), Trails B: 73" (51 %ile)

IV. Language
Boston Naming Test: 55/60, with phonemic cues: 59/60
Controlled Word Association Test: F (17) + A (14) + S (17) + Age Corr. = 48 (80-84 %ile)

V. Perceptual/Organizational
Rey-Osterrieth Complex Figure Copy: 33 /36 (60 %ile)

VI. Memory

VERBAL		NONVERBAL	
WMS Logical Memory	8 (48 %ile)	WMS Visual Repro.:	10 (70 %ile)
30 min. delay:	3.5	30 min. delay:	2
Percent retention:	44	Percent retention:	20
		Rey-Osterrieth Fig:	33/36 (70-80 %ile)
		3 min. delay:	12 (<10 %ile)

Rey Auditory Verbal Learning Test (15 items):
T1:3 T2:7 T3:8 T4:8 T5:11 Recall after Interference: 7
Recognition: 15 Hits, 0 False Identifications

VII. Motor Exam

	Dominant Hand	%ile	Nondom. Hand	%ile
Finger Tapping:	45	83	31.5	7

VIII. Frontal Systems
Stroop A: 47", Stroop B: 61", Stroop C: 177"

IX. Personality
MMPI: 2871**3*45"6'910-F'L/K:

Commentary on Head Injury Cases

The collection of cases in this chapter represents a broad sampling of many of the types of head injuries commonly referred to neuropsychologists for evaluation. Certainly, they represent the range of cases referred to us from behavioral neurologists, neurologic clinics, and attending psychiatrists, though it should be noted that neuropsychologists functioning in trauma centers may be referred more acute or serious cases than we have included here.

Several important observations may be made about the cases included in this chapter. First, it should be noted that all the cases showed residual deficits from their injuries, whether they were sustained three weeks or even 20 years ago. Second, many of the cases showed some recovery of function, especially when test-retest data were compared. This is particularly true within the first year following the injury, as was the case with Ms. B.

An emphasis in the introduction to this chapter was the importance of including a range of tests sensitive to higher level "executive" tasks dependent upon intact frontal lobe functioning even in seemingly minor head injury cases because of the vulnerability of these structures to injury. In fact, most cases in this chapter reflect significant compromise in tasks traditionally associated with frontal lobe functioning—response inhibition, divided attention, and cognitive flexibility. And in fact, Case 4 illustrates the dramatic behavioral changes that can occur post head injury, including impulse control and personality alteration. The case of Mr. A. also illustrates well how lateralized findings may be found (together with less severe but more general compromise in many domains) in a head injury case, despite the passage of some 20 years post injury.

Case 3 illustrates another aspect sometimes found in brain injury and, in particular, frontal lobe injury. Despite the number of cases in this chapter that have shown deficits in frontal systems tasks, this case is of known frontal lobe injury in which a portion of actual right frontal lobe tissue was surgically removed following the patient's trauma. In spite of this partial frontal lobectomy, the patient showed *remarkably* intact performance on many of the tests that are believed to be more sensitive to frontal systems dysfunction. This case is very important in illustrating that even our more sensitive indicators may not detect frontal lobe dysfunction, perhaps because of the high degree of structure imposed in the testing situation. That is, the patient is typically placed in a quiet room with little distracting stimulation and is directed on a one-to-one basis by a single examiner. The structure in the testing situation may compensate for deficient strategies from brain dysfunction. Thus, in addition to examination of cognitive tasks, it is very important for the examiner to incorporate behavioral indices of dysfunction, such as grossly inappropriate or disinhibited behavior or difficulties in planning or strategy formation, since they may document dysfunction not found in formal testing.

A final point should be made about many findings in these cases that are common to head injury. Most of the cases contained psychiatric disturbance (depression, anxiety, and seemingly psychotic disturbance) that are not uncommon sequelae of more serious head injury. Merely ascribing them as purely psychiatric in etiology would be a serious diagnostic error, we believe, and should be noted by those who evaluate head injury cases. A careful personal and family history will be important in such cases.

The cases presented here illustrate the complexity and variability in head injury, with often diffuse deficits present. A thorough and comprehensive examination may be necessary to tease out sometimes subtle deficits associated with such injuries.

2
Cerebrovascular Disease

Cerebrovascular diseases are a common cause of brain dysfunction providing a frequent reason for evaluation in neuropsychology, particularly in adults over 40 years of age. Such individuals are typically referred by neurologists or other primary-care physicians to obtain a neuropsychological evaluation of cognitive and emotional functioning. A thorough neuropsychological evaluation, particularly if repeated at intervals, may be useful in determining the degree and pattern of spared and impaired cognitive functions following such episodes and may aid in plans for rehabilitation. The results of the initial neuropsychological examination may also serve as a baseline from which to interpret future test performance. Because the area of pathology often dictates the pattern of neuropsychological deficit, the study of cerebrovascular disease and its consequences affords an opportunity to increase our understanding of brain-behavior relationships.

It is important for the neuropsychologist to carefully consider the neurological findings in cerebrovascular diseases because behavioral patterns differ depending on the specific etiology. Also, specific focal signs may be associated with occlusion of particular arteries. This chapter provides only a basic overview of this information, but we encourage the reader to become familiar with the excellent books by Adams and Victor (1985) and Chusid (1979).

Cerebrovascular accidents (CVA), which are also referred to as apoplexy or stroke, are disorders of the central nervous system resulting from pathology involving the blood vessels. During a CVA, the blood flow to an area of the brain is disrupted, thereby interfering with the brain's supply of nutrients—oxygen and glucose. Damaged or dead tissue, an infarct, results from the disruption of normal blood flow. Ischemic infarctions are caused by abnormal blood flow resulting in tissue starvation.

The primary mechanisms that can account for the tissue starvation are cerebral *hemorrhage* and obstruction of blood vessels by either *thrombosis* or *embolism*. Cerebral hemorrhage results from rupture of one of the cerebral blood vessels and can be described as a "bleed" within the brain. A thrombosis is a sclerotic plaque attached to a vessel wall that obstructs the flow of blood and is usually caused by arteriosclerosis and hypertension. Cerebral embolism is most commonly caused by heart disease and is defined as the occlusion of a vessel in the brain by a small piece of blood clot, tumor, air, fat, or other substance (Chusid, 1979).

There are a variety of behavioral changes that may occur following a CVA. The nature of such changes may differ as a function of the site and extent of pathology, the age of the patient, the premorbid level of functioning, and the patient's laterality, among other factors. Regardless of which hemisphere is implicated, common sequelae of CVA include impairments in general intellectual ability, attentional processing, and memory; disturbances in emotional functioning; as well as hemiplegia or hemiparesis contralateral to the site of pathology.

In addition to generalized impairments in cognitive function, there is often accompanying focal dysfunction. Focal cerebral lesions are typically associated with a specific pattern of deficits that differ depending upon which hemisphere is implicated in the CVA. It has been generally established that lesions involving the left hemisphere may result in language disturbance (aphasia), whereas lesions involving the right hemisphere often result in disturbances in visuo-spatial and temporal-spatial relations and may produce a syndrome of hemispatial neglect (see Heilman, Watson, & Valenstein, 1985). Neuropsychological test performance may be impaired in patients with left hemisphere stroke, particularly on measures sensitive to language function such as the verbal subtests of the WAIS-R, Boston Naming Test, Verbal Fluency, and Token Test, as well as aphasia examination batteries such as the Boston Diagnostic Aphasia Examination and Western Aphasia Battery. Verbal memory test performance may also be impaired and may be assessed by the Rey Auditory Verbal Learning Test, the California Verbal Learning Test, and the verbal memory portions of the Wechsler Memory Scale. Left hemisphere lesions may also lower Performance IQ, although Verbal IQ is usually most affected (Reitan & Fitzhugh, 1971). Patients with right hemisphere CVA may evidence impairment on perceptual measures such as the performance subtests of the WAIS-R (particularly Block Design and Object Assembly), Hooper Visual Organization Test, Street Visual Gestalt Test, Embedded Figures Test, Line Orientation, Line Bisection, and Visual Form Discrimination. Test performance of visual-motor integration/construction may also be compromised, such as on the Beery Visual Motor Integration Test and the Rey-Osterrieth Complex Figure. Whereas right-sided dysfunction tends to impair Performance IQ, Verbal IQ is relatively unaffected (Reitan & Fitzhugh, 1971). Motor function is typically impaired for the hand contralateral to the hemisphere with the cerebrovascular lesion (Brown, Baird, & Shatz, 1986; Haaland & Delaney, 1981), though abnormal findings on motor tests without supporting evidence from other cognitive tasks must be interpreted with caution (Bornstein, 1985). Motor impairment can usually be detected using tasks of motor performance such as the Finger Tapping Test, Grooved Pegboard, and Grip Strength, where a greater than expected asymmetry between performance of each hand may implicate impairment of the hand contralateral to hemispheric dysfunction.

Perhaps the most common finding associated with a CVA affecting the left hemisphere is the presence of aphasia as most right- and left-handers are believed to have speech mediated in the left hemisphere. Aphasia most frequently results from lesions in the middle cerebral artery; lesions of the anterior cerebral artery rarely cause aphasia. The major types of aphasia are *Broca's aphasia*, which involves a disturbance in speech output producing nonfluency, *Wernicke's aphasia*, which involves a fluent but often meaningless speech output and impaired comprehension, and *Global aphasia*, which encompasses both Broca's and Wernicke's aphasia. Broca's aphasia commonly results following a lesion of the posterior portion of the frontal operculum, which may be either cortical or subcortical (Geschwind, 1970). Hemiplegia is a common concomitant of Broca's aphasia. Wernicke's aphasia, which is less often accompanied by hemiplegia, results from a lesion involving the posterior-superior temporal region. Global aphasia is produced by destruction of both Broca's and Wernicke's areas and results from infarctions of the entire opercular region. It is commonly associated with hemiplegia. Other types of aphasia include Conduction aphasia, Transcortical Sensory aphasia, Transcortical Motor aphasia, and Subcortical aphasias. (For more detail see Benson & Geschwind [1971] and Goodglass & Kaplan [1983].)

Emotional changes often accompany cerebral infarctions involving either the left or right hemisphere. They may be found with an aphasic disturbance and typically differ depending on the nature of the neurological disorder. The patient with Broca's aphasia often responds in a depressed and even anguished manner to his or her disability and typically become distressed when confronted with his or her cognitive limitations, particularly in a testing situation. In contrast, the patient with Wernicke's aphasia is generally unaware of his or her deficits and may even appear euphoric. Agitation and anger toward others may also be present in the Wernicke's patient and, when combined with seemingly meaningless speech in the absence of neurological signs, have historically posed a problem in the differential diagnosis between this illness and an acute psychotic state. Emotional changes may also be seen in patients with right hemisphere involvement. In fact, right hemisphere infarctions have been associated with disturbance in the comprehension and/or expression of affect, and indifference to illness (Heilman, Bowers, & Valenstein, 1985).

The pattern of neuropsychological deficits following hemorrhages tends to differ from that following ischemic cerebral vascular accidents; in the former they are typically more widespread and are usually not associated with well-defined anatomic findings. Patients with cerebral hemorrhages tend to show serious disturbances in attention and memory and are more irritable (Walton, 1977). In contrast, the behavioral effects of ischemic infarctions are more apt to lateralize to the left or right hemisphere, and depending on the specific arteries involved, focal deficits are more commonly found.

Transient ischemic attacks (TIAs) are episodes of transient, focal neurologic deficit secondary to temporary obstruction of a blood vessel. Similar to full strokes, they are also believed to be caused by atherosclerosis and are considered warning signals to major strokes. TIAs generally last from several minutes to several hours and are associated with complete neurologic recovery within 24 hours of the event (Brust, 1977). Although the neurologic signs appear to recover relatively quickly, mild cognitive deficits may persist over time. Delaney, Wallace, and Egelko (1980) studied 15 patients with TIAs two to five days after the clinical signs had cleared and found them to be more impaired than a control group on measures of memory, perceptual-motor integration, concept formation, and verbal fluency, though not on measures of simple motor or sensory functioning.

Recovery patterns tend to differ among stroke victims. Factors such as age, education, premorbid competence, social support, handedness, etiology, and amount and type of rehabilitation are all important in predicting prognosis for recovery from stroke. Recovery processes following stroke include changes in regional blood flow, reduction in edema, restoration of normal neurotransmitter activity, and reorganization of brain systems (Brown et al., 1986). A considerable amount of spontaneous recovery of function can occur as early as one month following stroke. Hartman (1981) administered the Porch Index of Communicative Abilities (PICA) to 44 right-handed aphasics two weeks after stroke onset and again approximately two weeks later. Results at repeat testing showed improvement in 42 of the patients although none had received speech therapy, providing evidence for spontaneous recovery at one month post stroke. Meier and his colleagues developed a battery of neuropsychological tests to predict recovery from stroke (Meier, 1970; Meier & Okayama, 1969; Meier & Resch, 1967). They administered neuropsychological tests to 93 patients with recent onset of stroke (one month or less) including the Trail Making Test, Porteus Maze Test, Sequin-Goddard Formboard Test, and Visual Space Rotation Test. They found a high correlation between test performance and neurologic status that subsequently allowed accurate prediction of recovery patterns among patients. In an investigation of the prediction of patient outcome after stroke rehabilitation, Novak, Haban, Graham, and Satterfield (1987) found that psychological screening of motor persistence and verbal memory are good predictive factors of functional outcome. Their findings suggest that patients who display poor ability to store and recall information and who do not spontaneously persist with repetitive tasks are not as likely to show benefit from rehabilitation.

Recent studies suggest that CT scan findings may also be useful in predicting stroke recovery. Pieniadz, Naeser, Koff, and Levine (1983) have found correlations between atypical CT scan cerebral hemispheric asymmetries (i.e., the left posterior region is *not* wider or longer) and recovery from stroke. They reported that right-handed male global aphasic patients with atypical cerebral hemispheric asymmetries showed better recovery of specific language functions (one-word level in comprehension, repetition, and naming) than those with typical hemispheric asymmetries. Other types of patients who generally show a better prognosis include left-handers. Interestingly, individuals who show a left-handed preference typically recover more fully and more quickly from aphasia than right-handers (Hecaen & Sauguet, 1971; Subirana, 1958). This is believed to occur due to the more symmetric hemispheric organization of speech and language functions in the left-handed.

Also of note, it has been suggested that right hemisphere stroke patients who exhibit hemispatial neglect may show poor functional outcome (Kinsella & Ford, 1980). In fact, patients with inferred right hemisphere dysfunction (left-side motor weakness) have been found to be more functionally impaired following rehabilitation efforts than patients with inferred left hemisphere dysfunction (right-side motor weakness) (Novak, Haban, Graham, & Satterfield, 1987). Other frequent concomitants of right hemisphere dysfunction secondary to stroke, such as apparent unawareness of deficit (anosognosia) and emotional lability, may also serve as poor prognostic signs.

In sum, focal dysfunction along with generalized cerebral involvement frequently occurs secondary to cerebrovascular disease. The neuropsychological evaluation therefore should initially emphasize the assessment of functional deficits implicated by the areas of pathology as determined by the neurologic examination. Such information may aid in the care of the patient and in plans for rehabilitation. Elucidation of the patient's cognitive and motor limitations and capabilities will certainly lead toward better care of the stroke victim.

References

Adams, R.D., & Victor, M. (1985). *Principles of neurology* (3rd ed.). New York: McGraw-Hill.

Benson, D.F., & Geschwind, N. (1971). The aphasias and related disturbances. In A.B. Baker & L. Baker (Eds.), *Clinical neurology, Vol. 1*. New York: Harper and Row.

Bornstein, R. (1985). Normative data on selected neuropsychological measures from a nonclinical sample. *Journal of Clinical Psychology, 41*, 651–659.

Brown, G.C., Baird, A.D., & Shatz, M.W. (1986). The effects of cerebral vascular disease and its treatment on higher cortical functioning. In I. Grant & K.M. Adams (Eds.), *Neuropsychological assessment of neuropsychiatric disorders* (pp. 384–414). New York: Oxford University Press.

Brust, J. (1977). Transient ischemic attacks: Natural history and anticoagulation. *Neurology, 27*, 701–707.

Chusid, J.G. (1979). *Correlative neuroanatomy and functional neurology* (17th ed.). CA: Lange Medical Publications.

Delaney, R.C., Wallace, J.D., & Egelko, S. (1980). Transient cerebral ischemic attacks and neuropsychological deficit. *Journal of Clinical Neuropsychology, 2*, 107–114.

Geschwind, N. (1970). Language disturbances in cerebrovascular disease. In A.L. Benton (Ed.), *Behavioral changes in cerebrovascular disease*. New York: Harper and Row.

Goodglass, H., & Kaplan, E. (1983). *The assessment of aphasia and related disorders* (2nd ed.). Philadelphia: Lea and Febiger.

Haaland, K.Y., & Delaney, H.D. (1981). Motor deficit after left or right hemisphere damage due to stroke or tumor. *Neuropsychologia, 19*, 17–27.

Hartman, J. (1981). Measurement of early spontaneous recovery from aphasia with stroke. *Ann Neurol, 9*, 89–91.

Hecaen, H., & Sauguet, J. (1971). Cerebral dominance in left-handed subjects. *Cortex, 7*, 19–48.

Heilman, K.M., Bowers, D., & Valenstein, E. (1985). Emotional disorders associated with neurological diseases. In K.M. Heilman & E. Valenstein (Eds.), *Clinical neuropsychology* (2nd ed.) (pp. 377–402). New York: Oxford University Press.

Heilman, K.M., Watson, R.T., & Valenstein, E. (1985). Neglect and related disorders. In K.M. Heilman & E. Valenstein (Eds.), *Clinical neuropsychology* (2nd ed.) (pp. 243–294). New York: Oxford University Press.

Kinsella, G., & Ford, B. (1980). Acute recovery patterns in stroke patients. *Med J Aust, 2*, 663–666.
Meier, M.J. (1970). Objective behavioral assessment in diagnosis and prediction: Presentation 14. In A.L. Benton (Ed.), *Behavioral change in cerebrovascular disease.* New York: Harper and Row.
Meier, M.J., & Okayama, M. (1969). Behavioral assessment. *Geriatrics, 24*, 95–110.
Meier, M.J., & Resch, J.A. (1967). Behavioral prediction of short-term neurologic change following acute onset of cerebrovascular symptoms. *Mayo Clinic Proc, 42*, 641–647.
Novak, T.A., Haban, G., Graham, K., & Satterfield, W.T. (1987). Prediction of stroke rehabilitation outcome from psychologic screening. *Archives of Physical and Medical Rehabilitation, 68*, 729–734.
Pieniadz, J.M., Naeser, M.A., Koff, E., & Levine, H. (1983). CT scan cerebral hemispheric asymmetry measurements in stroke cases with global aphasia: Atypical asymmetries associated with improved recovery. *Cortex, 19*, 371–391.
Reitan, R.M., & Fitzhugh, K.B. (1971). Behavioral deficits in groups with cerebral vascular lesions. *Journal of Consulting and Clinical Psychology, 37*, 215–223.
Subirana, A. (1958). The prognosis in aphasia in relation to cerebral dominance and handedness. *Brain, 81*, 415–425.
Walton, S.N. (1977). *Brain's diseases of the nervous system* (8th ed.). Oxford, England: Oxford University Press.

Case 1: Bilateral Occipitotemporal Hemorrhage

Reason for Referral

Mr. M.K. was referred by his neurologist in order to evaluate possible changes in neuropsychological status post stroke.

Presenting Situation and Background Information

Mr. K. is a 69-year-old, Caucasian male who is a semi-retired real estate broker with three years of college. The patient is predominantly right-handed, though uses his left hand for many sports activities. He has no family history of left-handedness. He suffered acute onset of visual difficulties, memory loss, and gait disturbance two months ago. At that time he was found by his wife on the floor in a confused state asking, "Where am I?" He complained of a mild bifrontal headache, difficulty standing, and problems with his vision. Neurologic examination at the time of hospitalization revealed a profound memory impairment involving anterograde and retrograde memory loss, a bilateral superior quadrantanopia, and problems with recognizing famous faces. The results of a CT scan indicated a bilateral occipitotemporal hemorrhage. Over the course of his hospital stay, his memory and vision gradually improved. Past history is negative for head trauma or neurologic symptoms but positive for atherosclerotic heart disease. The patient is a heavy tobacco smoker and uses alcohol only occasionally. He is not taking any medications currently. There is no history of medical difficulties encountered at birth or in early development.

Behavioral Observations

Mr. K. appeared his stated age. He was well groomed and casually though neatly dressed. The patient was alert and oriented to person and place although he was incorrect by five days on the date. He was friendly and cooperative throughout the testing, and his frustration tolerance was good. He denied neurovegetative symptoms, and there were no signs of a formal thought disorder, hallucinations, delusions, or suicidal or paranoid ideation. His insight and judgment appeared to be poor to fair. For example, the patient denied any memory problems, despite his difficulty recalling facts during the interview, and stated that he felt almost completely recovered from his stroke.

Tests Administered

See data summary sheet.

Test Results

Attention/Concentration

Selective concentration skills were found to range from average to high average. Mr. K. could repeat six digits forward and four digits backwards, which is in the average range for his age although lower than expected in relation to other verbal skills. He was able to count backwards from 20 in nine seconds without error and to count serially by 3s up to 40 in 17 seconds without error; his performance on each of these tasks is above average for his age. Performance on tasks that required more active and sustained attention were also in the normal range. For example, Mr. K. performed at the 75th percentile for his age when asked to mentally compute arithmetic problems (Arithmetic subtest of the WAIS-R). The patient displayed difficulties on a visual motor task requiring conceptual tracking and sustained attention (Trail Making Test) though they were attributed to perceptual rather than attentional problems. Overall, no significant impairments in attention or concentration were found on this examination.

Intelligence

Mr. K. is currently functioning overall in the average range of intelligence with a Full Scale IQ of 109. He obtained a Verbal IQ of 115 (84th percentile) and a Performance IQ of 104 (61st percentile). With the exception of a subtest of immediate span of attention (Digit Span), which was normal but slightly lower than expected, there was little variability among his verbal subtests, which were in the average to above average range. No problems were found on subtests measuring general fund of information, range of vocabulary, abstract reasoning, or social judgment. Mild variability was noted among his performance subtests which ranged from average to high average. His ability to visually detect missing details was above average (Picture Completion subtest). He performed less well, though within the average range, on a motor test of visual spatial analysis (Block Design subtest).

Sensory/Motor

Mr. K. prefers to write with his right hand although he uses his left hand for several sport activities. On a test of fine motor coordination (Grooved Pegboard Test), he demonstrated an expected right hand advantage with no significant motor slowing. On a sensory perceptual examination, no lateralizing signs were found using simple tactile and visual stimuli. Tests for finger agnosia, fingertip number writing, and astereognosia were negative. However, on an auditory simultaneous stimulation exam, responses from the left ear were suppressed consistently.

Language

Spontaneous speech was grossly unremarkable except for an occasional word finding problem, though no problems in confrontational naming were confirmed on the Boston Naming Test. No gross signs of aphasia were noted on the Reitan-Indiana Aphasia Screening Test. Expressive language and fluency were above average as measured by both the Vocabulary subtest of the WAIS-R and the Verbal Fluency Test.

Perceptual Organizational Abilities

Test performance revealed a visual perceptual disturbance. Borderline performance was found on a visual closure test (Street Test) and on a visual organization task (Hooper Test). Problems in visual-motor integration were also observed and were particularly prominent when Mr. K. was asked to copy a key, which resulted in a distorted version. In spite of these significant visual perceptual and spatial impairments, there was no evidence of hemispatial neglect on either the Line Orientation Test, the Cancellation Test, or in drawings. Also, the problems in famous faces recognition noted on the neurologic examination completed earlier were not evident on current evaluation. It is unlikely that these results are caused by visual difficulties, as primary visual functioning was reported to be intact at the time of the evaluation.

Memory

Significant difficulty was found in the acquisition and retention of both verbal and nonverbal material. These problems were found on the WMS–Associate Learning subtest in which the patient's ability to learn common and uncommon word associations was significantly below average levels. His ability to learn word lists was also depressed as evidenced by his performance on the AVLT and the Shopping List Test. His performance on both of these tests was marked by frequent confabulations (i.e., extralist intrusions). In addition, his recall on the

AVLT was signficantly depressed after an interference condition. His immediate recall of material that was contextual and emotionally laden (WMS–Logical Memory subtest) was average, although his delayed recall of this material was severely impaired with many confabulations and intrusions.

Similarly, Mr. K.'s nonverbal memory was impaired. His immediate recall performance on the WMS–Visual Reproduction subtest was in the low average range, but he was only able to retain a small portion of it (33%) following a delay. His poor nonverbal memory performance may be confounded by problems in visuo-spatial functioning.

It is also important to note that Mr. K. appeared unaware of his severe memory deficits.

Summary and Impressions

Mr. K. is a 69-year-old man who sustained a bilateral occipitotemporal hemorrhage two months earlier. The pattern of neuropsychological findings is consistent with significant, though selective, impairment in higher information processing functions in an individual with average intelligence. Specifically, there is evidence of a significant memory impairment, a disturbance in perceptual functioning including visuo-perceptual functioning and visuo-motor integration, sensory extinction to simultaneous auditory stimulation on the left, and a mild attentional decline.

Most significant is the presence of a profound memory impairment involving the acquisition and retention of both verbal and nonverbal material. Pathognomonic signs were noted in his performance on verbal learning tests such as frequent confabulations. His recall was significantly depressed following a time delay with distraction. It is noteworthy that his memory was mildly facilitated by providing information in a context that was emotionally laden. However, he was not able to retain even this material over time. The patient's immediate memory span was average but lower than expected in relation to other verbal skills.

The presence of an auditory extinction to simultaneous stimulation on the left side coupled with anosognosia (i.e., the apparent unawareness of one's deficits) raise the possibility of the neglect syndrome. The neglect syndrome is characterized by the failure to respond to meaningful stimuli presented to the side contralateral to the lesion. The patient's extinctions on the left side would be compatible with right hemisphere dysfunction. It should be noted that other features of the neglect syndrome, such as hemispatial neglect for visual stimuli, were not evident on examination.

Additional signs of possible right hemisphere dysfunction included lowered visuo-perceptual ability and a relative lowering of Performance IQ. Problems in visuo-motor integration tasks were also observed, particularly when Mr. K. was asked to copy simple line drawings. However, these problems may be secondary to his depressed perceptual abilities. Since visual acuity was reported intact at the time of the evaluation, this was not an issue.

Overall, Mr. K.'s deficits are consistent with the areas of the brain implicated in his hemorrhage. The constellation of symptoms including memory loss, initial problems with facial recognition of historically famous faces (found on an earlier neurologic exam), and visual perceptual problems are consistent with bioccipitotemporal lesions that were diagnosed in his neurologic report. Other symptoms, such as features of the neglect syndrome and perceptual organization disability, emphasize right hemisphere involvement.

Due to the recency of the brain insult and the progress already noted in terms of regaining functions, additional recovery is expected. However, because he does not appear to have insight into his memory impairment, we feel that his family should be aware of this and take adequate precautions. We are most concerned about his lack of awareness of his memory deficit. His memory impairment coupled with his denial render this individual somewhat dependent on the help of others in daily living. Reevaluation in six to eight months is recommended to assess for possible changes in cognitive functioning.

NEUROPSYCHOLOGY TEST SCORE SUMMARY SHEET

Patient: M.K. Age: 69 Sex: M Handedness: R

I. Intelligence WAIS-R Age-Corrected Scores

VERBAL			PERFORMANCE		
Information	14	(91 %ile)	Picture Completion	13	(84 %ile)
Digit Span	8	(25 %ile)	Picture Arrangement	12	(75 %ile)
Vocabulary	13	(84 %ile)	Block Design	10	(50 %ile)
Arithmetic	12	(75 %ile)	Object Assembly	--	(%ile)
Comprehension	12	(75 %ile)	Digit Symbol	10	(50 %ile)
Similarities	12	(75 %ile)			
VERBAL IQ =	115	(84 %ile)	PERFORMANCE IQ =	104	(61 %ile)

FULL SCALE IQ = 109 (73 %ile)

II. Attention/Concentration
Digit Span: 6 forward + 4 backwards = 10 Total (25 %ile)
Mental Control, WMS: 9, (89 %ile)
Trails A: 46" (15 %ile), Trails B: 120" (5 %ile)

III. Language
Boston Naming Test: 57/60
Controlled Word Association: F(14) + A(11) + S(13) + Age Corr.=45 (75-79 %ile)
Aphasia Screening Exam: intact

IV. Perceptual/Organizational
Hooper Visual Organization Test: 19/30 Street Test: 6 /13
Line Orientation Test: 24/30 Famous Faces: intact
Cancellation Test: intact

V. Memory

VERBAL			NONVERBAL	
WMS Logical Memory	6	(32 %ile)	WMS Visual Repro.:	3 (21 %ile)
45 min. delay:	0		45 min. delay:	1
Percent retention:	0		Percent retention:	33

WMS Associate Learning: Easy 2, 2, 2; Hard 0, 1, 1; Score: 5 (6 %ile)

Rey Auditory Verbal Learning Test (15 items):
T1:2 T2:5 T3:7 T4:9 T5:9 Recall after Interference: 3

Shopping List Test (10 items):
T1:2 T2:3 T3:3 T4:4 T5:3 15 min. delay: 2

VI. Motor Exam

	Dominant Hand	%ile	Nondom. Hand	%ile
Grooved Pegboard:	60"	13	65"	10

VII. Sensory
Finger Gnosis: intact Fingertip writing: intact
Sensory Perceptual Exam: intact
Auditory Simultaneous Stimulation: 5 L, 0 R

Case 2: Wernicke's Aphasia

Reason for Referral

Mrs. S.M. was referred for neuropsychological evaluation of a severe language disturbance. She was brought to the clinic by her sister. The patient was unable to provide historical information due to the presence of an aphasia. Hence, such information was gleaned from interviews with her sister and review of medical records.

Presenting Situation and Background Information

Mrs. M. is a 79-year-old, widowed, right-handed Caucasian woman who lives at home with the aid of a companion. She was in good health until a year and a half ago when she experienced an abrupt onset of loss of speech associated with right-sided facial weakness. No other neurologic symptoms were evident at that time. The patient experienced an additional episode one year later with increasing difficulties in expression of speech, again associated with right-sided facial contortion. A CT scan at that time revealed no abnormalities. However, a repeat CT scan performed approximately four months later showed a low density area in the left temporoparietal region consistent with an old infarction. Also, a focal area of enhancement was found in the right parietal lobe. On neurological exam, the patient was unable to write, copy simple line drawings, or copy words accurately, in addition to other difficulties, including verbal expressive problems.

Mrs. M.'s sister reported that the patient's speech has improved through rehabilitation therapy, although she still experiences difficulties in verbally expressing herself effectively.

Since the initial episode, Mrs. M. has experienced some major changes in lifestyle. Before the episode, she reportedly had been a very active, independent, bright woman who worked as a court stenographer and engaged in volunteer work as well as other activities. Currently, Mrs. M. is severely limited in her activities. She is still able to care for activities of daily living, but she requires a live-in companion to keep house for her. The patient now spends much of her time playing cards by herself or hook-latching rugs. She has lost 15 pounds within the past year and a half and denies changes in her sleep habits. Mrs. M. reports that she is not able to do much and is very sad and scared about what has happened to her.

Mrs. M. is a high school graduate with no history of previous neurologic or psychological problems. She denies alcohol and tobacco intake and is not taking any medications currently. Family history is positive for cardiac disease and negative for left-handed immediate family members. The patient denies any significant medical trauma experienced at birth or in early development.

Behavioral Observations

Mrs. M. was alert and cooperative but presented with obvious expressive language difficulties. Her speech was fluent but marked by literal and verbal paraphasias, as well as severe word finding difficulties. Her ability to comprehend the examiner was severely restricted. Her affect was anxious, and she evidenced great frustration with the ability to make herself understood and to understand other's requests. She was acutely aware of her inaccuracies in attempting to communicate and was noticeably distraught when confronted with her limitations. The patient appeared agitated and frightened and became easily frustrated on evaluation. Testing was abbreviated due to the patient's marked comprehension deficits coupled with time constraints.

Tests Administered

See data summary sheets.

Test Results

Intelligence

Formal evaluation of intellectual functioning was not undertaken due to the patient's severe receptive and expressive language deficits.

Language

Significant impairments were found in various aspects of language functioning as measured by selected portions of the Boston Diagnostic Aphasia Examination (Figure 2.1). Mrs. M. was severely restricted in terms of her language comprehension. Her speech was fluent, though marked by phonemic transpositions (literal paraphasias) and word substitutions (verbal paraphasias). She was unable to read or spell words. Mrs. M. was able to read numbers if she first counted aloud up to the number. She was able to write her name and address, but she was unable to generate a written sentence. In addition, she displayed significant difficulty in word repetition. Severe deficits in comprehension were also found using the Token Test, a tool that is sensitive to disrupted linguistic comprehension processes. The patient evidenced severe naming difficulties as measured by the Boston Naming Test, with frequent literal paraphasic errors, and phonemic cueing was of little help.

Perceptual Organizational Abilities

The patient was able to copy simple geometric drawings on the Reitan-Indiana Aphasia Examination. This is most significant because she was unable to do so one month earlier on neurological exam. These results point to recovering visuospatial functioning. Mrs. M. was also now able to draw a cube and a clock. Right/left discrimination was impaired but appeared to be secondary to comprehension deficits.

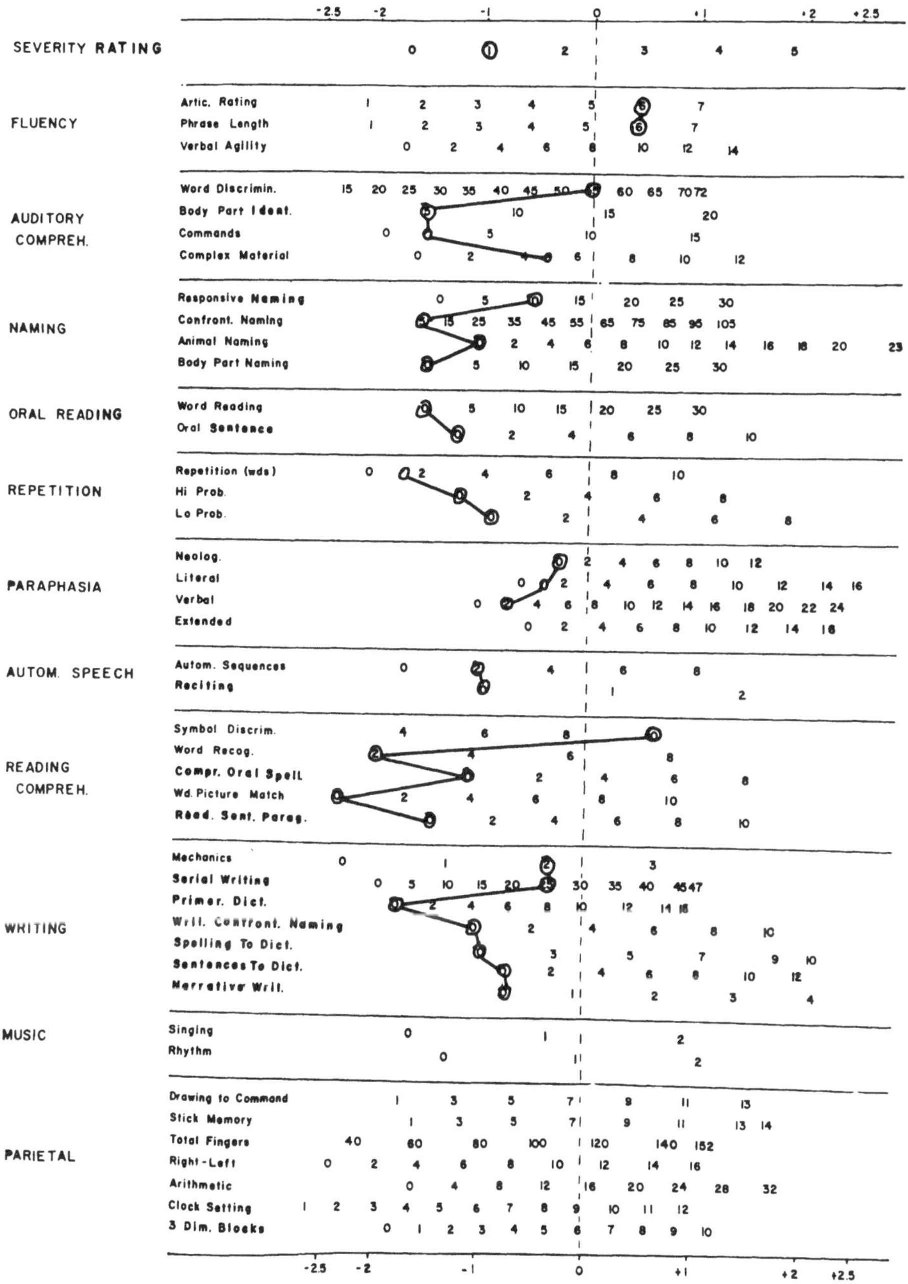

FIGURE 2.1. Case S.M. Z-score profile of aphasia subscores on the Boston Diagnostic Aphasia Examination.

Motor

The patient's history is negative for injury to arms, hands, or shoulders. Motor function was measured with the Finger Tapping Test, which revealed results that were essentially within normal limits, although a greater dominant-hand (right) advantage was found (20%) than expected (10%) suggesting possible left-sided motor weakness (right = 37, left = 30).

Memory

Visual memory functioning was grossly intact. On informal testing of visual memory, the patient was able to recognize three figures following a brief delay. Unfortunately, verbal memory functioning could not be assessed reliably because of her language disturbance.

Summary and Impressions

The pattern of neuropsychological test results obtained for this patient indicates a Wernicke's aphasia. Her symptoms of fluent but empty speech, impaired auditory comprehension, literal and verbal paraphasias, anomia, and difficulties in reading, writing, and repetition are all consistent with a posterior aphasia (Wernicke's). However, her acute awareness of her speech difficulties is unusual. The presence of recovering visuo-spatial dysfunction is not inconsistent with lesions of the left hemisphere and is commonly associated with aphasia. The results of a recent CT scan document left and right hemisphere lesions. It is likely that the left temporoparietal region lesion may account for her aphasia as well as visuo-spatial dysfunction, although the old infarction in the right parietal lobe may also be tied to her impairments in visuo-spatial functioning.

The fact that Mrs. M. is aware of her speech difficulties may be considered a motivator in rehabilitation of her aphasia. She is agitated and frightened of the changes that have been imposed in her life as a result of her problem. She wants very much to regain her independence and active involvement in social and work events and is thus motivated to improve her speech handicap. We strongly recommend that speech therapy, which has been helpful in the past, be resumed with careful attention to emotional factors to prevent a major depression. Also, because she is showing significant signs of emotional distress and displays the neurovegetative symptom of a considerable weight loss, further evaluation of depressive affect may be warranted. Reevaluation in six months is strongly recommended to determine the course of her cognitive functioning over time.

NEUROPSYCHOLOGY TEST SCORE SUMMARY SHEET

Patient: S.M. Age: 79 Sex: F Handedness: R

I. Language

Boston Diagnostic Aphasia Exam: see profile
Boston Naming Test: 3 /60, with phonemic cues: 12 /60
Token Test: 10.5

II. Perceptual/Organizational

Copy-A-Cube: intact Draw-A-Clock: intact
Letter Cancellation Test: intact

VI. Motor Exam

	Dominant Hand	%ile	Nondom. Hand	%ile
Finger Tapping:	37.0	79	30.0	34

Case 3: Multiple CVAs

Reason for Referral

Mr. D.F. is an 86-year-old, widowed, right-handed black male who was referred for neuropsychological evaluation to assess cognitive deficits and depressive features.

Presenting Situation and Background Information

Upon recent hospital admission, the patient presented with left-sided weakness and left homonymous hemianopsia secondary to a right temporoparietal CVA. Past history is remarkable for a left hemispheric CVA sustained 19 years ago and controlled hypertension. Information regarding the left hemispheric CVA is not available. The patient reported getting average grades with no particular school-related problems, though he dropped out of school in the ninth grade. He is a retired chauffeur and past field superintendent. Prior to his admission, he was functioning independently and living alone in his apartment. He currently is taking several medications, including Digoxin. Previous medical history is negative for head trauma and seizures, and birth and developmental history is also unremarkable. The patient denies significant alcohol intake and tobacco use at present.

Behavioral Observations

Mr. F. was cooperative and polite and showed no signs of fatigue on either of the two testing sessions. He admitted to feelings of depression and expressed concern for not being able to care for his daily needs or continue with previous recreational activities.

Tests Administered

See data summary sheet.

Test Results

General Cognitive Functioning

Mr. F.'s score of 20/30 on the MMSE was suggestive of cognitive impairment. Errors were noted on orientation items requiring the patient to determine the date, day of the week, and the season. He was, however, able to correctly provide the year and month. Mr. F. was unable to calculate serial 7s backwards or spell the word "world" backwards. He was unable to write a complete sentence upon command or reproduce a simple geometric design. These results are suggestive of mild to moderate deficits in general cognitive functioning.

Intelligence

The patient's intellectual functioning, as assessed using the WAIS-R (Satz-Mogel format), yielded a Verbal IQ of 82 (12th percentile), a Performance IQ of 68 (2nd percentile), and a Full Scale IQ of 76 (6th percentile), placing him overall in the borderline range of intelligence. Based upon this patient's educational and vocational history, these findings are suggestive of probable intellectual decline, with nonverbal intellectual functioning more seriously affected than verbal intellectual functioning. The patient showed marked impairment on those subtests of the WAIS-R that most heavily tap visuo-spatial abilities (i.e., Block Design and Object Assembly), on which he scored below the first percentile. On a task particularly sensitive to the effects of brain damage, the Digit Symbol subtest, the patient was able to accurately reproduce only one of the matching symbols. Although some loss in visuo-spatial abilities is expected with aging, these results suggest a more severe loss than can be explained by an age factor alone. However, it should be noted that age-corrected scores extend only to age 74 on this test. Thus, current scores, especially nonverbal scores, no doubt reflect an underestimation of ability.

Attention/Concentration

No significant problems were noted on tests measuring attention and concentration. Digit span performance was within normal limits for his age and commensurate with overall verbal intellectual functioning. Performance on the Arithmetic subtest of the WAIS-R, though low in relation to other verbal subtest scores, is not appreciably lower than expected given his limited educational attainment. In fact, the patient was able to attend quite well to verbal material presented in the form of a word list (SLT) or short story (WMS-LM). His performance on Trail Making A, a task requiring vigilance to nonverbal stimuli and visual tracking, suggests marked impairment but is believed to be tied largely to problems in visual perception (as noted below).

Language

Impairments were also found in the language domain. Mr. F. scored below expected levels on the Boston Naming Test, a task measuring confrontational naming abilities; he was unable to identify pictures of a seashore, dart, globe, or beaver—words believed to have been in his active vocabulary premorbidly. Phonemic cueing was only helpful in aiding the patient on 5 of 14 items. Literal paraphasias were also noted, such as substituting the word "compastic" for compass. Errors in visual perception confounded test performance (e.g., labeling a harmonica a "ferry"). Problems in word list generation were found on the Verbal Fluency task in which the patient was only able to generate a total of 11 words that begin with three specific target letters in three minutes. Mr. F. was able to repeat a complex phrase and follow a three-step command but was unable to write a self-generated sentence. Overall, problems in language functioning were found that could be tied, in part, to visual perceptual dysfunction.

Perceptual Organizational Abilities

Marked deficits in visuo-spatial and visuo-perceptual abilities were found. The patient demonstrated significant impairment on subtests of the WAIS-R that tap visuo-spatial analysis such as the Block Design and Object Assembly subtests (< 1st percentile). It was observed that Mr. F. was unable to form the 2 × 2 block matrix required on even the most simple of the Block Designs, and on Object Assembly he was able to form only one constructional match out of the designs presented, despite being given ample time past the standard limit imposed by the test. The patient was able to match and reproduce only one of the symbols of the Digit Symbol subtest of the WAIS-R (< 1st percentile), a test particularly sensitive to brain damage. Additionally, as noted above, perceptual errors were found on a confrontational naming test (Boston Naming Test).

Impairment in paper and pencil constructions was also noted. On the Rey-Osterrieth Complex Figure (copy format), the patient performed below the 10th percentile. Qualitatively, Mr. F. retained many of the inner details of the design; however, he was unable to represent the gestalt of the design. On the VMI, a copy task of simple line drawings, the patient was able to correctly reproduce only 9 of 24 designs, and his performance deteriorated markedly with increasing complexity of the designs. Evidence of left-sided hemispatial neglect was found on both the VMI and, more dramatically, on the Line Bisection Test (LBT). On the LBT, his line bisections were mostly all on the right half of the page.

Verbal (Auditory) and Nonverbal (Visual) Learning and Memory

No impairment was found on verbal memory testing beyond the effects of normal aging. Mr. F. performed at an average level on an associated word list learning test, the Shopping List Test. He was able to recall seven of the 10 items on each of the five trials and again after a 15-minute delay. Although no learning curve was noted, he was able to recognize all 10 items following the delay. Mr. F. performed at the 33rd percentile on the WMS-AL subtest, which is a word-pair learning task. He was able to recall all six easy word pairs and 1 of 4 unassociated word pairs by the third trial. His verbal memory performance was facilitated by presenting material in a form more analogous to conversational language. Mr. F.'s performance was above average in his immediate recall on the WMS-LM subtest (90th percentile). Moreover, he was able to retain 67% of the material over 30 minutes, which is within the average range for his age.

Nonverbal memory functioning was not assessed due to the patient's marked deficits in visual spatial processing.

Motor Functioning

The patient denied any history of injury to his arms, hands, or shoulders. Assessment of motor speed was conducted using the Finger Tapping Test. Results with each hand were within normal limits for his age (right = 33.0, left = 26.6), but a slightly greater than expected discrepancy between hands was noted. This discrepancy, though slight, raises the question of a possible mild impairment of nondominant (left) hand motor speed from estimated premorbid levels.

Personality Functioning

Brief assessment of personality functioning was conducted. Testing with the Beck Depression Inventory suggests the presence of mild to moderate depressive features. The patient indicated problems with sleeping, appetite loss, fatigue, and anxiety related to his physical problems. He also admitted to feeling sad and experiencing decreased enjoyment of activities. These results are certainly compatible with the patient's self-report of depression.

Summary and Impressions

Mr. F. is an 86-year-old man with a history of a recent right temporoparietal CVA and a past left hemispheric CVA sustained approximately 19 years ago. Interpretation of test scores was problematic due to the patient's advanced age and low educational level. Normative test data are rarely available for individuals in their 80s. Also, individuals with low educational levels are frequently found to perform more poorly on neuropsychological tests despite normal brain functioning.

Overall, the results of neuropsychological evaluation suggest bilateral hemisphere involvement with impairment of right hemispheric functions appearing more severe at this time. Findings consistent with right hemisphere dysfunction are marked deficits in visuo-spatial and visuo-perceptual functioning, pronounced left-sided hemispatial neglect, lowered performance IQ, and possible slight motor slowing of the nondominant (left) hand. The observed impairment in visuo-perceptual functioning is believed to be beyond the typical decline noted with advanced aging. Abilities typically mediated by the left hemisphere appear more intact. Verbal memory functioning was remarkably intact; his performance was above average for his age. However, significant impairments were noted in naming abilities, such as in confrontational naming and verbal productivity and generation. Although some of the naming errors could be attributed to perceptual dysfunction, the majority were tied to word substitutions.

The overall pattern of neuropsychological test results are compatible with his medical history of bilateral CVAs with compromise of functions mediated by both hemispheres, resulting in a probable multi-infarct dementia. Evidence of a dementia is found with deficits in general cognitive ability, selective language functioning, visuo-spatial and visuo-perceptual processing, and a suspected decline in intelligence, particularly affecting Performance IQ. It should be noted that the present test results may be influenced by his current drug regimen, and this possibility should be explored. The patient is aware of his deficits and appears to be exhibiting some signs of a reactive depression. Mr. F. is no longer able to care for his daily needs, though this may be a result of his depressed affect. We recommend psychotherapy with attention to his mild to moderate depressive condition.

NEUROPSYCHOLOGY TEST SCORE SUMMARY SHEET

Patient: D.F. Age: 86 Sex: M Handedness: R

I. Gross Cognitive Functioning
Mini-Mental State Exam: 20/30

II. Intelligence WAIS-R Age-Corrected Scores

VERBAL			PERFORMANCE		
Information	9	(37 %ile)	Picture Completion	7	(16 %ile)
Digit Span	7	(16 %ile)	Picture Arrangement	7	(16 %ile)
Vocabulary	7	(16 %ile)	Block Design	2	(.4 %ile)
Arithmetic	5	(5 %ile)	Object Assembly	2	(.4 %ile)
Comprehension	10	(50 %ile)	Digit Symbol	1	(.1 %ile)
Similarities	5	(5 %ile)			

VERBAL IQ = 82 (12 %ile) PERFORMANCE IQ = 68 (2 %ile)
FULL SCALE IQ = 76 (5 %ile)

III. Attention/Concentration
Digit Span: 6 forward + 3 backwards = 9 Total (16 %ile)
Trails A: 373", 1 error (< 1 %ile)

IV. Language
Boston Naming Test: 30/60, with phonemic cues: 35/60
Controlled Word Association: F (1) + A (4) + S (6) + Age Corr.= 20 (<4 %ile)

V. Perceptual/Organizational
Rey-Osterrieth Complex Figure Copy: 8 /36 (<10 %ile)
Beery VMI: 9 /24

VI. Memory VERBAL
WMS Logical Memory 8.25 (90 %ile)
30 min. delay: 5.5
Percent retention: 67

WMS	I	Easy	3	4	6
Associate	I	Hard	0	1	1
Learning	I	Score: 8.5 (33 %ile)			

Shopping List Test (10 items):
T1: 7 T2: 7 T3: 7 T4: 7 T5: 7 15-min. Delayed Recall: 7
Recognition: 10 Hits, 0 False Identifications

VII. Motor Exam	Dominant Hand	%ile	Nondom. Hand	%ile
Finger Tapping:	33.0	13	26.6	5

VIII. Personality
Beck Depression Inventory: 23

Case 4: Right Hemisphere CVA

Reason for Referral

Mr. R.M. was referred by his neurologist for neuropsychological evaluation following a recent syncopal episode.

Presenting Situation and Background Information

Mr. M. is a 64-year-old, right-handed Caucasian male who sustained a right hemorrhagic CVA with an accompanying left hemiplegia approximately three months ago. He recently sustained a syncopal episode. While walking, he reportedly developed spasms in his left arm and felt light-headed. After sitting down, he lost consciousness for an unknown period of time. On regaining consciousness, he discovered he had bowel and bladder incontinence, though he experienced no confusion, tongue biting, weakness, numbness, or paralysis. He subsequently was hospitalized and placed on Dilantin. A CT scan revealed a shift in the midline structures. The patient's hemiplegia has resolved for the most part, and he is able to walk with the aid of a cane. His history is positive for sleep apnea and negative for other neurological or psychological disturbances. There is no history of head trauma. He is not taking any medication currently and denies significant alcohol or tobacco use. Birth and developmental history are unremarkable.

Mr. M. has had four years of schooling at a large state university but did not complete his B.A. degree, though he reportedly did well in his courses. He is currently vice-president of a small electrical company.

It is noteworthy that significant signs of left-sided neglect were evident during his hospitalization following the syncopal episode. For example, Mr. M. was noted to have fully dressed himself with the exception of his left shoe. Moreover, when the shoe was provided for him, he was unable to put it on correctly without assistance. Also noteworthy were signs of anosognosia, the seeming indifference to his disability or failure to recognize his deficits. He also displayed problems with spatial disorientation and was reported to have gotten lost on his way back to his ward. Furthermore, his daughter reported that he often gets lost on his way to a frequently visited restaurant.

Behavioral Observations

The patient was oriented for time, person, and place. He appeared mildly disheveled on evaluation. His hair was not well groomed, and he had missed areas while shaving, more noticeable on the left than right side of his face. Additional signs of left-sided neglect were evident on examination; specifically, on motor construction tasks such as the Block Design subtest of the WAIS-R, Line Bisection Test, and figure drawings.

Tests Administered

See data summary sheet.

Test Results

Intellectual Functioning

Mr. M. is currently functioning overall in the low average range of intelligence with a WAIS-R Full Scale IQ of 88. There was a significant difference between his Verbal IQ of 104 (average range) and his Performance IQ of 70 (borderline range). This discrepancy, which is significantly larger than expected, is suggestive of visuo-spatial dysfunction.

Performance subtest age-corrected scores ranged from the impaired (2) to the low average range (7). Among his Performance subtests, the patient encountered the most difficulty on the Block Design subtest in which signs of left hemispatial neglect precluded him from successfully completing any of the designs. For example, Mr. M. tended to assemble only the right side of the 2 × 2 array and ignored the left side. Other times, he would only assemble the top two blocks in the array. Despite his obvious difficulty with this subtest, the patient denied having any problems with it. There was also a moderate degree of intersubtest scatter among the Verbal subtests from the average to the high average range (age-corrected scaled scores ranged from 8 to 13). The patient performed best on subtests measuring his vocabulary range, fund of general information, and judgment; he performed relatively more poorly though in the normal range, on tasks tapping attentional processes.

Attention/Concentration Processes

Attention and concentration processes were found to be intact. The patient was able to count forward by serial 3s, backwards from 20, and to recite the alphabet without error. His digit span performance was average for digits successfully recited forward (7) and backwards (4). Although he displayed significant problems in his Trail Making Part A performance, this can be attributed mostly to perceptual rather than attention problems because he exhibited difficulty in locating numbers due to neglect.

Language Functioning

No significant problems in language functioning were noted on examination. His speech was fluent, with adequate volume and speed. There was no evidence of paraphasias or dysarthria. No language-related errors were noted on the Aphasia Screening Test. Expressive language and range of vocabulary were in the high average range as measured by the verbal subtests of the WAIS-R. Writing and reading abilities were grossly intact as was sentence repetition. It should be noted, however, that the patient tended to neglect words on the left side of the page when reading a paragraph. This latter problem is related to a perceptual rather than to a language disturbance.

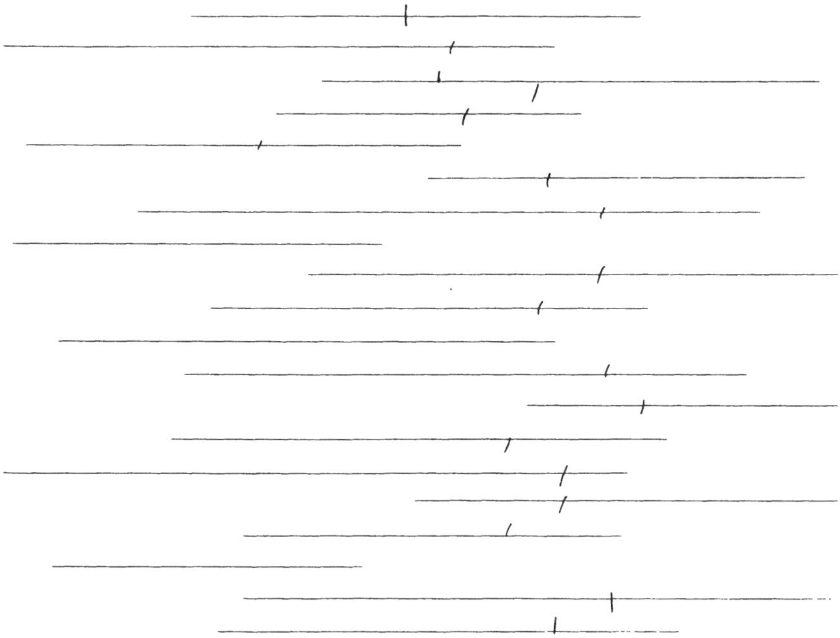

FIGURE 2.2. Case R.M. Line Bisection Test. Reduced by 60%.

Perceptual Organizational Functioning

As noted above, the patient displayed a significant problem in perceptual functioning and a prominent left-sided neglect. Evidence of his hemispatial neglect was most salient on the Line Bisection Test in which the patient's bisections were incorrectly placed off to the right of the page (Figure 2.2). Moreover, he tended to utilize only the right half of the page when drawing or writing. This pattern was also observed on the Performance subtests of the WAIS-R in which a left-sided neglect contributed to his low Performance IQ relative to his Verbal IQ. A significant problem secondary to hemispatial neglect was also observed on the Hooper VOT in which he scored in the impaired range. On the Hooper, he tended to make "isolate" errors in which he incorrectly guessed the objects based on a small detail on the right side of the figure. For example, he responded that the mouse (item #22) was a "pipe" and that the broom (item #30) was a "salt shaker."

A disorder in visual-motor integration was also noted, particularly in his copy of a complex figure (Rey-Osterrieth) in which the patient exhibited significant difficulty with the organizational structure of the design (Figure 2.3). Also, as noted above, perceptual dysfunction was found on the Trail Making Test.

Verbal (Auditory) and Nonverbal (Visual) Learning and Memory

Results of verbal memory testing were variable. The patient demonstrated superior ability in the acquisition and retention of short stories on the WMS-LM

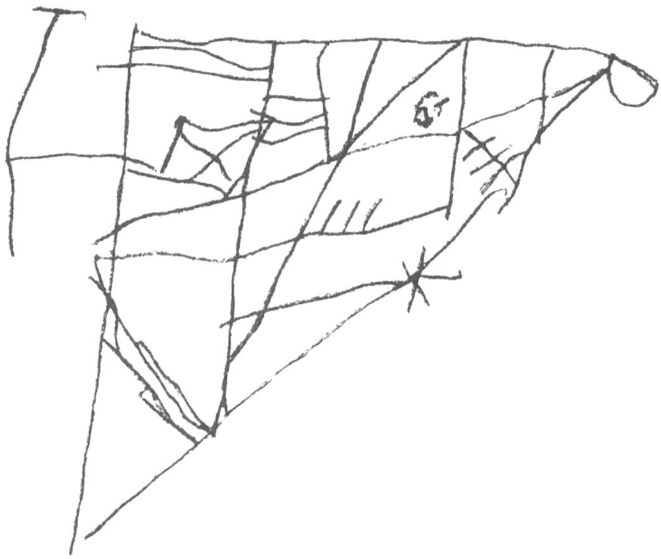

FIGURE 2.3. Case R.M. Rey-Osterrieth Complex Figure: copy. Reduced by 10%.

subtest (95th percentile). Moreover, he was able to retain 83% of the material following a 45-minute delay, which is above average retention for his age. The patient was also able to learn and retain related and unrelated word associations without difficulty (WMS-AL).

In striking contrast, the patient displayed significant difficulty in learning an unrelated word list (AVLT). His performance on the 15-item list revealed intact recall following the initial presentation of the list (Trial 1 = 5) but no evidence of further learning over the next four trials in which the list was re-presented. Moreover, he was unable to recall any of the words following a distracter list or after a 30-minute delay. He was only able to immediately recognize two of the 15 words, with no false-positive errors. Whereas compliance to task demands is a possible factor in explaining task performance, another possibility is that he displays difficulty with unorganized word lists although his memory for semantically related verbal material is intact.

Visual memory testing was confounded by the patient's significant perceptual difficulties and could not be reliably measured. His significantly below average performance on the WMS-VR subtest, on both immediate and delayed reproduction, was believed to be secondary to his perceptual motor dysfunction. Due to the extent of the severity of his impairment in copying the Rey-Osterrieth figure, the memory condition was not administered.

Summary and Impressions

Mr. M. is a 64-year-old male who recently sustained a hemorrhagic CVA involving the right hemisphere and a subsequent syncopal episode. The results of neuropsychological testing reveal the presence of significant, though selective, impairment in higher-level information processing abilities. Significant impairments were found in perceptual processing, visual spatial analysis, spatial orientation, and visuo-motor integration. There was strong evidence of a unilateral neglect for the left side of space accompanied by an apparent unawareness of his deficits. Also, there was some evidence of difficulty in learning unorganized verbal material (i.e., unrelated word lists). In contrast to these significant impairments, other types of functioning were preserved, such as intact verbal abilities and language functioning, verbal intelligence, attention and concentration processes, and semantically organized verbal memory. Thus, profound deficits implicit of right hemisphere dysfunction were found in the face of relatively intact functions typically mediated by the left hemisphere. Overall, it appears that the pattern of deficits are consistent with the cerebral area implicated by the brain lesion.

Most striking was the patient's neglect for the left side of space. It was observed in the manner in which the patient was groomed; he had missed areas on the left side of his face while shaving, and he had difficulty putting on his left shoe. Additional signs of hemispatial neglect were evident on examination, specifically on motor-construction tasks such as the Block Design subtest of the WAIS-R, the Line Bisection Test, and figure drawings. Evidence of neglect was also found on a visual perceptual task (the Hooper VOT) in which the patient tended to make "isolate" errors characterized by incorrectly guessing the objects based on a small detail on the right side of the figure. Other signs of right hemisphere dysfunction, in addition to the left spatial neglect, were present, such as spatial disorientation and an apparent unawareness of his deficits. This latter problem, also referred to as anosognosia, was most striking, particularly in light of the severity of the patient's impairments.

It is unclear to what extent his history of sleep apnea has contributed to his presenting cognitive difficulties; however, it certainly would not account for the marked lateralized findings.

Due to the recency of the stroke, continued recovery of function is expected to occur. Mr. M. has already demonstrated some recovery as reported by his physician and family members, and further recovery is expected, with the time of greatest recovery falling within the first year following the stroke. Repeat assessment in one year is strongly recommended to provide a more accurate estimate of the patient's ability level, which will be helpful in rehabilitation planning. At his present ability level, he could not be expected to sufficiently resume his job responsibilities as vice-president of a small electrical company, particularly in light of his failure to recognize his deficits at this time. However, because of his anosognosia, he may attempt to return to work. His relatively intact verbal skills may make it appear that he is more capable of functioning in the work force than he in fact is. Only if his hemi-neglect and anosognosia resolve will he be able to adequately return to his employment. His spatial neglect and significant visual spatial deficits may also pose possible dangers in operating machinery or driving a car. His family should be well advised of these issues. Therapeutic intervention for the patient and his family members is recommended to help them cope with these issues.

NEUROPSYCHOLOGY TEST SCORE SUMMARY SHEET

Patient: R.M. Age: 64 Sex: M Handedness: R

I. Intelligence WAIS-R Age-Corrected Scores

VERBAL			PERFORMANCE		
Information	12	(75 %ile)	Picture Completion	7	(16 %ile)
Digit Span	10	(50 %ile)	Picture Arrangement	7	(16 %ile)
Vocabulary	13	(84 %ile)	Block Design	2	(.4 %ile)
Arithmetic	8	(25 %ile)	Object Assembly	4	(2 %ile)
Comprehension	12	(75 %ile)	Digit Symbol	4	(2 %ile)
Similarities	11	(63 %ile)			
VERBAL IQ =	104	(61 %ile)	PERFORMANCE IQ =	70	(2 %ile)

FULL SCALE IQ = 88 (21 %ile)

II. Attention/Concentration
Digit Span: 7 forward + 4 backwards = 11 Total (75 %ile)
Mental Control, WMS: 7 (63 %ile)
Trails A: 287" (<1 %ile)

III. Language
Aphasia Screening Exam: intact

IV. Perceptual/Organizational
Hooper Visual Organization Test: 9.5/30
Line Bisection Test

V. Memory

VERBAL		NONVERBAL	
WMS Logical Memory	11.5 (95 %ile)	WMS Visual Repro.:	0
45 min. delay:	9.5	45 min. delay:	0
Percent retention:	83	Percent retention:	0

WMS Associate Learning
I Easy 3 , 5 , 6
I Hard 1 , 2 , 1
I Score: 11 (42 %ile)

Rey Auditory Verbal Learning Test (15 items):
T1: 5 T2: 5 T3: 6 T4: 3 T5: 4 Recall after Interference: 0
30-min. Delayed Recall: 0
Recognition: 2 Hits, 0 False Identifications

Commentary on Cerebrovascular Disease Cases

The preceding cases have been presented to provide examples of different profiles of neuropsychological functioning following cerebrovascular accidents. Unfortunately, we could not provide examples of all syndromes that can occur following a CVA, such as Broca's aphasia or Gerstmann's syndrome. However, the cases presented illustrate many of the cardinal neuropsychological features following a stroke. Each of the patients exhibited common sequelae of CVA, including disturbances in specific areas of intellectual functioning, attentional processing, learning and memory, and perceptual and emotional functioning.

The case presentations help illuminate the relationship between location of lesion and pattern of neuropsychological deficit. CVAs that were lateralized were associated with a specific pattern of deficits. For example, lesions localized in the left hemisphere were associated with language disturbances. S.M.'s case revealed a significant language disturbance following a recent left temporoparietal infarct. Unfortunately, this case could not be evaluated in greater detail, but existing data showed striking evidence of a Wernicke's aphasia. There was evidence of fluent speech output with impaired comprehension.

Lesions involving the right hemisphere were associated with perceptual dysfunction. In fact, some of the patients exhibited features of the neglect syndrome including hemispatial neglect, sensory extinction to simultaneous stimulation, and anosognosia. The case of R.M. depicts quite clearly the presence of hemispatial neglect and anosognosia (apparent unawareness of one's deficits) following a right hemisphere hemorrhage. In R.M.'s case, the observed hemispatial neglect was sufficiently severe as to interfere with adaptive functioning. It was most striking that these impairments were found in the face of intact left hemisphere mediated functions. The case of D.F. also revealed hemispatial neglect following a recent right hemisphere infarct. However, D.F. did not display anosognosia; rather, the patient was painfully aware of his deficits, and a clinical depression was noted. M.K. evidenced apparent unawareness of his deficits but no hemispatial neglect following a bilateral bleed.

Another point to consider is the importance of serial neuropsychological assessment in evaluating quality and extent of recovery following stroke. Repeated testing following stroke can monitor the amount and rate of recovery of function. This can help to provide the patient and his or her family with realistic expectations of potential gains over time and help in goal setting. Many of the patients, such as M.K., R.M., and S.M., were found to have recovered some of their cognitive functioning at the time of evaluation. This is not unusual because a considerable amount of spontaneous recovery of function can occur as early as one month following stroke. The time at which recovery is most rapid tends to be in the first year following the stroke.

Each of the cases illustrates how understanding the nature of the presenting behavioral sequelae following a CVA can help in the care of the patient. For example, in the case of M.K., there is an apparent unawareness of memory disturbance despite a profound memory loss sufficiently severe to interfere with adaptive functioning. Identification of the quality and severity of such a deficit can help family members to better manage the patient. In addition, consideration of this impairment, together with other areas of cognitive weakness and preservation, can be reflected in more effective rehabilitation planning.

3
Dementia

Increased attention is being given by the popular press and by professionals alike to aging and the "graying of America"—a reference to the rising mean age of the U.S. population. With this attention has come a heightened awareness of patterns of both normal and abnormal aging, such as the dementias, and particularly Alzheimer's disease. It is not uncommon for the neuropsychologist to receive referrals from other professionals requesting testing for an elderly patient to help determine whether or not a dementia syndrome is present, or to determine whether the patient's cognitive functioning is consistent with normal aging.

In large urban areas in particular, multi-specialty geriatric clinics with knowledgeable geriatric neuropsychologists are often able to offer very specialized services to the elderly population and are well equipped to answer many of these referral questions. However, many clinical-generalist psychologists have been less prepared to answer these referrals. One primary aim of this chapter is to provide the nonspecialist with some essential concepts of geriatric neuropsychology so as to be able to perform a dementia *screening examination* and interpret the results, knowing when to refer for more specialized, in-depth assessment. The interested reader is referred to the work of Albert (1981), Cummings and Benson (1983), Kazniak (1986), Birren and Schaie (1985), and Van Gorp and Satz (in press) for more extensive information on aging and cognition, in addition to techniques of evaluating the demented patient.

Neuropsychology and Normal Aging

Before any attempt can be made to detect abnormal decline in the elderly, the practitioner must first be acquainted with normal changes associated with the aging process. This issue is more difficult than it appears at surface level because a good deal of controversy exists in the literature as to exactly what cognitive changes occur as a function of the normal aging process (and how they can best be explained). Conflicts over cross-sectional (which are believed to potentiate cohort differences) versus longitudinal designs (which are affected by selective attrition) in the study of the elderly make interpretation and generalization of many studies difficult. Also, the dearth of normative data on many neuropsychological tests for the elderly further impedes test interpretation. Finally, most studies investigating neuropsychological changes in the elderly have studied only *one* cognitive domain at a time, making it difficult to understand how a variety of functions in the same elderly subjects changes over the older adult life span. Clearly, there is a need for more extensive research studying a number of cognitive domains in the same subjects.

With the vast complexity of research pitfalls and the paucity of normative data for older adults, one might even wonder how any assessment of the cognitive status of older adults might be attempted. Fortunately, there has been sufficient work to date to allow an adequate assessment of the older adult, but the clinician must be aware of the relevant pitfalls.

As noted above, there is at present a dearth of information in neuropsychology as to what constitutes "normal" or "expected" patterns of performance on cognitive measures in the elderly. Considerable controversy exists on whether aging is best explained by an irreversible decrement model, a stability model, a "frontal lobe" decrement model, or some combination of these. The *irreversible decrement* model (Horn and Donaldson, 1976; Botwinick, 1977) assumes that a maximal level of functioning is reached at some point in adulthood and that the characteristic age function thereafter involves a linearly accelerating decline. Proponents of the more recent *stability* model propose the preservation of certain abilities (e.g., verbal comprehension, word knowledge, and creative thought) with advancing age (e.g., Baltes & Schaie, 1976) and argue that past reports of decline in many cognitive functions were the result of research artifacts, such as cohort differences in cross-sectional designs (Schaie, Labouvie, & Buech, 1973). Still others have proposed alternative models, and Albert and Kaplan (1980) have compared the performance of normal elderly on many neuropsychological tests with the performance of patients who have sustained frontal systems dysfunction. They noted the similarity in performance of normal elderly and much younger patients with damage to frontal systems structures. Albert and Kaplan then postulated that the selective decline in these functions in the elderly is the result of subcortical/frontal systems changes during aging.

Because the clinician must take into account whether or not performance on a test is a function merely of normal aging versus a demonstrable pathologic process, the use of age-appropriate normative data to compare with the patient's performance is crucial. For example, reliance on WAIS-R standard scores in an older patient (in lieu of age-corrected scores) will often give the false impression of deficits particularly in timed visuo-spatial abilities and/or on the Digit Symbol subtest. For this reason, we strongly urge that all intelligence test raw data from older patients be compared with *age-equivalent norms* before any conclusions are reached regarding the level of the individual's performance. Inattention to this will result in a gross misinterpretation of the test findings and a high percent of false-positive identifications. The same holds true in terms of the need to interpret test results from other neuropsychological tests in light of age-appropriate normative data.

Pathologic Aging: Dementia

Many pathologic processes can cause cognitive impairment in older adults, such as a single stroke or the effects of chronic alcohol abuse. However, these conditions may not result in a full dementia syndrome, and they will be discussed elsewhere in this book. One of the immediate constraints facing the novice neuropsychologist in this area is the lack of a clear consensus of a precise definition of dementia. This is largely because the term is descriptive of a cluster of behavioral signs and symptoms (and thus a syndrome) and not reflective of one specific underlying etiology. Imprecise definitions serve only to blur the meaning of the dementia syndrome and further the notion that "dementia" implies a singular etiology (such as Alzheimer's disease, which is just one type of a dementia).

Because a precise definition of a syndrome is necessary for diagnostic specificity and accuracy, we prefer the operational definition proposed by Cummings and Benson (1983):

> Operationally, dementia can be defined as an acquired persistent impairment of intellectual function with compromise in at least three of the following spheres of mental activity: language, memory, visuo-spatial skills, emotions or personality, and cognition (abstraction, calculation, judgment, etc.). (p. 1)

In the above definition, assessment of the patient for a dementia requires a careful, methodic mental status examination covering various cognitive and affective domains, consistent with the recommendation of Albert (1981). In fact, it has been recommended by the National Institute of Neurological and Communicable Disorders and Stroke (NINCDS) and the Alzheimer's Disease and Related Disorders (ADRDA) joint task force that the *probable* diagnosis of Alzheimer's disease is a *behavioral* diagnosis based on behavioral observation and careful mental status examination as well as on specific exclusionary criteria. Thus, the diagnosis of many dementias (such as Alzheimer's disease) is made both on *exclusionary* grounds (such as the lack of focal lesions on CT scan, no metabolic imbalance, etc.), as well as on a specific pattern of mental status abnormalities on formal examination. Of course, definitive diagnosis of Alzheimer's disease awaits neuropathologic confirmation, usually on postmortem examination.

Although it is often naively thought that all dementias by definition are global disorders, various subtypes of the dementia syndrome may, in fact, affect various neuropsychological spheres differently. Thus, characteristic patterns of deficits and symptom clusters may well vary among the dementias, making it possible to evaluate for a subtype of a dementia. The task, then, for the clinician who is referred a patient for a "dementia workup" is to first determine whether the patient meets the criteria for a dementia. This can be accomplished by obtaining a full history and some estimate of the rate of progression of the illness, and then by carefully conducting a comprehensive neuropsychological assessment and

TABLE 3.1. Dementia classifications and common patterns of neuropsychological test results.

	Cortical	Subcortical	Mixed
Attention	Generally intact	Variable with some deficits present	+/−
Intelligence	Generally decreased globally	May be intact except for slowing, producing decline in speeded, timed tasks	Down, perhaps at an uneven rate
Language	Decreased naming, decreased word list (FAS), may resemble transcortical sensory aphasia, paraphasias common	Naming intact or down only slightly, word list often decreased, no paraphasias	+/−, aphasia common, naming often decreased
Visuo-Spatial	Poor constructions, impaired perceptual/analytic abilities	Mild deficits, largely due to poor planning	+/−
Memory	No new learning, impairment in initial acquisition	"Forgetful" – impairment in recall but not in initial acquisition	+/−
Mood	Indifferent, unconcerned, depression not common	Depression frequent, concern with and acknowledgment of deficits	+/−

examining the pattern of deficits to assist in clarifying the nature of the dementia if possible.

We have found it useful to conceptually organize our system of dementia classification into those disorders where the neuropathology *primarily* involves the cortex (*cortical dementias*), those where neuropathology mostly involves subcortical and frontal lobe structures (*subcortical dementias*), and those where pathology involves both cortical and subcortical structures (*mixed dementias*). This system of conceptualization is not without challenge, and many note that "cortical" disorders also involve significant neuropathology to select subcortical structures, and vice versa. Although this is true, we find the groupings to be heuristic in terms of the pattern of *clinical* neuropsychological compromise in these patient groups. Table 3.1 outlines the various types of dementia syndromes and common patterns of neuropsychological test results. First, however, the clinician must rule out gross cognitive impairment resulting from an acute confusional state before a diagnosis of dementia can be applied. This will now be addressed.

Acute Confusional State

An acute confusional state (or delirium) is usually a transient state that results most notably in an impairment of attention. Often lasting for hours to days, the confusional state typically begins suddenly and is followed by a fluctuating level of alertness or attention level. Because attention is so notably impaired, deficits are also evident on most other neuropsychological tests because the patient's alertness is severely altered. Visual, auditory, and/or tactile hallucinations may be present. Acute confusional states are often caused by systemic illness, toxic exposure, the effects of multiple medications (prescribed or over-the-counter medications), or metabolic disturbance. Clinically, these patients will present with diminished digit span performance (often with three or fewer digits forward), impaired mental control, and an inability to perform other simple attention tasks such as the A-test (a continuous performance task in which the patient is presented auditorially with a series of random letters of the alphabet and must respond when hearing a specific target letter). They will also typically present with an agraphia, and their speech may be fluent but incoherent. Once a confusional state has been diagnosed, prompt medical referral is indicated so that the etiology of the condition may be determined and medically treated. Most confusional states reverse when the underlying cause is treated.

Cortical Dementias

Cortical dementias generally produce notable deficits in language abilities, visuo-spatial skills, and memory, resulting in such clinical entities such as agnosia, apraxia, aphasia, and acalculia. The two primarily cortical dementias are Alzheimer's disease and Pick's disease. Of the two, Alzheimer's disease occurs much more frequently. Neuropathologic changes (characterized by neurofibrillary tangles and senile plaques) have been found in the brains of patients with Alzheimer's disease, occurring in the associative areas of the cortex as well as hippocampal structures. Patients with Pick's disease have pathologic findings mostly in the anterior temporal and frontal areas. Additionally, deficits in the choline transport system of patients with Alzheimer's disease have been noted. Because of the relative infrequency of the diagnosis of Pick's disease and the brief overview nature of this section, we will concentrate on clinical patterns of patients with Alzheimer's disease.

As noted earlier, the clinical diagnosis of "probable" Alzheimer's disease (definitive diagnosis entails neuropathologic confirmation) is based upon behavioral criteria, such as a neuropsychological assessment. In addition, specific exclusionary criteria must be met in order to rule out metabolic, neoplastic, and vascular causes. Though it was once thought that patients under age 65 with Alzheimer's disease were somehow different from those over 65, this division is generally viewed as arbitrary because both groups of patients share similar clinical characteristics and neuropathologic changes (Rocca, Amaducci, & Schoenberg, 1986). Interestingly, there has been some renewed interest in examining whether there are differences in "younger" elderly patients with Alzheimer's disease compared with "older" elderly patients with the disease, and

TABLE 3.2. Principal clinical findings in each stage of Alzheimer's disease.

Stage I (duration of disease 1 to 3 years)
Memory – new learning defective, remote recall impaired
Visuo-spatial skills – topographic disorientation, poor constructions
Language – poor word-list generation, anomia
Personality – apathy, occasional irritability or sadness
Motor system – normal
EEG – normal
CT – normal
Stage II (duration of disease 2 to 10 years)
Memory – recent and remote recall more severely impaired
Visuo-spatial skills – poor constructions, spatial disorientation
Language – fluent aphasia
Calculation – acalculia
Praxis – ideomotor apraxia
Personality – indifference and apathy
Motor system – restlessness
EEG – slowing of background rhythm
CT – normal or ventricular dilatation and sulcal enlargement
Stage III (duration of disease 8 to 12 years)
Intellectual functions – severely deteriorated
Motor – limb rigidity and flexion posture
Sphincter control – urinary and fecal incontinence
EEG – diffusely slow
CT – ventricular dilatation and sulcal enlargement

Note: From Cummings and Benson, 1983, p. 38. Reprinted by permission.

some preliminary findings raise the question of mildly variant clinical features in the two groupings.

Clinically, patients with Alzheimer's disease undergo a reasonably steady cognitive decline. Initially, others may notice the patient's memory to be failing – recent events may be forgotten, the patient may forget where he or she placed certain things, or may become lost in familiar surroundings. Poor judgment including affective or other personality changes, language errors such as paraphasias or word finding difficulty, and apathy/indifference to the illness may be evident. Because the patient may present differently depending on the stage of illness, we have reproduced a table (Table 3.2) that outlines the principal mental status findings in each stage of Alzheimer's disease (Cummings and Benson, 1983).

The following section describes common test findings for patients in the early to middle stages of Alzheimer's disease. It is difficult, at best, to determine the neuropsychological status of patients in the third stage because they are usually untestable. We emphasize Alzheimer's disease, both because of the frequency of referrals to "rule out Alzheimer's disease" as well as the frequent occurrence of Alzheimer's disease among the dementias.

Alzheimer's Disease

Gross Cognitive Functioning

A variety of gross cognitive screening measures are available to assess fairly quickly the overall level of functioning. Probably the most widely used (and one of the most economic in terms of time) is the Mini-Mental State Exam (MMSE) (Folstein, Folstein, & McHugh, 1975). Traditionally, a score of 23/30 is used as a cut-off for dementia though, when used clinically, it must be recognized that the individual's premorbid intelligence may result in higher or lower scores earlier in the dementia process. Another useful global screening measure is the Dementia Rating Scale developed by Mattis (1976), which although longer than the MMSE (it has 144 items compared with 30 on the MMSE) offers a slightly more extensive assessment of cognitive abilities and may be useful for patients who are so impaired that they are not readily testable on more traditional or extensive measures. The Blessed Dementia Rating Scale is unique in that its scores have been shown to significantly correlate with actual neuropathologic brain changes in demented patients, and because it includes assessment of functional abilities rather than on purely cognitive abilities (Blessed, Tomlinson, & Roth, 1968).

These examples of gross cognitive/adaptive screening measures offer the advantage of a brief and reliable assessment of overall level of functioning, but are insufficient in the clinician's attempt to more carefully document the specific pattern of cognitive deficits in various domains to assist with determination of subtype of dementia.

Intelligence

Central to the presence of a dementia is overall loss of intellectual abilities from estimated premorbid status. Certainly, the WAIS-R is most commonly used to assess current level of intellectual functioning, but others have reported supplementing assessment of intelligence with other measures (e.g., Kazniak, 1986, notes that he uses portions of the Stanford-Binet intelligence scale, such as Picture Absurdities). Although clinicians traditionally have used large discrepancies between subtest scores on traditionally viewed "hold" tests (such as Information, Vocabulary, and Similarities) to document intellectual decline, research (Larrabee, Largen, & Levin, 1985) has shown that Vocabulary subtest scores decline along with other WAIS-R subtest scores in patients with Alzheimer's disease, making its use inappropriate as an estimate of premorbid intelligence for demented patients. More predictive of premorbid intelligence is the individual's prior level of educational and occupational attainment (Larrabee et al., 1985), and formulas are available (Wilson, Rosenbaum, Brown, Rourke, Whitman, & Grisell, 1978; Barona, Reynolds, & Chastain, 1984) to actually compute an estimated premorbid IQ. Table 3.3 offers one formula (Barona et al., 1984) for calculating an estimated premorbid IQ.

TABLE 3.3. Demographic estimation of WAIS-R premorbid IQ.

FSIQ = 55 + 0.5 age + 1.8 sex + 4.7 race + 5.0 education + 1.9 occupation + 0.6 region (SEest = 12; R = .60)

VIQ = 54 + 0.5 age + 1.9 sex + 4.2 race + 5.3 education + 1.9 occupation + 1.2 U-R residence (SEest = 12; R = .62)

PIQ = 62 + 0.3 age + 1.1 sex + 5.0 race + 3.8 education + 1.5 occupation + 0.8 region (SEest = 13; R = .49)

Age	Sex	Race	Education	Region
16–17 = 1	F = 1	Black = 1	0–7 = 1	Southern = 1
18–19 = 2	M = 2	Other = 2	8 = 2	N. Central = 2
20–24 = 3		White = 3	9–11 = 3	Western = 3
25–34 = 4			12 = 4	Northeast = 4
35–44 = 5			13–15 = 5	
45–54 = 6			16+ = 6	U-R Residence
55–64 = 7				Rural = 1
65–69 = 8				Urban = 2
70–74 = 9				

Occupation

1 = farm laborers, farm foremen, laborers (unskilled workers)
2 = operatives, service workers, farmers, farm managers (semiskilled)
3 = not in the labor force
4 = craftsmen, foremen (skilled workers)
5 = managers, officials, proprietors, clerical and sales workers
6 = professional, technical

Note: In cases where premorbid FSIQ was >120 or <60, use of the above formuli might seriously under- or overestimate, respectively.

Finally, Fuld (1984; see also Brinkman & Brawn, 1984) has suggested a WAIS-R pattern that is more characteristic of patients' protocols who have Alzheimer's disease than those with multi-infarct dementia. The Fuld pattern from the WAIS-R is: $A>B>C\leq D$, $A>D$, where "A" is the mean of the age-corrected Information and Vocabulary subtest scores, "B" is the mean of the age-corrected Similarities and Digit Span subtest scores, "C" is the mean of the age-corrected Digit Symbol and Block Design subtest scores, and "D" is the Object Assembly age-corrected subtest score. Fuld reports that some 50% of Alzheimer's disease patients in her sample evidenced this pattern, whereas only some 8% of patients with multi-infarct dementia showed it; thus it may be one additional clinical marker of Alzheimer's disease. Satz, Van Gorp, Soper, and Mitrushina (1987) have shown—using Bayesian statistics and the estimated base rate for various types of dementia in various clinical settings—that the use of this formula in assisting to differentiate Alzheimer's disease cases from those with multi-infarct dementia may improve diagnostic accuracy above the base rate of occurrence for the two conditions.

Attention and Concentration

Thorough assessment of attention and concentration is very important for the patient referred for dementia evaluation because these processes typically remain relatively preserved until the later stages of decline. Certainly, digit span performance remains generally intact throughout the normal aging process (Birren & Schaie, 1985) and in the early and middle stages of dementia of the Alzheimer type (DAT). Not only are brief selective attention abilities necessary for confidence in the interpretation of performance in other areas, but performance on tests of attention may be diagnostically important in the differential between a dementia and a confusional state (see pp. 72–73).

Language

Language abnormalities are a critical component in the assessment to evaluate for a cortical dementia because certain language deficits can be sensitive as early indicators of cortical impairment. The spontaneous speech of the patient with Alzheimer's disease may vary, dependent on the stage of the illness. Early in the disease process, the most notable language deficit might be the patient's difficulty in word finding, and he or she may engage in much circumlocution or "talking around" the unretrieved word. On formal testing, perhaps an even earlier indication of subtle language disturbance is impaired word list generation, such as category naming (i.e., the patient is instructed to name as many animals as possible in one minute or generate as many novel words as possible beginning with a target letter) (Benson, 1979; Ober, Dronkers, Koss, Delis, & Friedland, 1986). However, after the earliest phases, clear deficits in confrontational naming usually occur, and impaired performance on such tests as the Boston Naming Test are usually evident. As the disease progresses, the patient's spontaneous speech remains fluent but becomes more "empty" and circumlocutory, and frank paraphasic errors are typically evident. Formal language examination (using standard aphasia batteries) often produces results characteristic of transcortical sensory aphasia or Wernicke's aphasia (Cummings & Benson, 1983; Cummings, Darkins, Mendez, Hill, & Benson, in press). Deficits in comprehension may be noted as the disease progresses and as language functions progressively decline until the patient presents with severe deficits in comprehension, word finding, pragmatics, etc., with frequent paraphasias and even echolalia. In the terminal stage the patient is often mute.

Visuo-Spatial Abilities

Often, relatives or caregivers of Alzheimer's disease patients early in the course of their disease will note that the patient will become lost in familiar surroundings or be unable to accurately follow a map or other visuo-spatial instructions. Formal assessment of constructional abilities will often reveal impairment, including deficits on copy of more complex figures such as the Rey-Osterrieth Complex Figure or a three-dimensional cube. Block Design and Object Assembly subtests from the WAIS-R that tap visuo-spatial abilities will likely reveal deficits from premorbid levels. Additionally, visuo-perceptual-analysis deficits are also often evident, such as impaired performance on such tests as the Benton Facial Recognition Test or the Benton Line Orientation Test (Brouwers, Cox, Martin, & Chase, 1984; Boller et al., 1984).

Learning and Memory

It has often been noted that memory deficits herald the cognitive decline in the patient early in the course of DAT. Formal assessment of memory will almost always reveal impairment in the acquisition and recall of information. Little or no learning curve will be evident in the patient with Alzheimer's disease, and deficits will not only be evident on measures of recall, but typically on measures of recognition as well. For example, performance on a list of unrelated items presented over five trials (e.g., AVLT) may not show a learning curve. If information is not learned, it cannot be stored, recalled, or recognized. In the assessment of nonverbal learning and recall, care must be taken in assessing dementia patients who also have a visuo-constructional impairment so as to not confound one deficit with the assessment of another ability. Nonconstructional visual memory tests (such as the Benton Visual Retention Test–multiple-choice form) will also reveal the nonverbal memory deficit in the patient with Alzheimer's disease. Several researchers (e.g., Wilson, Kazniak, & Fox, 1981; Albert, Butters, & Brandt, 1981) have demonstrated that Alzheimer's disease patients present with deficits in *both* recent and remote memory.

Motor Exam

Assessment using various motor measures such as the Finger Tapping Test or the Grooved Pegboard Test will reveal generally intact performance and usually no asymmetries beyond expected levels. However, caution must be urged in not overinterpreting an asymmetric finding (i.e., greater than 10% dominant-hand advantage) because Bornstein (1985) found that a substantial minority of normals also exhibited a greater than 10% dominant-hand advantage on motor measures such as the Finger Tapping Test.

Personality

This area has been relatively ignored by clinical neuropsychologists, but some recently conducted research (e.g., Kazniak, 1986) highlights clear personality and affective changes in patients with Alzheimer's disease. Most characteristic of the Alzheimer's disease patient (except for those very early in the course of the disease) is an unconcern or lack of awareness of any deficits. The patient with Alzheimer's disease will often state that he or she is in the hospital because of physical problems, such as back trouble or arthritis. When asked the date and the current year, one patient with DAT (who, premorbidly, had been a very successful attorney with a law degree from a prestigious university) said, "Oh, I don't know—when you're on vacation, you don't keep up with things like that." It should be noted that in the *very early stages*, one may see more mood changes, such as depression.

The Neuropsychology Behavior and Affect Profile (NBAP) from UCLA (Nelson, Satz, & Mitrushina, 1988) has been helpful in assessing changes in personality in these patients. In this questionnaire, a relative or significant other who has known the patient for some time rates the patient on various questions as they perceived them *before* their illness versus *now*. Changes are often found on constructs such as indifference, inappropriateness, and deficits in pragmatics (pragnosia), which is social/contextual appropriateness in communication.

Thus, we see that the patient with Alzheimer's disease typically presents with neuropsychological deficits in many, if not all, functional domains that represent definite loss from premorbid levels. We see widespread cognitive changes, including aphasia, apraxia, amnesia, and acalculia. This pattern is in contrast with patterns evident in many patients with other dementia syndromes, such as a subcortical dementia.

Pick's Disease

The patient with Pick's disease may be difficult to identify reliably on neuropsychological tests, largely because of the presumed infrequency of the disorder. However, there are certain salient characteristics of Pick's disease that can be identified on formal testing. Because the disease most severely affects frontal and temporal brain regions, clear behavioral and personality changes and abnormalities will be evident, and the patient may exhibit marked disinhibition and inappropriate behavior. In fact, these patients often will be initially diagnosed with psychiatric diagnoses or as having an organic personality syndrome. The patient with Pick's disease will also present with a definite language abnormality, most prominently a word-finding disturbance, and may even have a semantic anomia (in which the unidentified word has lost all meaning for the patient). Subtle deficits in comprehension may also be present. However, visuo-spatial functions are usually less affected until later stages, and memory may be largely preserved as well. Again, inappropriate, disinhibited, and frankly offensive or uncharacteristic behavior may be the most salient characteristic early in the course of the disease.

Subcortical Dementias

In contrast to the cortical dementias, pathologic states involving mostly subcortical structures do not typically result in frank agnosias, apraxias, confrontational naming deficits, paraphasic distortions, etc. Rather, the syndrome that typically characterizes a subcortical dementia is a marked *slowness* of mental processing together with a pattern of forgetfulness, altered mood, lowered attention, and difficulties with strategy formation (Cummings & Benson, 1984; Cummings, 1986; Freidenberg, Van Gorp, & Cummings, in press). Though first described by S.A.K. Wilson in 1912, more recent attention to this syndrome was initiated by Albert, Feldman, and Willis (1974), who described the dilapidation in cognition of patients with Progressive Supranuclear Palsy, and by McHugh and Folstein (1975), who described a similar dementia syndrome in patients with Huntington's disease. In fact, the syndrome may be evident in diseases that affect the deep gray-matter structures such as the thalamus, basal ganglia, and related brainstem nuclei, such as is found in Progressive Supranuclear Palsy, Parkinson's disease, Huntington's disease, and Wilson's disease. Dementia has become a frequently observed component in patients with AIDS, and recent neuropathologic evidence in patients with an AIDS-related dementia (Navia, Cho, Petito, & Price, 1986) has indicated that subcortical regions were most affected in their sample of 70 autopsied patients, with the cortex relatively spared. Navia and colleagues propose that the dementia associated with AIDS may indeed represent a subcortical dementia, though there is still controversy regarding the exact sites of predominant neuropathologic involvement in this syndrome.

Because of the many connections between subcortical structures and other brain regions (particularly the frontal lobes), many have questioned the accuracy of the term "subcortical dementia," and some have proposed alternate nomenclature, such as "frontal-subcortical dementia." Whatever terminology is used, the essential damage originates in subcortical brain regions producing a distinctly different neuropsychological syndrome than in mostly cortically based disorders.

Neuropsychologically, the subcortical syndrome is characterized by a notable *slowness* (not only motoric but also in speed of cognition [bradyphrenia] (Evarts, Teravainen, & Caine, 1981; Brouwers et al., 1984). Thus, these patients will obtain lower scores on the WAIS-R timed Performance subtests. However, given sufficient time, many of these patients will eventually be able to solve the task. They will produce decreased performance on other measures of visual scanning and tracking as well as on measures of selective and sustained attention such as Digit Span, Arithmetic subtests of the WAIS-R, the Trail Making Test, and Number Cancellation Tests. Assessment of intelligence may reveal relatively preserved intellectual abilities (relative to the degree of decrement found in cortical dementias), with more notable deficits on timed tests, as well as subtests tapping attention, as noted above. Learning and recall will be impaired; though in sharp contrast to patients with a cortical dementia, these patients typically benefit from cueing and will perform better on recognition portions of the exam. That is, they can *acquire* knowledge but cannot freely *recall* it—they show a pattern of forgetfulness, but careful probing using cues or a recognition format will indicate that learning has indeed taken place. Both recent and remote memories appear equally impaired, and the temporal gradient for more remote memories (such as that found in Korsakoff's syndrome) is not evident (Freedman, Rivoria, Butters, Sax, & Feldman, 1984). Visual-perceptual-organizational as well as constructional abilities are impaired in these patients, though typically cortically demented patients have demonstrably greater impairment on visuo-constructional tests (Gainotti, Caltagirone, Masullo, & Miceli, 1980; Brouwers et al., 1984). Again in contrast to cortical dementias, these patients will produce intact or very mild deficits in confrontational naming, though word list generation (such as on the FAS test) is often impaired. Frank deficits in repetition and comprehension, for example, are typically not present, nor are paraphasic distortions. Finally, altered mood is typically present in these patients, with depression and apathy common (Albert et al., 1974; McHugh & Folstein, 1975; Cummings, 1986). For a more complete discussion, we recommend the comprehensive review by Cummings (1986).

Mixed Dementias and Multi-Infarct Dementia

Common types of "mixed dementia" include post traumatic dementia and dementia resulting from multiple vascular occlusions involving both cortical and subcortical regions, with corresponding infarctions to correlated brain regions. Typically, multi-infarct dementia produces a stepwise, deteriorating course (though in reality, this is often difficult to determine from history provided by family members) and occurs in individuals with a history of hypertension, stroke, atherosclerosis, and other vascular disease. These patients will often be found to have focal neurologic signs and symptoms on formal exam, although it has been noted by Roberts, McGeorge, and Caird (1978), that CT scans, by themselves, were helpful in identifying multi-infarct dementia patients in only 20% of the cases studied. Loring, Meador, Mahurin, and Largen (1986) studied 12 patients with a diagnosis of Alzheimer's disease and 12 age- and education-matched patients with multi-infarct dementia. They found differences between the two groups for only several Performance subtests of the WAIS, but no differences for other tests, including tests of memory, visuo-spatial functions, or measures of sustained attention. Because multi-infarct dementia, by definition, varies in severity and clinical presentation—depending on where the infarctions occur—it will likely be difficult to establish one neuropsychological pattern that characterizes this state. Certainly Fuld's formula from the WAIS and WAIS-R has shown demonstrable utility in the discriminant classification of patients with DAT (versus multi-infarct dementia). Use of Hachinski's Ischemia Scale has also been documented to help separate those individuals with a vascular dementia from those with DAT. Motor asymmetries may also be evident on neuropsychological testing (Lezak, 1983) and "pockets" of preserved functioning may be apparent relative to patients with a purely cortical or subcortical dementia.

The Dementia Syndrome of Depression

Sometimes mistakenly referred to as "pseudodementia" (in actuality, there is nothing "false" about the dramatic but reversible cognitive deficits shown by these patients), the dementia syndrome of depression most frequently occurs in older adults, though it has been known to occur in younger patients as well. The patients qualifying for the diagnosis of a dementia syndrome of depression present with disturbances in overall cognition, as well as deficits in attention, learning and memory, visuo-spatial disorders, and clear personality alterations that are similar to patients with subcortical dementias.

Few investigations have compared neuropsychological test performance of these patients with other dementia patients. In a recent study, LaRue, D'Elia, Clark, Spar, and Jarvik (1986) systematically compared: (1) elderly adults with major depression with (2) a group of patients diagnosed as having Alzheimer's disease and (3) healthy aged controls. They found the two patient groups to have equally severe performance on most all cognitive measures – including immediate recall reproduction of line drawings, among others. Only a test of selective reminding (Fuld Object Memory Examination) was successful at differentiating the two groups. Unfortunately, a comprehensive neuropsychological battery including assessment of confrontational naming and purely constructional abilities (not confounded by immediate recall) was not included. In another interesting study, Houlihan, Abrahams, La Rue, and Jarvik (1986) found that cognitively impaired, depressed patients gave more elaborate and more accurate responses to the WAIS-R Vocabulary subtest using a more refined scoring procedure than patients with Alzheimer's disease, even though the two groups were equated for overall WAIS-R Vocabulary standard subtest scores.

Other researchers have noted deficits in attention and processing speed (Frith et al., 1983; Caine, 1986; Sternberg & Jarvik, 1976), memory, and other abilities. Qualitative observations may be equally helpful. It has often been noted that the depressed patients will respond with "I don't know" answers and are aided by prompts to continue or guess. Less common are errors of comission, and instead, the patient often simply leaves out relevant information in the response. Details may be omitted on constructional tasks, word list generation may be impaired, and abstract thought processes impaired. Thus, standard neuropsychological tests will reflect the cognitive impairment in the patient with the dementia syndrome of depression. However, personality assessment will reveal a self-deprecatory stance, feelings of worthlessness, despair about the future, and often, much concern about their current, abject state. This is in contrast to many cortically demented patients in later stages, where indifference to the illness is more common. However, the similarities with subcortical dementias are great, and often the two coexist. We have included the case of Mr. D. B. to illustrate a subcortical dementia where depression was a factor in his cognitive deficits. In reality, the distinction between the dementia syndrome of depression and a progressive cortical dementia often is not a simple determination, and qualitative observations must be combined with quantitative measures.

Summary

In summary, we have attempted to show that the determination of a dementia should be made using well-defined criteria in an assessment of multiple cognitive domains. Many dementia syndromes produce characteristic neuropsychological deficit patterns, and a thorough, careful assessment can aid in the determination of the type of dementia syndrome present. Table 3.1 illustrates the key neuropsychological differences among the primary types of the dementia spectrum.

References

Albert, M. (1981). Geriatric neuropsychology. *Journal of Consulting and Clinical Psychology, 49*, 835–850.

Albert, M., Butters, N., & Brandt, J. (1981). Patterns of remote memory in amnestic and demented patients. *Archives of Neurology, 38*, 495–500.

Albert, M.L., Feldman, R.G., & Willis, A.L. (1974). The 'subcortical dementia' of progressive supranuclear palsy. *Journal of Neurology, Neurosurgery, and Psychiatry, 37*, 121–130.

Albert, M.S., Kaplan, E.F. (1980). Organic implications of neuropsychological deficits in the elderly. In L.W. Poon, J. Fozard, L. Cermak, D. Arenberg, & L.W. Thompson (Eds.), *New directions in memory and aging: Proceedings of the George A. Talland Memorial Conference* (pp. 403–432). Hillsdale, N.J.: Lawrence Erlbaum.

Baltes, P.B., & Schaie, K.W. (1976). On the plasticity of adult and gerontological intelligence. Where Horn and Donaldson fail. *American Psychologist, 31*, 720–725.

Barona, A., Reynolds, C.R., & Chastain, R. (1984). A demographically based index of premorbid intelligence for the WAIS-R. *Journal of Consulting and Clinical Psychology, 52*, 885–887.

Benson, D.F. (1979). *Aphasia, alexia, and agraphia*. London: Churchill Livingstone.

Birren, J., & Schaie, K.W. (1985). *The handbook of the psychology of aging*, (2nd ed.). New York: Van Nostrand Reinhold.

Blessed, G., Tomlinson, B., & Roth, M. (1968). The association between quantitative measures of dementia and of senile change in the cerebral grey matter of elderly subjects. *British Journal of Psychiatry, 114*, 797–811.

Boller, F., Passafiume, D., Keefe, N., Rogers, K., Morrow, L., & Kim Y. (1984). Visuospatial impairment in Parkinson's disease. *Archives of Neurology, 41*, 485–490.

Bornstein, R.A. (1985). Normative data on selected neuropsychological measures from a nonclinical sample. *Journal of Clinical Psychology, 41*, 651–659.

Botwinick, J. (1977). Intellectual abilities. In J.E. Birren and K.W. Schaie (Eds.), *Handbook of the psychology of aging* (pp. 580–605). New York: Van Nostrand Reinhold.

Brinkman, S.D., & Brawn, P. (1984). Classification of dementia patients by a WAIS profile related to central cholinergic deficiencies. *Journal of Clinical Neuropsychology, 6*, 393–400.

Brouwers, P., Cox, C., Martin, A., & Chase, T. (1984). Differential perceptual-spatial impairment in Huntington's and Alzheimer's dementias. *Archives of Neurology, 41*, 1973–1976.

Caine, E.D. (1986) The neuropsychology of depression: The pseudodementia syndrome. In I. Grant and K. Adams (Eds.), *Neuropsychological assessment of neuropsychiatric disorders* (pp. 221–243). New York: Oxford University Press.

Cummings, J. (1986). Subcortical dementia: An analysis of the contributions of subcortical brain structures to human thought and emotion. *British Journal of Psychiatry, 149*, 682–697.
Cummings, J., & Benson, D.F. (1983). *Dementia: A clinical approach*. Boston: Butterworths.
Cummings, J., & Benson, D.F. (1984). Subcortical dementia: Review of an emerging concept. *Archives of Neurology, 41*, 874–879.
Cummings, J., Darkins, A., Mendez, M., Hill, M.A., & Benson, D. (in press). Alzheimer's disease and Parkinson's disease: Comparison of speech and language alterations. *Neurology*.
Evarts, E., Teravainen, H., & Caine, D. (1981). Reaction time in Parkinson's disease. *Brain, 104*, 167–186.
Folstein, M., Folstein, S., & McHugh, P. (1975). "Mini-mental state": A practical method for grading the mental state of patients for the clinician. *Journal of Psychiatric Research, 12*, 189–198.
Freedman, M., Rivoria, P., Butters, N., Sax, D., & Feldman, R. (1984). Retrograde amnesia in Parkinson's disease. *Canadian Journal of Neurological Science, 11*, 297–301.
Freidenberg, D., Van Gorp, W., & Cummings, J. (in press). Subcortical dementia. In A. Katona (Ed.), *Senile dementia: Advances and prospects*. London: Croom & Helm.
Frith, C.D., Stevens, M., Johnstone, E.C., Deakin, J., Lawler, P., & Crow, T. (1983). Effects of ECT and depression on various aspects of memory. *British Journal of Psychiatry, 142*, 610–617.
Fuld, P. (1984). Test profile of cholinergic dysfunction and of Alzheimer-type dementia. *Journal of Clinical Neuropsychology, 6*, 380–392.
Gainotti, G., Caltagirone, C., Masullo, C., & Miceli, G. (1980). Patterns of neuropsychologic impairment in various diagnostic groups of dementia. In L. Amaducci, A.N. Davison, & P. Antuono (Eds.), *Aging of the brain and dementia* (pp. 245–250). New York: Raven Press.
Horn, J.L., & Donaldson, G. (1976). On the myth of intellectual decline in adulthood. *American Psychologist, 31*, 701–709.
Houlihan, J., Abrahams, J., LaRue, A., & Jarvik, L. (1986). Qualitative differences in vocabulary performance of Alzheimer versus depressed patients. *Developmental Neuropsychology, 1*, 139–144.
Kazniak, A. (1986). The neuropsychology of dementia. In I. Grant and K. Adams (Eds.), *Neuropsychological assessment of neuropsychiatric disorders* (pp. 172–220). New York: Oxford University Press.
Larrabee, G., Largen, J., & Levin, H. (1985) Sensitivity of age-decline resistant ("hold") WAIS subtests to Alzheimer's disease. *Journal of Clinical and Experimental Neuropsychology, 7*, 497–504.
LaRue, A., D'Elia, L., Clark, E., Spar, J., & Jarvik, L. (1986). Clinical tests of memory in dementia, depression, and healthy aging. *Psychology and Aging, 1*, 69–77.
Lezak, M. (1983). *Neuropsychological assessment*. New York: Oxford University Press.
Loring, D., Meador, K., Mahurin, R., & Largen, J. (1986). Neuropsychological performance in dementia of the Alzheimer type and multi-infarct dementia. Paper presented at the Fourteenth Annual Meeting of the International Neuropsychological Society, Denver, Colorado, February 1986.
Mattis, S. (1976). Mental status examination for organic mental syndrome in the elderly

patient. In L. Bellack and T.B. Karasu (Eds.), *Geriatric psychiatry* (pp. 77–121). New York: Grune and Stratton.
McHugh, P.R., & Folstein, M.F. (1975). Psychiatric syndromes of Huntington's chorea: A clinical and phenomenologic study. In D.F. Benson and D. Blumer (Eds.), *Psychiatric aspects of neurologic disease* (pp. 267–286). New York: Grune and Stratton.
Navia, B., Cho, E., Petito, C., & Price, R.W. (1986). The AIDS dementia complex: II. Neuropathology. *Annals of Neurology, 19*, 525–540.
Nelson, L.D., Satz, P., & Mitrushina, M.N. (1988). Validation of a test to measure personality and affective change in a brain-impaired population: Preliminary results. *Journal of Clinical and Experimental Neuropsychology,* (abstract), *10*, 59.
Ober, B., Dronkers, N., Koss, E., Delis, D., & Friedland, R. (1986). Retrieval from semantic memory in Alzheimer-type dementia. *Journal of Clinical and Experimental Neuropsychology, 8*, 75–92.
Roberts, M.A., McGeorge, A.P., & Caird, F.I. (1978). Electroencephalography and computerized tomography in vascular and non-vascular dementia in old age. *Journal of Neurology, Neurosurgery and Psychiatry, 41*, 903–906.
Rocca, W., Amaducci, L., & Schoenberg, B. (1986). Epidemiology of clinically diagnosed Alzheimer's disease. *Annals of Neurology, 19*, 415–424.
Satz, P., Van Gorp, W., Soper, H., & Mitrushina, M. (1987). A WAIS-R marker for dementia of the Alzheimer type? An empirical and statistical induction test. *Journal of Clinical and Experimental Neuropsychology, 9*, 767–774.
Schaie, K.W., Labouvic, G., & Buech, V.U. (1973). Generational and cohort-specific differences in adult cognitive functioning: A 14-year study of independent samples. *Development Psychology, 9*, 151–166.
Sternberg, D., & Jarvik, M. (1976). Memory functions in depression. *Archives of General Psychiatry, 33*, 219–224.
Van Gorp, W., & Satz, P. (in press). Neuropsychological assessment of the older adult. In H. Kaplan and B. Sadock (Eds.), *Comprehensive textbook of psychiatry, V.*
Van Gorp, W., Satz, P., & Mitrushina, M. (1987). Neuropsychological processes associated with normal aging and the early detection of "at risk" elders. Paper presented at the 10th annual meeting of the International Neuropsychological Society, Washington, DC.
Wilson, R.S., Kazniak, A.W., & Fox, J.H. (1981). Remote memory in senile dementia. *Cortex, 17*, 41–48.
Wilson, R.S., Rosenbaum, G., Brown, G., Rourke, D., Whitman, D., & Grisell, J. (1978). An index of premorbid intelligence. *Journal of Consulting and Clinical Psychology, 46*, 1554–1555.

Case 1: Basal Ganglia Calcification Producing Subcortical Dementia

Reason for Referral and Presenting Situation

Mr. D.B. is a 55-year-old, right-handed, Caucasian male with a 12th-grade education who recently presented to the clinic for evaluation of cognitive difficulties and "slowing down," which have forced him to leave his job and require medical disability leave. The patient and his wife report that his "thinking has slowed" and that the onset of his symptoms began approximately two years ago when he was no longer able to function at his job for local government as an overseer of workers on county projects.

Neurobehavioral examination confirmed his slowed behavior and altered mental status, and a CT scan revealed a calcification of the basal ganglia, consistent with a diagnosis of Fahr's disease, a subcortical disorder characterized by idiopathic calcification of the basal ganglia that can result in a subcortical dementia syndrome.

The patient's work history, in addition to his most recent position, includes his employment as a supervisor in a boy's club and similar types of work over the years. There is no history of alcohol or drug abuse, hypertension, or other risk factors for stroke and he achieved an Hachinski Ischemia Score of 2. The patient is taking no medication currently, and physical examination and laboratory studies revealed no other abnormalities.

Behavioral Observations

Mr. B. appeared as a soft-spoken, friendly, and cooperative man who was dressed casually for the examination. The most striking feature of his presentation was his *profound* slowness, both motoric and cognitive. For instance, the Satz-Mogel short form of the WAIS-R was administered, and though it normally takes 30 to 45 minutes to complete, Mr. B. required two hours just to complete this abbreviated test. Likewise, he required 41 minutes to copy a complex two-dimensional figure and 7½ minutes to copy the simple line drawings from the Wechsler Memory Scale. Despite his excruciating slowness, he persevered on all tasks given him and emphatically stated that he did not wish to stop any task until he had completed it. Though he presented with a docile demeanor, he seemed moderately concerned about his condition and, at the conclusion of the testing, stated that he hoped that he would not be any worse the next time he was evaluated for follow-up testing. Because of his very slow performance, a brief battery of tests was administered as each test required substantial time for the patient to complete.

Tests Administered

See data summary sheet.

Test Results

Gross Cognitive Functioning

Mr. B. received a score of 26/30 on the Mini-Mental State Exam, revealing grossly intact cognitive functioning. He had difficulty spontaneously recalling the date, could not correctly spell "world" backwards, nor compute serial 7 subtractions. He could recall two out of three words after a brief distraction and was able to name the third after a cue.

Attention and Concentration

Borderline to impaired performance was evident in Mr. B.'s attention abilities. He performed at the second percentile on both the Digit Span subtest (4F, 3B) and the Arithmetic subtest of the WAIS-R, both measures of attention. He performed at the eighth percentile on a rote task requiring him to count backwards from 40, recite the alphabet, and count forward by 3s (WMS–Mental Control). Despite his lowered performance in this realm, he appeared alert and able to visually fixate well on the examiner. Together, these results reveal moderate deficits in attention and concentration.

Intelligence

Results of intellectual assessment reveal a Verbal IQ of 80, a Performance IQ of 74, and a Full Scale IQ of 77, placing Mr. B. overall in the borderline range (6th percentile) of intellectual functioning. These results likely represent a moderate overall loss in general intellectual abilities from estimated premorbid levels based upon education and occupation. There was a nonsignificant six-point discrepancy favoring verbal abilities over performance, though his slow performance and time penalties for this slowness contributed to his lowered score in this realm. Within the verbal domain, Mr. B. consistently performed much lower on tasks of attention and concentration with his best performance (average range) occurring on tasks measuring his knowledge of the world about him (Information) and average performance appearing in his knowledge of word usage (Vocabulary), and judgment and understanding of social conventions (Comprehension). Within the performance domain, Mr. B. performed best on a task that required him to discriminate the essential from the nonessential elements of a series of pictures (Picture Completion), with notably poor performance on a timed task requiring a rapid problem-solving approach to a novel task (Digit Symbol) and on other visual spatial tasks in which speed of performance is a factor.

Language

The patient's spontaneous speech was somewhat hypophonic but otherwise fluent and with meaning. He showed no evidence of word-finding difficulties on the Boston Naming Test and evidenced no impairment on gross screening of repetition, comprehension, writing to dictation, and reading written material. In sharp contrast, a notable decrement in word list generation was observed (FAS = <4th percentile). Thus, language abilities appear intact except for greatly diminished word list generation.

Perceptual Organizational Abilities

Mr. B.'s copy of a complex two-dimensional figure was well below expected levels (Rey-Osterrieth Complex Figure = <10th percentile), although he used an appropriate strategy when copying the figure. He could complete all the 2 × 2 Block Design tasks (though it took him up to 5½ minutes to complete one of them), though he could not complete any of the more complex 3 × 3 arrangements. Unfortunately, no motor free visuo-spatial measures were administered. Thus, many of the patient's lowered scores in this domain reflect time penalties for slow performance. Even so, mild to moderate compromise was noted in this domain.

Learning and Memory

The patient's immediate recall of verbal material in paragraph story format (WMS–Logical Memory) was within the average range for his age (32nd percentile), though he evidenced a greater than expected 66% loss of the information following a 30-minute delay. On a serial-selective reminding task of 10 animal names (Buschke Selective Reminding Test), Mr. B. learned six of the names by the fourth trial, but his performance over the five trials was erratic. On a recognition portion of the test, Mr. B. correctly recognized all 10 of the names with two false-positive identifications, indicating generally intact acquisition of the information. Assessment of nonverbal memory revealed average immediate recall reproduction (60th percentile) of simple line drawings (WMS–Visual Reproduction), but he could only recall 29% of this information after a 30-minute delay, well below expected levels. He also exhibited difficulty recognizing any of the figures on the Benton Visual Retention Test–multiple-choice form (1st percentile). It is also noteworthy that the patient became lost when attempting to find his way back to the office from a nearby restroom and he was found walking in the opposite direction as he left the restroom. This provides additional evidence of a nonverbal, visuo-spatial learning deficit.

Personality

Personality assessment (Beck Depression Inventory and clinical interview) revealed a mild depression in an individual with little energy, who tends to be anxious and somewhat ruminative. Because of his slowness, a formal true/false personality questionnaire was not attempted, though clinical interviews revealed slightly depressed mood and a preoccupation with bodily concerns and his slowed movements.

Summary and Conclusions

Mr. B. presents with significant though selective deficits of higher cognitive functioning. Most striking was his profoundly slowed performance, requiring up to 10 times the amount of time an unimpaired person would need to complete a task. Additionally, he evidenced a moderate loss of overall intellectual abilities (borderline range) with no significant disparity between verbal and nonverbal abilities, borderline performance in attention, decreased word list generation with otherwise intact language functioning, visuo-spatial disturbance, and decreased recall of verbal and nonverbal information. Together, these results are consistent with a subcortical dementia process, and consistent with his documented calcification of the basal ganglia.

Could these deficits be the result of depression? Certainly, depressed mood can affect cognitive functioning and speed of performance. It is indeed likely that his mild depression has impacted to some extent on his level of cognitive functioning. However, it is not believed that his mild depression is solely or even largely responsible for the serious deficits and profound slowness that this gentleman exhibits. Of course, only retesting following appropriate treatment of his mood disturbance will enable us to tease out the effects of depression from the effects of his basal ganglia calcification.

On a practical level, the test results confirm Mr. B.'s inability to perform successfully in a work situation. He not only has diminished general intellectual capacity, but his deficits in learning, memory, and planning and strategy formation will cause him serious difficulties in many situations. He will need frequent assistance in many activities of daily living, and it is recommended that the family be counseled regarding community resources to provide them with assistance in caring for this gentleman.

It is also recommended that the patient be retested in six months to follow any possible progression in his cognitive status over time.

NEUROPSYCHOLOGY TEST SCORE SUMMARY SHEET

Patient: D.B. Age: 55 Sex: M Handedness: R

I. Gross Cognitive Functioning
Mini-Mental State Exam: 26 /30

II. Intelligence WAIS-R Age-Corrected Scores

VERBAL			PERFORMANCE		
Information	9	(37 %ile)	Picture Completion	9	(37 %ile)
Digit Span	4	(2 %ile)	Picture Arrangement	8	(25 %ile)
Vocabulary	8	(25 %ile)	Block Design	5	(5 %ile)
Arithmetic	4	(2 %ile)	Object Assembly	5	(5 %ile)
Comprehension	8	(25 %ile)	Digit Symbol	4	(2 %ile)
Similarities	6	(9 %ile)			

VERBAL IQ = 80 (9 %ile) PERFORMANCE IQ = 74 (4 %ile)
FULL SCALE IQ = 77 (6 %ile)

III. Attention/Concentration
Digit Span: 4 forward + 3 backwards = 7 Total (2 %ile)
Mental Control, WMS: 3 (8 %ile)

IV. Language
Boston Naming Test: 57 /60
Controlled Word Association: F (4) + A (3) + S (8) + Age Corr.=20 (<4 %ile)

V. Perceptual/Organizational
Rey-Osterrieth Complex Figure Copy: 19 /36 (<10 %ile)

VI. Memory

VERBAL		NONVERBAL	
WMS Logical Memory	6 (32 %ile)	WMS Visual Repro.:	7 (60 %ile)
30 min. delay:	2	30 min. delay:	2
Percent retention:	33	Percent retention:	29

Buschke Selective Reminding Test (10 items):
T1: 4 T2: 5 T3: 5 T4: 6 T5: 5
Recognition: 10 Hits, 2 False Identifications

VII. Personality
Beck Depression Inventory: 12

Case 2: Progressive Dementing Disorder

Reason for Referral and Presenting Situation

Mr. L.S. is a 56-year-old, married, right-handed, Caucasian male who was referred for neuropsychological assessment as part of his comprehensive evaluation for a dementia and to rule out Alzheimer's Disease. He presents with a three-year history of progressive memory and general cognitive decline. For the past six years he has worked as a minister who received a master's degree in theology some 15 years ago. Before this, the patient was very successful in sales. He first noticed problems when he got lost taking a walk three years ago. Shortly thereafter, he was taken to a church hospital and was told that his problems were the result of repression. He retired from his church work approximately one year ago because of supposed doctrinal differences. He has no past psychiatric history and no known history of neurologic disorder, substance abuse, or past history of hypertension. Neurologic exam and imaging studies were all within normal limits, and the patient is currently on no medications.

Behavioral Observations

Mr. S. appeared as a well-dressed, well-groomed man with carefully styled white hair, wearing an attractive tie and sport jacket. The patient was accompanied to the evaluation by his wife, who drove him to the session and helped him locate the office. He stated that he was not sure why he was referred for the evaluation, and when asked why he was at the clinic, his language disturbance (characterized by largely empty speech with a paucity of meaningful content words) was readily apparent. He had obvious word-finding difficulty and evidenced considerable circumlocution and paraphasic output. He denied any significant memory or other cognitive problems and, though compliant with the testing, stated he did not need medical care because he had no problems.

Tests Administered

See data summary sheet.

Test Results

Gross Cognitive Functioning

Mr. S. obtained a score of 17/30 on the Mini-Mental State Exam, indicating grossly impaired cognitive functioning. He failed many orientation items and thought he was in Cincinnati, Ohio (even though he was in Los Angeles, California). He could not recall any of the three words following a distraction and was not able to compute serial 7 subtractions. He spelled 3 of the 5 letters of "world" backwards correctly.

Intelligence

On the WAIS-R, Mr. S. obtained a Verbal IQ of 69, a Performance IQ of 74, and a Full Scale IQ of 71, placing him overall in the borderline range of intellectual functioning. This represents an obvious moderate to severe decline from estimated premorbid levels in an individual with post-graduate education. The patient evidenced low performance across virtually all subtests, with his best performance (though still significantly below average) on tasks measuring his knowledge of the world about him (Information), his long-known vocabulary (Vocabulary), attention to visual details (Picture Completion), and his ability to sequentially arrange a series of pictures to tell a meaningful story (Picture Arrangement). Notably poor performance was seen on tasks measuring concentration, calculation, and judgment.

Attention and Concentration

Borderline to impaired performance was noted in this domain. Mr. S. was able to repeat four digits forward and three backwards (Digit Span). He performed at the eighth percentile on an attentional task requiring him to count backwards from 20, recite the alphabet, and count forward by 3s (WMS–Mental Control). He was not able to spell "world" backwards (three of five letters correct).

Language Functioning

Mr. S.'s spontaneous speech was fluent with a paucity of meaningful content words. He evidenced an obvious anomia and circumlocutory speech with multiple paraphasic errors, such as saying "movie spar" for "movie star." Assessment of confrontational naming confirmed his word-finding disturbance (Boston Naming Test = 34/60). Likewise, word-list generation was notably depressed (FAS = 9, <4th percentile). Assessment of comprehension revealed generally intact performance for simple material, and he was able to follow all steps of a five-step command. However, he evidenced notably impaired performance on more complex ideational material. His repetition was grossly intact except for an inability to repeat "Methodist Episcopal," and he was accurate on high probability phrases but less accurate on low probability phrases, such as repeating the phrase, "The Chinese fan had a rare emerald." His writing to dictation was intact for simple material, and he was able to read simple written material. Body part identification was intact, as was right/left orientation. Thus, language assessment indicated a fluent aphasic disturbance.

Visuo-Spatial Abilities

Significant impairment in this domain was apparent. Mr. S. performed well below the 10th percentile on a task in which he was required to copy a complex two-dimensional figure (Rey-Osterrieth), and he performed in the borderline to impaired range (fifth percentile) on a task requiring him to put a number of blocks together to match a design (Block Design), and also at the fifth percentile on a task requiring him to put puzzle-like pieces together to make a familiar object (Object Assembly). His drawing of a clock was grossly adequate except for his omission of the number 11. However, he was not able to set the hands as requested at "10 past 11" (he set one hand at 10 and left out the other hand).

Learning and Memory

Mr. S. was not able to immediately recall any elements of two stories read to him (WMS–Logical Memory). On a serial list learning test (Shopping List Test), the patient was able to learn only two of the 10 words by the fifth learning trial, and he showed a pronounced recency effect, recalling only the last two items on each trial. He also had multiple intrusions of extra-list items on most of the five trials. Following a 15-minute delay, the patient was unable to recall any of the words that he had been given earlier. On a recognition portion, the patient correctly identified all 10 words, though he also had eight false-positive identifications. This indicates a disturbance in the acquisition of verbal material, which is affected by his attentional disturbance. Assessment of nonverbal memory revealed similar deficits. The patient was unable to completely reproduce any of the simple line drawings shown him (WMS–Visual Reproduction); no doubt his constructional deficits interfered with performance on this task.

Summary and Conclusions

Together, these test data reveal marked decline in virtually all cognitive spheres in a man with a graduate degree, who once functioned well above the average range in intelligence. He has impairment of gross cognitive functioning, intellectual functioning (borderline range), decreased attention ability, notable language impairment characterized by fluent output, anomia, and diminished word-list generation, with intact repetition, perceptual organizational disturbance, and a notable inability to learn new information, either verbal or nonverbal. These results, combined with the patient's reported steadily progressive course, are wholly consistent with a diagnosis of probable Alzheimer's disease.

It is recommended that the family be counseled regarding the nature of this patient's probable illness and that community support services be made available to them as they attempt to care for their relative. He will require substantial caregiving and assistance with activities of daily living, and the family will require support in coping with this patient's illness and the progressive decline in his cognition and ability to care for himself.

NEUROPSYCHOLOGY TEST SCORE SUMMARY SHEET

Patient: L.S. Age: 56 Sex: M Handedness: R

I. Gross Cognitive Functioning
Mini-Mental State Exam: 17 /30

II. Intelligence WAIS-R Age-Corrected Scores

VERBAL			PERFORMANCE		
Information	6	(9 %ile)	Picture Completion	6	(9 %ile)
Digit Span	4	(2 %ile)	Picture Arrangement	6	(9 %ile)
Vocabulary	6	(9 %ile)	Block Design	5	(5 %ile)
Arithmetic	2	(0 %ile)	Object Assembly	5	(5 %ile)
Comprehension	3	(1 %ile)	Digit Symbol	5	(5 %ile)
Similarities	5	(5 %ile)			

VERBAL IQ = 69 (2 %ile) PERFORMANCE IQ = 74 (4 %ile)
FULL SCALE IQ = 71 (3 %ile)

III. Attention/Concentration
Digit Span: 4 forward + 3 backwards = 7 Total (2 %ile)
Mental Control, WMS: 3 (8 %ile)

IV. Language
Boston Naming Test: 34 /60
Controlled Word Association: F (5) + A (2) + S (2) + Age Corr.=10 (<4 %ile)
Aphasia Screening Exam

V. Perceptual/Organizational
Rey-Osterrieth Complex Figure Copy: 17.5/36 (<10 %ile)

VI. Memory

VERBAL		NONVERBAL		
WMS Logical Memory	0	WMS Visual Repro.:	2	(14 %ile)
		30 min. delay:	0	

Shopping List Test (10 items):
T1: 3 T2: 2 T3: 2 T4: 2 T5: 2 15 min. delay: 0
Recognition: 10 Hits, 8 False Identifications

Case 3: Multi-Infarct Dementia

Reason for Referral and Presenting Situation

Mr. N.T. is a 67-year-old, widowed, right-handed, Caucasian male who was referred for neuropsychological evaluation by his neurologist as part of the patient's current in-patient diagnostic evaluation. In particular, a chief complaint of deterioration in cognitive abilities and memory is presented, as well as personality changes, which have progressively worsened during the past six months. Mr. T. is a retired professor of mathematics. The patient has a personal and family history of cardiac problems, and he underwent a pacemaker implant approximately two and one-half years ago. Mr. T. was admitted at this time for a comprehensive evaluation to determine the etiology of cognitive and behavioral changes that have taken place since approximately two years ago and that have increased within the past six months. The patient is an extremely poor historian, with disorientation and notable memory deficits; hence, background information was primarily obtained from hospital medical records.

Mr. T. is currently in treatment with a psychiatrist, who noted that he suffered a stroke with resultant transient bilateral hemiparesis 14 months ago. This infarct reportedly occurred in the brainstem, with evidence of bilateral involvement. However, according to his sister, he began experiencing difficulty teaching and answering questions in the classroom approximately one to two years previously. Currently, the patient requires direction and supervision in most activities, including maintaining personal hygiene and dressing. He reportedly wanders from the home, and this year required psychiatric admission when he became delusional and was found urinating on his front lawn while wearing only a pajama top. His sister reports that his door is padlocked in order to keep him from wandering.

Recently, psychotic symptomatology has been manifested, including delusions of persecution, as well as auditory (hearing his deceased wife's voice) and visual hallucinations. In addition, he is incontinent of urine. Mr. T. is unable to drive or manage his finances and demonstrates impaired judgment. For example, it was reported that he gave a considerable amount of money and property to a casual female acquaintance; his sister is currently involved in legal proceedings to regain these assets. Past psychiatric history and substance or alcohol abuse were denied and there is no history from interviews with family members to indicate these were ever present.

Mr. T. received a master's degree in mathematics, and is a recently retired professor of a college mathematics department. He was married for 32 years, and his wife died of a CVA three years ago. The patient's sister indicated that he experienced prolonged grief following her death.

Personality changes reportedly began to be observed by family members two years ago. For example, it was noted that he no longer took interest in his great-grandchildren, who previously had been very close to him. It is noted that deterioration in memory and cognitive functioning, as well as agitation and abusive behavior, have been particularly evidenced in the last six months.

Medical history includes at least one known CVA (with left and right transient hemiparesis), cardiomyopathy with congestive heart failure, second degree atrial valve heart block, tachycardia and permanent transvenous demand pacemaker, and diabetes mellitus. Current medications include: Klotrix 10 mEq, one tab p.o., q.d.; Diabeta 2.5 mg 9 day; Procardia 10 mg d.q.; Lasix 40 mg q.d.; digoxin .375 mg q.d.

Previous evaluation 3 months ago has included a CT scan with contrast, which was reportedly normal. An EEG was read as "mildly abnormal compatible with mild generalized disturbance of a cerebral function." A more recent CT scan was obtained, but the results were unavailable at the time of this writing. The current hospitalization was recommended in order to further explore and clarify the diagnostic picture.

Behavioral Observations

Mr. T. appeared disheveled during the testing sessions. Test administration was five-and-one-half hours in length, and took place over the course of two days. During the entirety of the testing, Mr. T. was quite disorganized and confused, with poor memory. Behavior was cooperative. Mood was generally inappropriately pleasant, as was affect. Speech was often tangential. Mr. T. evidenced orientation difficulties and, on the second testing, was unable to recall the date.

Tremor was observed in Mr. T.'s hand movements. Perseverative tendencies were evidenced on a number of the objective tests (e.g., Rey-Osterrieth Complex Figure recall, AVLT). In addition, a very concrete and somewhat illogical cognitive style was frequently exhibited. For example, when the WRAT-R test was placed in front of him, he read the title and asked, "That's not a real rat is it?" On another occasion, he asked how he had arrived at the testing room ("Did I walk?"), and at midmorning he was uncertain whether he had yet eaten his lunch.

The patient was cooperative and appeared to attempt each of the tests to the best of his abilities. On the basis of behavioral observations, it is concluded that the current findings are an accurate representation of Mr. T.'s present level of intellectual, cognitive, and behavioral functioning.

Tests Administered

See data summary sheet.

Test Results

Intelligence

Mr. T. is currently functioning with the average range (34th percentile) of general intellectual ability, as exhibited by performance on the WAIS-R, with a Verbal IQ of 115, a Performance IQ of 68, and a Full Scale IQ of 94, placing him in the average range overall. A 47-point differential is observed between Verbal and Performance IQ's suggesting that he exhibits significantly better efficiency in the verbal domain. Given the significant disparity between the Verbal and Performance domains, it is postulated that the Full Scale IQ is a misrepresentation of Mr. T.'s current level of overall functioning.

More specifically, on verbal abilities, the patient performed quite efficiently (very superior range) in vocabulary skills (Vocabulary) and knowledge of long-term information (Information). However, only average performance was evidenced in oral arithmetic reasoning (Arithmetic), verbal abstraction (Similarities), and comprehension of social situations (Comprehension). Mr. T.'s arithmetic ability evidences a notable deficit, given his past level of occupational functioning. On Performance items, Mr. T. demonstrated impaired performance on block construction (Block Design, 2nd percentile) and impaired ability in analysis and synthesis skills when confronted with an object assembly task (Object Assembly, 1st percentile).

It is hypothesized, on the basis of previous occupational, academic, and scholastic history, that the patient's present level of intellectual functioning is significantly lower than premorbid levels. Premorbid intelligence is postulated to have been in the superior to very superior range of functioning.

Academic Achievement

In order to further quantify the patient's deficits in arithmetic abilities, the WRAT-R was administered. Mr. T.'s arithmetic ability on a written test was approximately comparable to students entering the seventh grade. Hence, these results clearly reflect significant decline in Mr. T.'s current oral and written arithmetic abilities, based on predicted premorbid levels.

Gross Cognitive Functioning

On the Mini-Mental State Exam, Mr. T. scored 26/30, with errors notable in memory tasks. For example, Mr. T. was unable to name the floor of the hospital and evidenced variable difficulty identifying the date. In addition, even with cueing, he was unable to recall any of the names of three objects presented to him three minutes earlier. Tremor was evidenced in the copy of two overlapping objects.

Attention and Concentration

On the Digit Span subtest of the WAIS-R, Mr. T. obtained scores of seven forward and five backward (75th percentile). He scored within the average range (63rd percentile) on a verbal task requiring active concentration (Arithmetic). In addition, he evidenced average performance on the Mental Control subtest of the Wechsler Memory Scale (46th percentile) and Stroop—section A. Stroop B was within the low average range. However, significantly impaired performance was exhibited when confronted with tasks that required both sustained and divided attention/concentration, visual scanning, and cognitive flexibility. For example, on Trails A and B, extremely impoverished performance was manifested, and he fell below the first percentile. Stroop C, requiring speed of performance and response inhibition was also significantly impaired (310 seconds, < lst percentile).

Thus, we find that the patient manifests intact abilities for brief, passive, and selective attention. However, visual scanning and sustained attentional tasks also involving shift of set and cognitive flexibility are dramatically impaired.

Language

As previously noted, Mr. T.'s level of vocabulary knowledge (Vocabulary) was in the very superior range (98th percentile) and is an area of particular strength. The patient performed within the average range (55th–59th percentile) on a word-list generation task (FAS) and named 10 animals in one minute. He performed within the average range on the Boston Naming Test (54/60), but evidenced one paraphasic naming error when he called a "harness" a "hames." Gross assessment of comprehension and repetition revealed intact performance. Overall, we find generally intact naming and other language functions, though diminished word-list generation given his verbal intellectual level.

Perceptual Organizational Abilities

An opthamology exam revealed normal vision with no visual field defects. However, Mr. T. performed within the impaired range (2nd percentile) on a task involving alertness to detail (Picture Completion). He also exhibited impaired ability on constructional tasks with blocks (Block Design, 2nd percentile), and scored in the impaired range (Rey-Osterrieth, < 10th percentile) in the drawing of a complex geometric design. Performance on a task in which he had to construct puzzle pieces to form an object was likewise impaired (Object Assembly, lst percentile). Thus, overall, we find dramatically impaired abilities within this domain.

Verbal Auditory Memory

Mr. T.'s performance on rote, verbal memory tasks was generally lower than expected, given his Verbal IQ performance and predicted premorbid intelligence. For example, on an auditorily presented task, although Mr. T. was able to learn five of six related word pairs, he was unable to learn any of the unrelated word pairs (WMS–Associate Learning).

Mr. T. demonstrated significant encoding and retrieval difficulties in the learning of a 15-item list of unrelated words (AVLT). He exhibited no learning curve, and in fact, his pattern of recall revealed distinct primacy and recency effects. Following an interference task, he recalled none of the 15 words, and was able to recall only one of the words following a 30-minute delay. On a reading recognition task, he recognized two of the words but with two false positive responses as well. Thus, the patient evidenced a pattern of learning and retrieval that was significantly different from that expected given his age reference group and predicted premorbid level of occupational functioning.

The patient's immediate memory for logical prose (WMS–Logical Memory) was examined by having him recall paragraphs read to him (analogous to conversational language). Mr. T. evidenced low-average performance on immediate recall (WMS–Logical Memory, 24th percentile), which was lower than expected premorbidly. Following a 30-minute delay, he also performed within the low average range.

In sum, Mr. T. demonstrated variable performance in verbal memory, which was less than expected given his previous level of predicted intellectual functioning. In particular, he evidenced difficulty in the learning of unrelated word pairs and unstructured word lists. Low average ability was evidenced in the recall of logical prose.

Visual Nonverbal Memory

Mr. T.'s performance on the learning and recall of nonverbal material was significantly lower than expected, though assessment of this domain is confounded by his visuo-spatial deficit described above. For example, his ability to recall and draw simple geometric designs after a 10-second exposure (WMS–Visual Reproduction) was in the borderline range (9th percentile). His memory drawing of these designs after a 30-minute delay was in the impaired range; he was unable to recall any of the 4 previously presented drawings. Moreover, the patient was unable to recognize any of the four figures when presented to him in a multiple-choice selection format. Furthermore, memory drawing of a complex geometric figure after a three-minute delay was also significantly impaired (Rey-Osterrieth, < 10th percentile), and a perseverative response pattern was evidenced.

In sum, we find that Mr. T. exhibits significant impairment in his ability to immediately copy and reproduce geometric designs and recall nonverbal material. Impaired memory recall was demonstrated in each of the nonverbal areas that were tested, although assessment was confounded by the patient's grossly deficient constructional skill.

"Frontal Systems" Tasks

Another area of performance inefficiency was demonstrated in ability to shift perceptual sets, abstract reasoning, and hypothesis-generating skills. For example, compromised performance from predicted premorbid levels was manifested on the Similarities subtest of the WAIS-R (average range), and behaviorally, perseveration, poor judgment and a concrete style were apparent. In addition, impaired performance was evidenced on Trails B (500 seconds), and Stroop C (< 1st percentile). These contrast sharply with predicted premorbid levels of functioning.

Motor

Mr. T. noted a preference for the use of his right hand for the majority of activities, and no peripheral injuries are known. The patient does have a bilateral peripheral neuropathy in both upper extremities, however. On a finger tapping test, the patient displayed extremely variable performance, making interpretation somewhat difficult. For example, he was unable to maintain a consistent tapping speed, and numerous trials were required. The test was discontinued after 10 trials with each hand, when he was unable to achieve the requisite scoring criterion. Thus, although Mr. T. obtained an overall level of dominant-hand tapping performance that was within normal limits (55th percentile), significant variability was evident, perhaps exacerbated by his peripheral neuropathy. Nondominant-hand performance was slower than expected (7th percentile), however, and in fact, there was a 31% superiority of the dominant versus nondominant hand. Dominant-hand superiority was evidenced on both the strength of grip and Grooved Pegboard tasks, although performance on each of these tests was impaired (<1st percentile).

Personality

An invalid profile was obtained on the MMPI, which was generally due to the patient's level of overall confusion, with an inability to answer many of the items. Each of the items was read to the patient by his sister. On the Sentence Completion Test, themes of loneliness and fear of death were evident.

Summary and Impressions

Neuropsychological test results portray a man who has sustained moderate to severe compromise in numerous cognitive domains when compared with predicted premorbid levels. Such decline was evident in overall intelligence (from very superior to average range), visuo-spatial/constructional skills, executive frontal lobe skills, and verbal (and probably nonverbal) memory. Thus, we find evidence of compromise in functions believed to be mediated by each hemisphere; however, far more dramatic impairment is evidenced in tasks traditionally associated with right-hemispheric functioning. This is corroborated by the demonstration of a dramatic differential between Verbal and Performance IQ scores (47 points). Furthermore, this conclusion is supported by particular inefficiencies in nondominant finger tapping performance and visuo-spatial deficits.

Other areas of dysfunction included arithmetic (an area of previous specialization), personality judgment, and word-list generation. Taken together, these features are consistent with a dementia syndrome of moderate severity.

What may be the etiology of these notable deficits in a man who once functioned successfully as a professor of college mathematics? Essentially, the results are difficult to interpret owing to chronic medical difficulties, his current medication regimen, and a history of significant depression 3 years ago. However, the findings described above would be consistent with a multi-infarct dementia given the motor asymmetries, variable performance pattern, islands of preserved abilities (e.g., naming) and dramatic decrement in nonverbal versus verbal tasks. It is likely that his medical difficulties, such as cardiovascular abnormalities and diabetes, and medications, however, have contributed to his overall cognitive deficits.

As described above, the data indicate that tasks requiring nonverbal-information processing are extremely difficult for this patient. This compounds difficulties in executive functions and in self-care (such as personal hygiene). It will be necessary for the patient to have caregivers continue to attend to his daily activities and provide close supervision. Social service involvement will be useful in assisting Mr. T. and his sister. Continued supportive psychiatric care is recommended for the patient and his family in light of his history of depression, grief, and current fear of death. In addition, it is recommended that the patient receive neuropsychological testing in approximately six to 12 months, in order to reevaluate his neuropsychological status at that time and compare it with the present level of functioning.

NEUROPSYCHOLOGY TEST SCORE SUMMARY SHEET

Patient: N.T. Age: 67 Sex: M Handedness: R

I. Intelligence WAIS-R Age-Corrected Scores

VERBAL			PERFORMANCE		
Information	17	(99 %ile)	Picture Completion	4	(2 %ile)
Digit Span	12	(75 %ile)	Picture Arrangement	4	(2 %ile)
Vocabulary	16	(98 %ile)	Block Design	4	(2 %ile)
Arithmetic	11	(63 %ile)	Object Assembly	3	(1 %ile)
Comprehension	8	(16 %ile)	Digit Symbol	8	(25 %ile)
Similarities	10	(25 %ile)			
VERBAL IQ =	115	(84 %ile)	PERFORMANCE IQ =	68	(2 %ile)

FULL SCALE IQ = 94 (34 %ile)

II. Attention/Concentration
Digit Span: 7 forward + 5 backwards = 12 Total (75 %ile)
Mental Control, WMS: 6 (46 %ile)
Trails A: 60" (<1 %ile), Trails B: 500" (<1 %ile)

III. Language
Boston Naming Test: 54/60
Controlled Word Association: F (11) + A (11) + S (14) + Age Corr.= 39 (55-59 %ile)

IV. Perceptual/Organizational
Rey-Osterrieth Complex Figure Copy: 14.5/36 (<10 %ile)

V. Memory

VERBAL		NONVERBAL	
WMS Logical Memory	5.25 (24 %ile)	WMS Visual Repro:	1 (9 %ile)
30 min. delay:	3.5	30 min. delay:	0
Percent retention:	67		

WMS I	Easy 4, 5, 5	Rey-Osterrieth Fig:	14.5 (<10 %ile)
Associate I	Hard 0, 0, 0	3 min. delay:	2 (<10 %ile)
Learning I	Score: 7 (14 %ile)		

Rey Auditory Verbal Learning Test (15 items):
T1:5 T2:4 T3:4 T4:5 T5:3 Recall after Interference: 0
30-min. Delayed Recall: 1
Recognition: 2 Hits, 2 False Identifications

VI. Motor Exam	Dominant Hand	%ile	Nondom. Hand	%ile
Finger Tapping:	43.6	55	30	7
Grip Strength:	26.67	<1	24.33	<1
Grooved Pegbd.:	116	<1	134	<1

VII. Frontal Systems
Stroop A: 57", Stroop B: 87", Stroop C: 310"

Commentary on Dementia Cases

The cases included in this chapter, though limited in number, represent somewhat typical cognitive changes for subcortical, cortical, and mixed dementias. Case 1, the gentleman who was found to have an idiopathic calcification of the basal ganglia, is interesting from several perspectives. First, his behavioral and cognitive abnormalities illustrate the slowing, forgetfulness, and affective changes commonly associated with subcortical dementia. Second, this case is interesting because he was first seen by a local mental health private practitioner not trained in neurobehavior or neuropsychology. Because of his profound slowness and forgetfulness without the presence of amnesia, aphasia, or apraxia, for example, he was diagnosed as "obsessive compulsive disorder" and was denied disability leave. It was not until several months later, when still unable to effectively perform his job, that his employer obtained a second opinion, and laboratory studies and this neuropsychological evaluation revealed his true dementia syndrome. This illustrates the potential harm that can come to patients when they are evaluated or treated by practitioners not trained in a specialty related to the presenting complaint.

Case 2 represents findings common in Alzheimer's disease in a patient with a mild to moderate dementia. In this case, it was important to consider three things: (1) the pattern of neuropsychological deficits was consistent with Alzheimer's disease, with deficits across many cognitive domains; (2) the course was consistent with a *progressive* decline in both cognitive and adaptive functioning; and (3) other causes of his dementia could be excluded by negative findings on neurologic exam, laboratory studies, and imaging measures. This illustrates the need to obtain a careful history to determine if the dementia is steadily progressive or stepwise in course, as well as collaborating with the neurologist who would interpret laboratory and neurologic exam findings.

Finally, Case 3 illustrates the "patchy" findings that can be found in a patient who has sustained one or more strokes and how the examiner must interpret current performance in light of premorbid level of functioning (in this case, a professor of mathematics performed at the seventh grade equivalency level in arithmetic).

Thus, the neuropsychological assessment of the elderly must consider whether or not the patient's pattern of performance deviates from the changes associated with normal aging and whether the pattern of deficits and domains of preserved functioning are consistent with various conditions. Close collaboration with a neurologist or geriatric psychiatrist is also important to exclude or confirm focal findings or metabolic or structural abnormalities that may be present.

4
Epilepsy

A voluminous literature is available on the neuropsychological correlates of epilepsy. We will precede our discussion of this literature with a definition of relevant terms and concepts.

A seizure is defined as a sudden, excessive, and disorganized discharge of cerebral neurons that may result in changes in consciousness and sensory and motor activity. The term "epilepsy" refers to the presence of recurrent seizures. The term "ictal" is used to designate the seizure event, whereas "interictal" refers to the time period between seizures. Status epilepticus is a condition of continuous seizure activity or consecutive seizures that do not allow for normalization of brain functioning.

Seizures are classified into two major types: *partial* and *generalized* (Bancaud et al., 1981). Partial seizures refer to seizures with onset confined to one cerebral hemisphere, whereas generalized seizures involve widespread neuronal discharge in both hemispheres. Partial seizures (also frequently referred to as temporal lobe seizures or psychomotor seizures) usually appear to arise from temporal lobe or fronto-temporal areas. Partial seizures are categorized as simple or complex dependent upon whether consciousness (ability to respond normally to external stimuli) is compromised. If consciousness is intact, the seizure is described as simple; if it is impaired the seizure is referred to as complex. Partial seizures may be associated with a wide variety of motor, somatosensory, autonomic, and psychic symptoms. For example, it is common to observe movement localized to discrete parts of the body (e.g., one side of the face, head turning, chewing motions, movement of an arm or leg). In addition, patients frequently report gustatory hallucinations, visual illusions, feelings of fear, and perceptions of déja vu.

Generalized seizures may be triggered from a cortical lesion, but it is the subsequent involvement of subcortical structures that leads to the development of the seizure (Adams & Victor, 1985). Generalized seizures include absence (petit mal) and tonic-clonic (grand mal, major motor) seizures. Absence seizures are characterized by a brief episode of altered consciousness with staring and eye blinking. Tonic-clonic seizures involve a sudden loss of consciousness and marked contraction of muscles throughout the body, followed by convulsive movements.

The most common etiologic factors in the development of seizures appearing at birth or shortly thereafter include toxemia and infections during pregnancy, fever, congenital defects, and inherited neurological disorders. The most frequent causes of epilepsy during the school-age years include head trauma, fevers, and infections. The onset of seizures in adults is most typically the result of brain tumors or vascular disorders.

The neuropsychological findings in epilepsy vary depending upon seizure type, as well as on other variables such as presence of a known etiologic factor, age of onset of seizure disorder, frequency of seizures, duration of seizure disorder, location of the seizure onset, anticonvulsant levels, and occurrence of head trauma sustained as the result of loss of consciousness during seizure activity. Owing to the large number of publications on the cognitive functioning of epileptics, this brief review will focus on the most recent and representative studies. We refer the reader to the reviews of Brown and Reynolds (1981), Dodrill (1981), and Trimble and Thompson (1986) for more comprehensive information. Intellectual findings in epilepsy will be discussed first, followed by a summary of the representative neuropsychological correlates of epilepsy.

Intellectual Scores

Patients with generalized tonic-clonic seizures have usually been reported to exhibit intellectual scores on the Wechsler Adult Intelligence Scale (WAIS) within the low average to average ranges (Giordani et al., 1985; Klove & Matthews, 1974). Mean Performance IQs of tonic-clonic seizure patients consistently have been found to fall an average of two to six points below Verbal IQs. Lowered scale scores have been noted on subtests tapping attention, perceptual organization, and verbal abstraction (Arithmetic, Digit Span, Digit Symbol, Block Design, Object Assembly, and Similarities subtests) (Giordani, et al., 1985; Milberg, Greiffenstein, Lewis, & Rourke, 1980).

Dikmen and Matthews (1977) indicate that seizure frequency is inversely related to intellectual performance; their tonic-clonic seizure patients with more than one seizure per month had intellectual scores within the low average range, whereas patients with seizure frequency of only one seizure every one to six months obtained intellectual scores within the average range. Age of onset of seizures also appears to significantly impact intellectual performance of patients with major motor seizures (Dikmen, Matthews, & Harley, 1975). Patients developing a major motor seizure disorder between birth and five years of age were observed to obtain mean Full Scale IQs within the borderline range; patients with onset of seizures between 10 and 15 years of age exhibited low average intellectual scores. The most marked group differences in intellectual scores are obtained when patients with high seizure frequency, early age of onset, and longer duration of seizure disorder (25+ years) are compared with patients having low seizure frequency, later age of onset, and relatively short duration of disorder (up to 10 years), with the latter clearly obtaining normal intellectual scores and the former showing the most impairment (borderline intellectual scores).

Less information is available on patients who exhibit absence seizures. Some investigators indicate that patients with petit mal seizures show the least intellectual disruption of any seizure group (Lennox & Lennox, 1960) and do not exhibit the mildly lowered Performance IQ found in major motor seizure patients (Zimmerman, Burgemeister, & Putnam, 1951).

Patients with partial seizures have generally been reported to obtain intellectual scores well within the normal range. Relatively lowered performances have been noted on the Information and Vocabulary subtests of the WAIS in this population (Milberg et al., 1980). Some evidence suggests that patients with left hemisphere seizure onset may show slightly lower mean intellectual scores than patients with right hemisphere seizure onset, although the scores are still within the average range (Blakemore, Ettlinger, & Falconer, 1966). These findings may be an artifact of seizure onset and duration of seizure disorder because left temporal lobe seizure patients have been found to have an earlier age of onset (Taylor, 1975). Some investigators have observed that left temporal lobe seizure patients show relatively lower Verbal IQs (Ivnik, Sharbrough, & Laws, 1987) and that right temporal lobe seizure patients show lower Performance IQs (Milner, 1958; Fedio & Mirsky, 1969), although this pattern has not been consistently reported for right temporal lobe seizure patients (Ivnik et al., 1987). Blakemore, Ettlinger, and Falconer (1966) compared left versus right temporal lobe patients and reported that the left seizure patients scored significantly poorer on the Vocabulary, Similarities, and Digit Symbol subtests of the WAIS (the Information subtest was not administered).

Little data have appeared evaluating the effect of seizure frequency, age of onset, and duration of seizure disorder on intellectual functioning in partial seizure patients, but perhaps the same relationships as documented in major motor seizure patients (Dikmen & Matthews, 1977) are true of partial seizure patients. Blakemore, Ettlinger, and Falconer (1966) did document that seizure frequency rather than severity of neuropathological changes was more closely related to impairment in WAIS Verbal subtest performance in partial seizure patients.

Neuropsychological Findings

Investigations into the neuropsychological correlates of epilepsy have frequently used the Halstead Reitan Battery (HRB). Klove and Matthews (1974) report that patients with generalized tonic-clonic seizures of known etiology scored significantly lower than controls on all HRB measures except for the Finger Tapping Test. Patients with tonic-clonic seizures of unknown (idiopathic) etiology were noted to score more poorly than controls on only the Tactual Performance Test (TPT), Seashore Rhythm Test (SRT), and the Category Test. The mean scores reported by Dikmen, Matthews, and Harley (1975) on their tonic-clonic seizure patients on the TPT, SRT, Speech Sounds Perception Test (SSPT), Finger Tapping, Trailmaking, and Category Tests are clearly within the impaired range when compared to current HRB normative data (Bornstein, 1985; Reitan, 1985);

information regarding whether the seizure etiology was known or idiopathic was not provided. No significant differences in scores were noted between patients with early and late onset major motor seizures. Patients with higher seizure frequency tended to score more poorly than patients with low seizure frequency on the SRT, Trails B, and the Impairment Index (Dikmen & Matthews, 1977). Patients with longer duration of seizure disorder, higher seizure frequency, and early age of seizure onset showed the most impairment on the HRB variables.

Patients with idiopathic partial seizures have been reported to perform similar to normals on the HRB, although patients with partial seizures of known etiology performed more poorly than controls on the TPT, Trails A and B, and Category Test (Klove & Matthews, 1974). These findings highlight the limitations of the HRB as the careful work of several investigators using other tests has pointed to unique cognitive limitations in patients with partial complex seizures of known and unknown etiology localized to the temporal lobes. Patients with left temporal lobe seizures have been described as exhibiting mild deficits in the learning and, especially, the delayed recall of novel verbal material (Ivnik et al., 1987; Meyer & Yates, 1955; Delaney, Rosen, Mattson, & Novelly, 1980; Milner, 1958; Mungas, Ehlers, Walton, & McCutchen, 1985; Taylor, 1968). For example, Delaney and colleagues (1980) cited evidence that left and right temporal lobe seizure patients both performed slightly more poorly than normals in the immediate recall of paragraph details (WMS Form II, approximate mean score = 8). On 30-minute delay, the left temporal lobe patients were only able to recall 53% of the information, as compared to 74% by the right temporal lobe seizure patients, and 85% by the normals. Mungas and co-workers (1985) found that left and right temporal lobe seizure patients did not differ from normals on the five learning trials on a 16-word list learning task, but the left temporal lobe seizure patients performed significantly more poorly than the other groups on recall following an interference task (seven words recalled versus greater than nine in the other groups), and phonemic/graphemic cueing was not helpful in eliciting the items.

In contrast to the pattern of memory difficulties shown by the left temporal lobe seizure patients, right temporal lobe seizure patients have been reported to have difficulty in "pictoral comprehension" and complex visual perceptual integration, immediate tonal memory, and learning and recall of nonverbal material, although the observed deficits tend to be more mild and elusive than the deficits exhibited by left temporal lobe seizure patients (Dennerll, 1964; Milner, 1958, 1975). Milner (1958) reported that right temporal lobe seizure patients showed more difficulty in identifying incongruous aspects of pictured scenes (McGill Picture Anomaly Series) and in correctly reporting which notes had been changed in a series (Seashore Tonal Memory Test). Delaney and colleagues (1980) reported that right temporal lobe seizure patients performed normally in the immediate recall of nonverbal figural designs (WMS-Visual Reproduction) and scored minimally poorer than left temporal lobe seizure patients and controls on recall after 30-minute delay (72% retention versus 79% and 89% retention in the left temporal lobe and control groups). Right temporal lobe seizure patients may perform more poorly on more difficult nonverbal memory tasks, such as the Rey-Osterrieth Complex Figure. Taylor (1979) reported that left temporal lobe seizure patients recalled 70% of the Complex Figure following a 45-minute delay, whereas right temporal lobe seizure patients recalled less than half of the information.

Though not much literature is available on memory functioning in tonic-clonic seizure patients, the limited evidence fails to document any memory impairment that is poorer than expected for the intellectual level, and these patients typically perform better on memory testing than temporal lobe seizure patients (Glowinski, 1973). Tarter, in his 1972 review of the intellectual findings in epilepsy, points out that patients with tonic-clonic seizures perform most poorly on tasks involving sustained attention and perceptual organization, whereas patients with partial complex seizures perform poorly on memory tasks, and he concludes:

> Thus, where the seizure focus is telencephalic, the deficits are primarily cognitive and intellectual, and where the focus is mesencephalic, the impairment is specifically in attentional capacities. This latter finding is not too surprising considering the role played by the midbrain RAS in mediating arousal and attention. (p. 768)

Effects of Anticonvulsant Medication

No discussion of the cognitive performance of patients with epilepsy would be complete without reference to the possible disruptive effects of anticonvulsant medication on cognition. The most common types of anticonvulsants include phenytoin (Dilantin), barbiturates (phenobarb), valproate, benzodiazepine (Valium), ethosuximide (Zarontin), and more recently, carbamazepine (Tegretol). We refer the reader to the recent reviews by Reynolds and Trimble (1985) and Trimble and Thompson (1986) for a more comprehensive discussion of this issue.

In general, cognitive deficits due to medication are most likely to occur when the patient is at toxic levels, and when a combination of drugs is employed (polytherapy) rather than a single anticonvulsant. Typical symptoms of toxicity include lethargy, altered attention, drowsiness, and ataxia (gait disturbance). In patients who are tapered from several medications to monotherapy, frequent improvements in concentration, alertness and arousal, motor functioning, mood, and to a slight degree, memory, are reported, especially if Dilantin and phenobarb have been the drugs eliminated (Shovron & Reynolds, 1979) and if Tegretol is instituted in place of other drugs (Thompson & Trimble, 1982). The improvements are most detectable at least six months after the substitution.

Unfortunately, increasing evidence is emerging that suggests that subtle cognitive impairments can occur in patients who register therapeutic levels of anticonvulsants. Research conducted on nonpatients who have volunteered to take anticonvulsants has revealed that phenobarbitone reduces perceptual motor performance and vigilance (Hutt, Jackson, Belsham, & Higgins, 1968). In addition, Dilantin has been reported to impair memory, motor speed, concentration, reaction time, and mental processing (Thompson & Trimble, 1981a,b, 1982, 1983; Idestrom, 1972). Valproate has been associated with slowing of mental processing, and some evidence indicates that Tegretol may reduce motor but not mental speed (Thompson & Trimble, 1981a,b, 1982, 1983). Research conducted on patients with well-controlled seizures and medication levels that are subtoxic suggest that Tegretol interferes less than Dilantin in performance involving memory and tracking (Andrews, Tomlinson, Elwes, & Reynolds, 1984) and attention and problem-solving (Dodrill & Troupin, 1977).

Pseudoseizures

Another important area that deserves brief discussion involves the phenomenon of pseudoseizures. Pseudoseizures refer to events that may appear similar to the behavioral manifestations of seizure activity but are not accompanied by epileptiform EEG activity or postictal EEG changes. It has been estimated that 5% to 36% of patients treated for seizures may exhibit pseudoseizures rather than (or in addition to) true epileptic seizures (Pond, Bidwell, & Stein 1960; Desai, Potter, & Penry, 1979; Ramani & Gummit, 1982). Neuropsychological testing does not appear to be useful in discriminating patients with actual versus pseudoseizures because pseudoseizure patients frequently have positive neurological histories. Wilkus, Dodrill, and Thompson (1984) failed to find any differences between pseudoseizure and actual seizure patients on Dodrill's Neuropsychological Battery for Epilepsy (1978), and they indicate that 51% of the pseudoseizure patient scores were outside normal limits. They report that compromise of adaptive abilities frequently accompanied psychological and social problems, and they hypothesize that organic factors may in fact predispose to the presence of pseudoseizures. Personality testing (MMPI) was more useful in correctly classifying pseudoseizure patients. Specifically, pseudoseizure patients showed elevations on scales 1, 3, 4, and 8 relative to the patients with actual epilepsy, and they demonstrated a pattern typically seen in conversion hysteria (1 and 3 elevated and higher than 2).

Prediction of Future Functioning

Neuropsychological testing appears to have usefulness in predicting the presence of future deficiencies in life functioning in adolescents and young adults with seizures. Dodrill and Clemmons (1984) reported that neuropsychological scores were better predictors of future adjustment (employment, independence in living) than intelligence scores, personality test scores (MMPI), or other variables such as seizure frequency, medication, and seizure type. Ability tests that emphasize language functioning were the most predictive of future adjustment; for example, a cut-off of three or greater errors on the Aphasia Screening Test resulted in an 87% correct prediction rate of overall later adjustment.

Personality Functioning

It is beyond the scope of this chapter to present the comprehensive literature on psychological symptoms associated with epilepsy. We refer the interested reader to reviews by Blumer and Benson (1982) and Trimble (1982).

Changes in personality functioning have been most commonly reported in patients with partial complex seizures (Blumer & Benson, 1982), although this has not been a consistent finding (Herrman, Schwartz, Karnes, & Vahdat, 1980). Onset of partial complex seizures in adolescence may be particularly associated with development of psychopathology (Herrman, Schwartz, Karnes, et al., 1980). Patients with partial complex seizures, especially those with a left-sided focus, have been reported to exhibit a higher than expected incidence of interictal depression (Mendez, Cummings, & Benson, 1986) and schizophrenia-like psychosis (Sherwin, Peron-Magnan, Bancaud, Bonis, & Talairach, 1982). The incidence of depression in temporal lobe epilepsy has been reported to range from 45% to 65% as compared to a 24% to 42% depression rate in other epileptics (Roy, 1979; Dongier, 1959/60). The depression tends to be characterized by irritability, emotionality, humorlessness, and paranoia with minimal self-pity, brooding, guilt, somatization, and anxiety (Mendez et al., 1986).

Sherwin and colleagues (1982) estimate that 10% to 15% of patients with poorly controlled temporal lobe epilepsy exhibit psychosis, and left-handers with left-sided seizure focus are particularly at risk. Taylor (1975) further suggests that left-handed females with left hemisphere alien tissue lesions are most predisposed to develop psychosis. The psychosis differs from "true schizophrenia" in that affect is generally preserved and the symptoms are less socially disruptive in terms of need for antipsychotic medication and/or hospitalization (Sherwin et al., 1982). The psychiatric disorder typically develops approximately 14 years post seizure onset (Blumer & Benson, 1982).

In addition to the presence of higher rates of depression and psychosis, a distinct personality style has been documented in some temporal lobe epilepsy patients that is characterized by viscosity-circumstantiality, hypergraphia, deepened emotionality and religiousness, and hyposexuality (Blumer & Benson, 1982; Bear & Fedio, 1977).

A controversial topic involves the association between epilepsy and violence. Ictal violence is a very rare phenomenon, but postictal aggression can occur, for example, in confused patients who react aggressively when physically restrained (Blumer & Benson, 1982). Interictal explosive behavior has been reported in temporal lobe seizure patients (Blumer & Benson, 1982), although other researchers suggest that seizure type is not related to aggression (Hermann, Schwartz, Whitman, & Karnes, 1980).

Extent of neuropsychological deficit may be related to the presence of psychopathology (Hermann, 1981), although this hypothesis has not been consistently reported (Moehle, Bolter, & Long, 1984).

Summary

Cognitive performance is usually within the normal range in patients with epilepsy, although the presence of tonic-clonic seizures, frequent seizures, early age of onset of seizure disorder, and known etiology for the seizures tends to be associated with lowering of scores, particularly when these factors occur in combination. Patients with partial complex seizures are especially prone to demonstrate memory declines. Patients with left-sided seizure onset generally show verbal memory deficits; patients with right-sided foci demonstrate depressed nonverbal visual memory ability. Patients with tonic-clonic seizures frequently show lowering of attention and perceptual motor skills relative to other cognitive abilities. Patients with absence seizures generally demonstrate no neuropsychological dysfunction. Changes in personality functioning and development of psychopathology, particularly depression and psychosis, frequently are associated with epilepsy, especially in patients with partial complex seizures.

References

Adams, R.D., & Victor, M. (1985). *Principles of Neurology* (3rd ed.). New York: McGraw-Hill.

Andrews, D.G., Tomlinson, L., Elwes, R.D.C., & Reynolds, E.H. (1984). The influence of carbamazepine and phenytoin on memory and other aspects of cognitive function in new referrals with epilepsy. Communication to Memory Symposium, Gothenburg, 1983. *Acta Neurological Scandinavica, 69* (Suppl. 99), 23–30.

Bancaud, J., Henriksen, O., Rubio-Donnadieu, F., Seino, M., Dreifuss, F., & Penry, J.K. (1981). Proposal for revised clinical and electroencedpahlographic classification of epileptic seizures. *Epilepsia, 22*, 489–501.

Bear, D.M., & Fedio, P. (1977). Quantitative analysis of interictal behavior in temporal lobe epilepsy. *Archives of Neurology, 34*, 454–467.

Blakemore, C.B., Ettlinger, G., & Falconer, M.A. (1966). Cognitive abilities in relation to frequency of seizures and neuropathology of the temporal lobes. *Journal of Neurology, Neurosurgery, and Psychiatry, 29*, 268–272.

Blumer, D. & Benson, D.F. (1982). Psychiatric manifestations of epilepsy. In D.F. Benson & D. Blumer (Eds.), *Psychiatric aspects of neurologic disease* (Vol. II.) (pp. 25–48). New York: Grune & Stratton.

Bornstein, R.A. (1985). Normative data on selected neuropsychological measures from a nonclinical sample. *Journal of Clinical Psychology, 41*, 651–659.

Brown, S.W., & Reynolds, E.H. (1981). Cognitive impairment in epileptic patients. In E.H. Reynolds & M.R. Trimble (Eds.), *Epilepsy and psychiatry* (pp. 147–164). New York: Churchill Livingstone.

Delaney, R.D., Rosen, A.J., Mattson, R.H., & Novelly, R.A. (1980). Memory function in focal epilepsy: A comparison of nonsurgical, unilateral temporal lobe and frontal lobe samples. *Cortex, 16*, 103–117.

Dennerll, R.D. (1964). Cognitive deficits and lateral brain dysfunction in temporal lobe epilepsy. *Epilepsia, 5*, 177–191.

Desai, B.T., Potter, R., & Penry, J.K. (1979). The psychogenic seizure by videotape analysis: A study of 42 attacks in 6 patients. *Neurology, 29,* 602.

Dikmen, S., & Matthews, C.G. (1977). Effect of major motor seizure frequency upon cognitive-intellectual functions in adults. *Epilepsia, 18,* 21–30.

Dikmen, S., Matthews, C.G., & Harley, J.P. (1975). Effect of early versus late onset of major motor epilepsy on cognitive-intellectual performance: Further considerations. *Epilepsia, 16,* 73–81.

Dodrill, C.B. (1978). A neuropsychological battery for epilepsy. *Epilepsia, 19,* 611–623.

Dodrill, C.B. (1981). Neuropsychology of epilepsy. In S.B. Filskov & T.J. Boll (Eds.), *Handbook of clinical neuropsychology* (pp. 366–398). New York: John Wiley.

Dodrill, C.B., & Clemmons, D. (1984). Use of neuropsychological tests to identify high school students with epilepsy who later demonstrate inadequate performances in life. *Journal of Consulting and Clinical Psychology, 4,* 520–527.

Dodrill, C.B., & Troupin, A.S. (1977). Psychotropic effects of carbamazepine in epilepsy: A double-blind comparison with phenytoin. *Neurology, 27,* 1023–1028.

Dongier, S. (1959/60). Statistical study of clinical and electroencephalographic manifestations of 536 psychotic episodes occurring in 516 epileptics between clinical seizures. *Epilepsia, 1,* 117–142.

Dorland, S. (1974). *Illustrated medical dictionary* (25th ed.). Philadelphia: W.B. Saunders.

Fedio, P., & Mirsky, A.F. (1969). Selective intellectual deficits in children with temporal lobe or centrecephalic epilepsy. *Neuropsychologia, 7,* 287–300.

Giordani, B., Berent, S., Sackellares, J.C., Rourke, D., Seidenberg, M., O'Leary, D.S., Dreifuss, F.E., & Boll, T.J. (1985). Intelligence test performance of patients with partial and generalized seizures. *Epilepsia, 26,* 37–42.

Glowinski, H. (1973). Cognitive deficits in temporal lobe epilepsy. *Journal of Nervous and Mental Disease, 157,* 129–137.

Hermann, B.P. (1981). Deficits in neuropsychological functioning and psychopathology in persons with epilepsy: A rejected hypothesis revisited. *Epilepsia, 22,* 161–167.

Hermann, B.P., Schwartz, M.S., Karnes, W.E., & Vahdat, P. (1980). Psychopathology in epilepsy: Relationship of seizure type to age at onset. *Epilepsia, 21,* 15–23.

Hermann, B.P., Schwartz, M.S., Whitman, S., & Karnes, W.E. (1980). Aggression and epilepsy: Seizure-type comparisons and high-risk variables. *Epilepsia, 21,* 691–698.

Hutt, S.J., Jackson, P.M., Belsham, A., & Higgins, G. (1968). Perceptual-motor behavior in relation to blood phenobarbitone level: A preliminary report. *Developmental Medicine and Childhood Neurology, 10,* 626–632.

Idestrom, C.M., Schalling, D., Carlquist, U., & Sjoqvist, F. (1972). Acute effects of diphenylhydantoin in relation to plasma levels: Behavioral and psychophysiological studies. *Psychological Medicine, 2,* 11–120.

Ivnik, R.J., Sharbrough, F.W., & Laws, E.R. (1987). Effects of anterior temporal lobectomy on cognitive function. *Journal of Clinical Psychology, 43,* 128–137.

Klove, H., & Matthews, C.G. (1974). Neuropsychological studies of patients with epilepsy. In R.M. Reiten & L.A. Davison (Eds.), *Clinical neuropsychology: Current status and applications* (pp. 237–266). New York: John Wiley.

Lennox, W.G., & Lennox, M.A. (1960). *Epilepsy and related disorders,* (2 vols.). Boston: Little, Brown.

Mendez, M.F., Cummings, J.L., & Benson, D.F. (1986). Depression in epilepsy. *Archives of Neurology, 43,* 766–770.

Meyer, V., & Yates, A. (1955). Intellectual changes following temporal lobectomy for psychomotor epilepsy. *Journal of Neurology, Neurosurgery, and Psychiatry, 18,* 44–52.

Milberg, W., Greiffenstein, M., Lewis, R., & Rourke, D. (1980). Differentiation of temporal lobe and generalized seizure patients with the WAIS. *Journal of Consulting and Clinical Psychology, 48,* 39–42.

Milner, B. (1958). Psychological defects produced by temporal lobe excision. *Research Publication Association of Nervous and Mental Diseases, 36,* 244–257.

Milner, B. (1975). Psychological aspects of focal epilepsy and its neurosurgical management. In D.P. Purpura, J.K. Penry, & R.D. Walter (Eds.), *Advances in neurology* (Vol. 8) (pp. 299–321)

Moehle, K.A., Bolter, J.F., & Long, C.J. (1984). The relationship between neuropsychological functioning and psychopathology in temporal lobe epileptic patients. *Epilepsia, 25,* 418–422.

Mungas, D., Ehlers, C., Walton, N., & McCutchen, C.B. (1985). Verbal learning differences in epileptic patients with left and right temporal lobe foci. *Epilepsia, 26,* 340–345.

Pond, D.A., Bidwell, B.H., Stein, L. (1960). A survey of epilepsy in fourteen medical practices. I. Demographic and medical data. *Psychiatr Neurol Neurochir, 63,* 217–236.

Ramani, V., & Gummit, R.J. (1982). Management of hysterical seizures in epileptic patients. *Archives of Neurology, 39,* 78–81.

Reitan, R. (1985) *The Halstead-Reitan Neuropsychological Test Battery.* Neuropsychology Press.

Reynolds, E.H., & Trimble, M.R. (1985). Adverse neuropsychiatric effects of anticonvulsant drugs. *Drugs, 29,* 570–581.

Rickler, K.C. (1982) Episodic dyscontrol. In D.F. Benson & D. Blumer (Eds.), *Psychiatric Aspects of Neurologic Disease* (Vol. II) (pp. 49–74). New York: Grune & Stratton.

Roy, A. (1979). Some determinants of affective symptoms in epileptics. *Canadian Journal of Psychiatry, 24,* 554–556.

Sherwin, I., Peron-Magnan, P., Bancaud, J., Bonis, A., & Talairach, J. (1982). Prevalence of psychosis in epilepsy as a function of the laterality of the epileptogenic lesion. *Archives of Neurology, 39,* 621–625.

Shovron, S.D., & Reynolds, E.H. (1979). Reduction in polypharmacy for epilepsy. *British Medical Journal, 2,* 1023–1025.

Tarter, R.E. (1972). Intellectual and adaptive functioning in epilepsy: A review of 50 years of research. *Diseases of the Nervous System, 33,* 763–770.

Taylor, D.C. (1975). Factors influencing the occurrence of schizophrenia-like psychosis in patients with temporal lobe epilepsy. *Psychological Medicine, 5,* 249–254.

Taylor, L.B. (1968). Localisation of cerebral lesions by psychological testing. *Clinical Neurosurgery* (Vol. 16) (pp. 269–287).

Taylor, L.B. (1979). Psychological assessment of neurosurgical patients. In T. Rasmussen & R. Marino (Eds.), *Functional neurosurgery* (pp. 165–180). New York: Raven Press.

Thompson, P.J., & Trimble, M.R. (1981a). Sodium valproate and cognitive functioning in normal volunteers. *British Journal of Clinical Pharmacy, 12,* 819–824.

Thompson, P.J., & Trimble, M.R. (1981b). Clobazam and cognitive functions. Effects in healthy volunteers. In Royal Society of Medicine International Congress and Symposium Series (pp. 33–38). London: Academic Press.

Thompson, P.J., & Trimble, M.R. (1982). Anticonvulsant drugs and cognitive functions. *Epilepsia, 23,* 531–544.

Thompson, P.J., & Trimble, M.R. (1983). The effect of anticonvulsant drugs on cognitive function: Relation to serum levels. *Journal of Neurology, Neurosurgery and Psychiatry, 46,* 227–233.
Trimble, M.R. (1982). The interictal psychoses of epilepsy. In D.F. Benson & D. Blumer (Eds.), *Psychiatric aspects of neurological disease* (Vol. II) (pp. 75–92). New York: Grune & Stratton.
Trimble, M.R., & Thompson, P.J. (1986). Neuropsychological aspects of epilepsy. In I. Grant & K. Adams (Eds.), *Neuropsychological assessment of neuropsychiatric disorders* (pp. 321–346). New York: Oxford University Press.
Wilkus, R.J., Dodrill, C.B., & Thompson, P.M. (1984). Intensive EEG monitoring and psychological studies of patients with pseudoepileptic seizures. *Epilepsia, 25,* 100–107.
Zimmerman, F.T., Burgemeister, B.B., & Putnam, T.J. (1951). Intellectual and emotional makeup of the epileptic. *Archives of Neurology and Psychiatry, 65,* 545–556.

Case 1: Seizures Associated with Tuberous Sclerosis[1]

Reason for Referral

Ms. A.B. was referred for neuropsychological testing for evaluation of possible cognitive dysfunction secondary to a partial complex seizure disorder and tuberous sclerosis.

Presenting Situation and Background Information

This 25-year-old, right-handed female was diagnosed as having a seizure disorder at the age of 7 that was characterized at the time as a "lack of attention in school." The patient was placed on phenytoin and phenobarbital but has continued to exhibit seizures. Approximately one year ago, carbamazepine was added to her treatment regimen. Currently the patient's seizures are characterized by blank staring, heavy breathing, and fidgeting with her hands. Ms. B. is unresponsive during these episodes and postictally exhibits confusion and sleepiness for approximately 12 to 20 minutes. The patient's seizure frequency varies from no seizures for up to two weeks to as many as five seizures in one day. The patient denies any history of generalized tonic-clonic seizures or status epilepticus.

Ms. B.'s seizure disorder appears to be a consequence of the presence of tuberous sclerosis. A CT scan obtained six months ago revealed calcifications on the walls of the lateral ventricles typical of tuberous sclerosis. An EEG also obtained at that time revealed generalized slowing of the background frequencies and left mid- to fronto-temporal spikes. The patient's current medication regimen consists of carbamazepine and phenobarbital.

---

[1]Tuberous sclerosis is a congenital familial disease characterized by tumors on the surfaces of the lateral ventricles and sclerotic patches on the brain's surface, and marked clinically by progressive mental deterioration and epileptic convulsions (Dorland, 1974, p. 1390).

In addition to the seizure disorder, the patient is also presenting with episodes of poor impulse control and rage attacks, and she is currently being evaluated for the presence of episodic dyscontrol.

The patient's medical history is negative for birth abnormalities, chronic and/or serious illnesses, head trauma, hospitalizations or surgeries, alcohol or drug abuse, or psychiatric treatment. The patient's mother also reportedly has been diagnosed as having tuberous sclerosis and two years ago underwent surgery for a brain tumor and subsequently became blind. The patient has one brother who does not have any significant health problems. Her biological father's medical history is unknown.

Ms. B. completed 11½ years of formal schooling and states that she was "kicked out of school because of my temper." She reported that her best subject was math. The patient is currently unemployed and receiving disability compensation. She worked for a department store for two years but was terminated when she "told off a supervisor." She has also been employed as a cocktail waitress and, for approximately one week, was a product demonstrator for a grocery chain. Ms. B. stated that her only complaint about her functioning is difficulty in controlling her "temper." She states that she has difficulty interacting socially and has never had many friends. She has never married and has a boyfriend approximately 25 years her senior.

Behavioral Observations

Ms. B. is a 25-year-old, right-handed, Caucasian female of tall height and medium weight. She arrived at the testing session on time and was accompanied by her boyfriend. She was noted to be very belligerent and somewhat tearful, and she stated that she had been under the impression that she was to have an EEG rather than psychological testing. She was encouraged to participate in the testing, and her cooperation was gradually obtained. Ms. B. indicated that she felt nervous and anxious regarding her performance and several times asked how she was performing. The patient's most recent seizure was approximately one week ago.

Tests Administered

See data summary sheet.

Test Results

Intellectual Scores

Intellectual testing indicates that the patient is currently functioning within the average range of general intellectual ability (Full Scale IQ = 93, 32nd percentile). A moderate discrepancy was observed between overall Verbal and Performance IQs, with the Verbal IQ falling 12 points below the Performance IQ and within the low average range (VIQ = 89; PIQ = 101). Significant scatter was noted across individual Verbal subtests (2nd-84th percentiles), with scores within the impaired to high average ranges. Performance within the high average range was observed on Verbal subtests tapping attention abilities (Digit Span, Arithmetic), and average to low average scores were exhibited on subtests measuring ability to abstract commonalities between objects and knowledge of social norms and judgment (Similarities, Comprehension). Borderline to impaired scores were obtained on subtests assessing vocabulary range and fund of general information (Information, Vocabulary). Mild variability was noted across individual Performance subtests (25th-75th percentiles), with all scores within the average to high average ranges. The individual Performance subtest scores will be discussed in further detail in the section on perceptual organization skills.

Attention and Concentration

Ms. B.'s basic attention skills appeared to be intact. The patient's forward digit span was seven and her backward digit span was six, and she was able to rapidly and accurately count backward from 20, recite the letters of the alphabet, and count by 3s to 40 (9, 6, and 22 seconds, respectively).

Sensory Perceptual/Motor Examination

The patient reported a strong preference for the use of her right hand. No finger agnosia was observed on a brief sensory perceptual exam.

On a task of finger tapping speed, Ms. B. was observed to perform above the average range bilaterally, and the slight expected dominant hand advantage was present (R = 50.6; L = 47.6). Likewise, evaluation of grip strength revealed normal performance bilaterally, and again the expected dominant hand advantage was observed (R = 34; L = 28.5).

Language Functioning

The patient's speech was generally unremarkable, and no difficulties were observed in her comprehension of task constructions. On an aphasia screening examination, the patient was able to write to dictation, repeat words and phrases, demonstrate gestures, follow verbal commands, and discriminate right and left (Aphasia Screening Test). Performance on a confrontation naming test was within the impaired range (Boston Naming Test = 38/60), although this low score might to some extent be an artifact of the patient's restricted vocabulary range (Vocabulary subtest = 9th percentile). Ms. B. scored within the superior range for her age and education level on a word generation task; specifically, she was able to generate 48 words beginning with the letters "f," "a," and "s" within three minutes. Thus, language skills were intact on formal testing with the exception of word-retrieval difficulties.

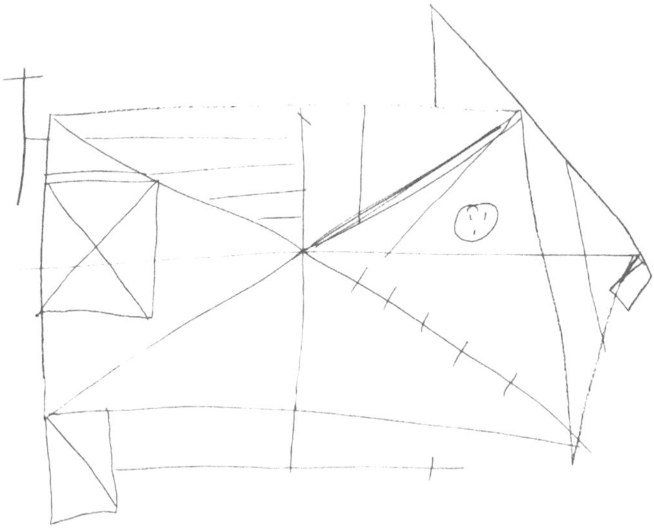

FIGURE 4.1. Case A.B. Rey-Osterrieth Complex Figure: copy. Reduced by 60%.

Perceptual Organizational Skills

Ms. B.'s perceptual organizational skills generally appeared to be intact. She scored within the high average range on a visual perceptual task involving identification of missing parts of pictured objects (Picture Completion = 75th percentile). Visual sequencing and tracking skills were consistently within the average range; the patient scored at the 25th percentile on a task involving sequencing of pictures into a logical story (Picture Arrangement), at the 50th percentile on a rapid visual motor tracking test (Digit Symbol), and well within the normal range on a task requiring the rapid drawing of lines between numbers, and between numbers and letters, in sequential order (Trails A = 24 seconds; B = 39 seconds). Scores on constructional tasks ranged from the low average to average range for pencil and paper copying of line drawings (Rey-Osterrieth = 20th percentile), puzzle-solving (Object Assembly = 37th percentile), and block arrangement (Block Design = 75th percentile). It should be noted that the patient's copying of a complex two-dimensional figure showed a poor organizational strategy and was rather imprecisely rendered, although accurate in detail placement. The drawing was also observed to be somewhat horizontally elongated (Figure 4.1).

Learning and Memory

Overall, the patient's learning and recall skills appeared to be intact, although some variability was observed on verbal learning tasks. The patient's rote learning of word pairs was within the average range for her age (WMS-AL = 61st percentile), and following a 45-minute delay, she was able to recall all 10 word pairs. Likewise, the patient's learning of a 15-item list of unrelated words was above the average range (AVLT; all 15 items recalled by the fifth learning trial). Following an interference task and a 30-minute delay, she was able to recall 14 and 12 of the items respectively, well within the normal range. On the other hand, the patient's immediate recall of paragraph details was within the borderline range for her age (WMS-LM = 6th percentile). She was allowed a second presentation of the material, and her performance improved dramatically (average of 13 details per paragraph). Following a 45-minute delay, she was able to recall 75% of the information, a normal retention rate.

Ms. B.'s immediate recall reproduction of relatively simple geometric figures was within the high average range for her age (WMS-VR = 77th percentile), and following a 45-minute delay, she was able to recall 77% of the information originally learned. The patient's recall of a complex two-dimensional line drawing following a three-minute delay was also within the high average range (Rey-Osterrieth = 80th percentile).

Categorization, Mental Flexibility, and Response Inhibition

The patient scored well within the average range for her education level on a task involving categorization and mental flexibility (ability to shift set). Specifically, the patient was able to complete four categories on the Wisconsin Card Sorting Test with 64 stimulus cards. Likewise, performance on the Stroop Test, a task involving the ability to screen out distracting stimuli and to inhibit habitual responses, was well within the normal range (A = 51 seconds; B = 62 seconds; C = 74 seconds). The patient scored slightly below the normal range on the Visual Verbal Test (TM = 13), a test that involves abstraction of commonalities between objects.

Achievement Scores

<u>WRAT-R</u>
Reading: 47th percentile, greater than 12th grade
Spelling: 50th percentile, 12th grade equivalent
Arithmetic: 32nd percentile, 10 grade equivalent

Achievement scores indicate that the patient is functioning academically well within the expected range for her intellectual and educational level.

Summary and Impressions

Intellectual scores suggest that Ms. B. is currently functioning within the average range of general intellectual ability (Full Scale IQ = 93, 32nd percentile). A moderate discrepancy was observed between overall Verbal and Performance IQ in favor of the Performance IQ (VIQ = 89; PIQ = 101).

Neuropsychological test scores revealed intact functioning in most domains, although selective difficulties were observed. Specifically, borderline to impaired performance was present on tasks measuring fund of general information, definition of vocabulary items, confrontational naming, immediate recall of paragraph details, and abstraction of commonalities between pictured objects. Intact performance was consistently observed on tasks assessing attention and concentration, overall intellectual level, visual perceptual and constructional abilities, rote verbal learning and recall, nonverbal learning and recall, word generation, motor functioning, and academic skills. The pattern of neuropsychological and intellectual scores is suggestive of mild dominant hemisphere dysfunction consistent with EEG findings. The patient's depressed fund of general information and lowered vocabulary range would suggest that she has suffered from long-standing difficulties in learning/processing verbal information such as was witnessed in her poor immediate recall of paragraph details on current testing. The influence of long-standing medication use on test performance is unclear.

Ms. B.'s neuropsychological and intellectual profile suggest that from a cognitive standpoint she is able to be gainfully employed at this time. Personality factors (poor impulse control, rage reactions), would appear to be her most debilitating symptoms in terms of occupational and social functioning. Personality testing was not completed because the patient had not expected to be tested on the examination day and was reluctant to remain, even for the cognitive testing. If personality testing is necessary, a second testing session certainly can be scheduled with the patient. Counseling may be useful in helping the patient learn to modulate her expression of anger and in providing an outlet for voicing of fears and concerns regarding current and future medical problems. Also, due to the progressive nature of tuberous sclerosis on cognitive function, neuropsychological reevaluation is recommended in one year.

NEUROPSYCHOLOGY TEST SCORE SUMMARY SHEET

Patient: A.B. Age: 25 Sex: F Handedness: R

I. Intelligence WAIS-R Age-Corrected Scores

VERBAL			PERFORMANCE		
Information	4	(2 %ile)	Picture Completion	12	(75 %ile)
Digit Span	12	(75 %ile)	Picture Arrangement	8	(25 %ile)
Vocabulary	6	(9 %ile)	Block Design	12	(75 %ile)
Arithmetic	13	(84 %ile)	Object Assembly	9	(37 %ile)
Comprehension	7	(16 %ile)	Digit Symbol	10	(50 %ile)
Similarities	8	(25 %ile)			
VERBAL IQ =	89	(23 %ile)	PERFORMANCE IQ =	101	(53 %ile)

FULL SCALE IQ = 93 (32 %ile)

II. Attention/Concentration

Digit Span: 7 forward + 6 backwards = 13 Total (75 %ile)
Mental Control, WMS: 9 (78 %ile)
Trails A: 24" (44 %ile), Trails B: 39" (79 %ile)

III. Language

Boston Naming Test: 38/60
Controlled Word Association: F (15) + A (14) + S (19) + Age Corr.= 54 (95 %ile)
Aphasia Screening Exam: intact

IV. Perceptual/Organizational

Rey-Osterrieth Complex Figure Copy: 30 /36 (20 %ile)

V. Memory

VERBAL		NONVERBAL	
WMS Logical Memory	4.5 (6 %ile)	WMS Visual Repro.:	13 (77 %ile)
2nd Presentation	13 (89 %ile)		
45 min. delay:	9.75	45 min. delay:	10
Percent retention:	75	Percent retention:	77

WMS Associate Learning
I Easy 5 , 6 , 6
I Hard 2 , 3 , 3
I Score: 16.5(61%ile)
45 min. delay: 6 easy, 4 hard, 100% retention

Rey-Osterrieth Fig: 30 (20 %ile)
3 min. delay: 27 (80 %ile)

Rey Auditory Verbal Learning Test (15 items):
T1: 5 T2: 11 T3: 11 T4: 14 T5: 15 Recall after Interference: 14
30-min. Delayed Recall: 12

VI. Motor Exam

	Dominant Hand	%ile	Nondom. Hand	%ile
Finger Tapping:	50.6	82	47.6	92
Grip Strength:	34	56	28.5	37

VII. Sensory

Finger Gnosis: intact

VIII. Frontal Systems

Stroop A: 51", Stroop B: 62", Stroop C: 74"
Wisconsin Card Sort: Categories: 4
Visual Verbal Test: SM = 11, DM = 1, TM = 13

IX. Achievement

		Grade Equivalent	Percentile Rank
WRAT-R:	Reading	>12	47
	Spelling	12	50
	Arithmetic	10	32

Case A.B.:

WMS-Logical Memory:

Story B:

Immediate Recall:

First Presentation: "Something about a guy that works in Liverpool. Something about a cave or a mine."

Second Presentation: "A guy was on a liner from New York, who found a mine in Liverpool Monday night. A very large snowstorm caused something to happen to the boats. A bunch of women...they were rescued in some manner."

45-Minute Delay:

"Somebody from New York gone to...I forgot, gone somewhere for a mine. There was a tragic snowstorm. A bunch of ladies got knocked over in their boat. They were being saved. What's the name of that place?...it's like food."

Boston Naming Test:

Could not spontaneously name pictures of a:

volcano	pyramid
seahorse	muzzle ("nozzle, gozzle")
globe	funnel ("drainer")
wreath	accordion
escalator	asparagus ("vegetable")
hammock ("cot")	compass
pelican ("goose")	scroll
stethescope	tongs

WAIS-R Information:

Presidents: "Henry, Reagan, Nixon"
Armstrong: "a boxer"
Panama: "no idea"
Labor Day: "March"
Brazil: "that way"
Hamlet: "Hamlet"

WAIS-R Vocabulary:

Commence: "to meet"
Ponder: "bigger pond,...I don't know"
Designate: "I don't know"
Reluctant: "I don't know"
Obstruct: "destroy"
Sanctuary: "some perfect land or something"

Case 2: Severe Seizure Disorder with Marked Cognitive Deterioration

Reason for Referral

Mr. R.A. was referred for neuropsychological testing for evaluation of level of cognitive functioning.

Presenting Situation and Background Information

This 35-year-old, right-handed male is currently presenting with a seizure disorder characterized by frequent complex partial seizures and occasional secondarily generalized major motor seizures. He often experiences one to two complex partial seizures per day and has exhibited up to 12 in one day. In addition, he suffers from several generalized tonic-clonic seizures per month. Of note, the patient has experienced several episodes of "back-to-back" generalized tonic-clonic seizures with only brief recovery of consciousness between seizures. Three of these repeated seizure events occurred within the last year.

The patient's partial complex seizures are characterized by head turning to the left, drooling and chewing movements, staring, flushing of his face, dilated pupils, and a frightened facial expression. He then ducks his head and rubs his nose. He also mumbles and may repeatedly say a name or phrase. The total episode lasts approximately two minutes. Post-ictally the patient is confused for five to 60 minutes.

The patient was apparently the product of a normal pregnancy and delivery, but at the age of three months he began experiencing periodic generalized seizures. At the age of 4 the patient suffered an episode of status epilepticus for eight to nine hours, accompanied by cardiac arrest with resultant cerebral anoxia. The patient was subsequently noted to have lost his language ability and toilet skills and required retraining in these areas. Up until this time the patient appeared to be left-hand dominant, but following this occurrence of status epilepticus, the patient was observed to become right-hand dominant.

At the age of 12 the patient began exhibiting partial complex seizures characterized by lapses in consciousness and repetitive speech and motor behavior, such as getting up and sitting down repeatedly. In addition, he would appear frightened and reach for his mother. During the ages of 12 to 18, the patient's seizures were well controlled with medication, but during the last 14 years the patient has experienced frequent partial complex seizures and occasional secondarily generalized seizures that have been intractable to medication. The patient's family has noted a deterioration in memory that corresponded to the increase in seizure activity.

The patient's medical history is also positive for possible mitral valve prolapse and head injury of unknown severity two years ago during a seizure. There is no apparent history of substance abuse, psychiatric symptoms, or chronic illnesses. Brain CT and MRI scans have been negative. The patient's current anticonvulsant regimen includes Tegretol, Mysoline, Dilantin, Tranxene, and Depakote. His seizures are now fairly well controlled, but he exhibits such side effects as excessive sedation, staggering gait, diplopia, and bleeding gums. The patient's most recent seizure occurred four days ago.

The patient's educational development has always been "very slow," and the patient attended special education classes in a school for the mentally handicapped for 12 years. He has held employment as a boxboy but was discharged because his seizures became very disruptive within the work setting. Family history is negative for seizures or other neurological disorders, and sinistrality. The patient has two siblings who performed normally in school and completed some college coursework.

Behavioral Observations

Mr. A. is a brown-haired, right-handed, Caucasian male of medium height and weight. He was brought to the testing session by his mother. He was observed to be appropriately groomed and casually attired. His facial features appeared to be somewhat coarsened and enlarged, and his tongue tended to mildly protrude between his lips most of the time. His behavioral presentation was prominent for signs of significant mental and social immaturity. For example, he was unable to answer such simple questions as the name of the city in which he lived (he responded with the name of the street on which he lived), and he would frequently reach over and quickly touch the examiner on her hands and shoulder in a teasing manner. Mr. A.'s speech was noteworthy for mild dysarthria and pronounced articulation difficulties. No seizure activity was observed during the lengthy testing session. The patient's test scores are judged to be an accurate estimation of his interictal functioning.

Tests Administered

See data summary sheet.

Test Results

Intellectual Scores

Intellectual testing indicates that Mr. A. is currently functioning within the mildly mentally retarded range of general intellectual ability (Full Scale IQ = 67, 1st percentile). A mild discrepancy was observed between overall Verbal and Performance IQs, with the Verbal IQ falling 10 points below the Performance IQ (VIQ = 64; PIQ = 74). Minimal scatter was noted across individual Verbal subtests (.1–5th percentiles), with all scores within the borderline to impaired ranges. Minimal scatter was also noted across individual Performance subtests (5th-16th percentiles), with all scores within the borderline range except for a low average score on the Object Assembly subtest.

Language Functioning

Measurement of the patient's receptive vocabulary range revealed performance consistent with his overall Verbal intellectual scores. Specifically, the patient performed below the first percentile on the Peabody Picture Vocabulary Test-Revised, obtaining an age equivalent of 7–5. Likewise, the patient scored within the very defective range on a measure of language comprehension ability (Token Test = 34/44).

Perceptual Organizational Skills

Perceptual organizational skills were generally within the borderline to impaired ranges and consistent with the patient's intellectual level. The patient scored within the borderline range on a visual perceptual task involving identification of missing parts of pictured objects (Picture Completion = 5th percentile). The patient's paper and pencil copying of line drawings revealed grossly deficient performance (Beery VMI = 6–10 age equivalent). Other constructional abilities were noted to fall within the borderline to low average range; the patient scored at the fifth and 16th percentiles respectively on the Block Design and Object Assembly subtests of the WAIS-R.

Motor Exam

The patient was reported to be right-hand dominant by his mother, and he corroborated this information. He and his family denied any history of significant injury to his hands, arms, or shoulders. On a task of finger tapping speed, the patient performed within the normal range bilaterally. However, it should be noted that he scored slightly better with his left hand than with his right hand (R = 44.8; L = 48). A left-hand superiority was also noted on a task involving the placing of pegs in a pegboard, although on this task the performance of both hands was within the impaired range (Grooved Pegboard: R = 104"; L = 94"). Evaluation of the patient's grip strength revealed low average performance bilaterally, and scores across hands were comparable (R = 35.7; L = 35.3).

Achievement Scores

<u>WRAT</u>
Reading: 0.9 percentile; 3.7 grade equivalent
Spelling: 3rd percentile; 3.3 grade equivalent
Arithmetic: 9th percentile; 3.3 grade equivalent

Results of achievement testing indicate that the patient is performing consistently at the third-grade level in sight reading, spelling, and mathematical abilities.

Summary and Impressions

Intellectual scores indicate that the patient is currently functioning within the mildly mentally retarded range of general intellectual ability (Full Scale IQ = 67, 1st percentile). A mild discrepancy was noted between overall Verbal and Performance IQs in favor of the Performance IQ (VIQ = 64; PIQ = 74), and minimal scatter was noted across individual subtest scores.

Assessment of basic language skills, constructional abilities, and academic skills consistently revealed deficient performance that was consistent with the patient's intellectual level. Memory testing was not attempted because it was judged that the patient's poor language comprehension and perceptual organizational abilities would render formal memory scores uninterpretable. Motor skills were variable, with some scores within the normal range and others within the impaired range. Of note, although the patient is described as right-hand dominant, he tended to perform better with his left hand on the motor tasks. The overall pattern of findings points to bilateral cerebral dysfunction, although possibly more extensive in the left hemisphere as suggested by the relatively lowered Verbal IQ and poorer dominant-hand motor performance.

The history of possible initial left-hand dominance with subsequent shift of hand preference at age 4 is difficult to integrate with the current test findings. Shift from left to right handedness in a genetic left-hander would be associated with right hemisphere damage, but current test results would appear to implicate more extensive left hemisphere dysfunction. Handedness is not a particularly stable trait before age 4, and thus the purported shift in hand dominance is of questionable utility in retroactively localizing the patient's brain insult at age 4.

In conclusion, the current test scores reveal a consistent picture of a low level of cognitive functioning apparently related to the severe disorder and history of anoxic encephalopathy. These results would appear to be a relatively accurate assessment of the patient's cognitive capabilities in that his most recent reported seizure occurred four days prior to the testing. It is not clear to what extent the patient's current medications are depressing his intellectual abilities, but they by themselves would not result in the observed severe cognitive impairment.

NEUROPSYCHOLOGY TEST SCORE SUMMARY SHEET

Patient: R.A. Age: 35 Sex: M Handedness: R

I. Intelligence WAIS-R Age-Corrected Scores

VERBAL			PERFORMANCE		
Information	4	(2 %ile)	Picture Completion	5	(5 %ile)
Digit Span	5	(5 %ile)	Picture Arrangement	5	(5 %ile)
Vocabulary	1	(.1 %ile)	Block Design	5	(5 %ile)
Arithmetic	4	(2 %ile)	Object Assembly	7	(16 %ile)
Comprehension	1	(.1 %ile)	Digit Symbol	6	(9 %ile)
Similarities	4	(2 %ile)			

VERBAL IQ = 64 (<1 %ile) PERFORMANCE IQ = 74 (4 %ile)
FULL SCALE IQ = 67 (1 %ile)

II. Attention/Concentration
Digit Span: 5 forward + 2 backwards = 7 Total (5 %ile)

III. Language
PPVT-R: Age Equivalent = 7-5, <1 %ile.
Token Test: 34/44.

IV. Perceptual/Organizational
Beery VMI: 13/24

V. Motor Exam	Dominant Hand	%ile	Nondom. Hand	%ile
Finger Tapping:	44.8	21	48	57
Grooved Pegbd.:	104"	<1	94"	3
Grip Strength:	35.7	10	35.3	15

VI. Achievement		Grade Equiv.	Percentile Rank
WRAT:	Reading	3.7	.9
	Spelling	3.3	3
	Arithmetic	3.3	9

Case 3: Seizure Disorder Associated with Psychosis

Reason for Referral

Ms. F.C. was referred for neuropsychological testing for evaluation of possible deficits in memory and cognition associated with the patient's seizure disorder.

Presenting Situation and Background Information

This 19-year-old, left-handed, college freshman began experiencing grand mal seizures one-and-one-half years ago that were associated with left-sided paralysis. The generalized seizures have been controlled with medication, but she has subsequently developed partial complex seizures. Despite increased doses of phenobarbital and phenytoin, she continues to have complex partial seizures one to two times per month and an occasional secondarily generalized seizure. She has also experienced two episodes of status epilepticus, most recently three weeks ago. The patient's complex partial seizures are characterized by autonomic, visceral, and vertiginous symptoms followed by staring spells and jaw movements. Absence, déja vu, jamais vu, the sensation of a "presence," and wandering episodes have also been reported by the patient. The patient indicates that she experiences "strange feelings" approximately 15 to 20 times per day.

Pre-ictally Ms. C. is described as angry and hostile and reportedly experiences Capgras-type delusions in which she believes that family members are imposters. During these episodes, the patient has sometimes struck her mother, denied her mother's identity, called her mother by another name, and insisted that she is not her mother's biological daughter. She also has denied the identity and relationship of her twin brother and her father. When in this state the patient has claimed that she is being detained in the house against her will and must be allowed to leave. The personality alteration often lasts for a few hours but can continue for several days. It is always followed by a seizure with subsequent recovery of personality functioning. The patient is amnesic for these episodes and denies formal hallucinations, paranoia, or other types of delusions. She has experienced the development of significant depression since the onset of her seizures and reportedly has made two suicide attempts, each just prior to a seizure and the most recent two months ago when she attempted to cut her wrists.

A recent neurological exam was normal except for mild bilateral dystonic posturing when asked to walk on the sides of her feet and an equivocal right plantar reflex. A CT scan showed a cavum septum pellucidum but was otherwise considered normal. An initial EEG showed nonfocal spike activity with bursts of high-voltage slow waves and bilateral central phase-reversing spike and sharp waves. A more recent EEG demonstrated a clear left anterior temporal spike focus.

Ms. C. was one of twins delivered by breech birth. The obstetrician apparently was not aware it was a twin birth, and the patient was discovered with the nuchal cord when the placenta was being delivered and may have suffered anoxia. The patient is left handed, and her twin brother is right handed, although the patient reports that he was originally left handed and was "trained" to be right handed. There is no other history of familial sinistrality. The patient's developmental history is unremarkable. Medical history is noteworthy for a closed head trauma with possible loss of consciousness and several minutes of post traumatic amnesia at age 14. The patient and her family deny any history of alcohol or drug abuse, psychiatric history prior to seizure onset one-and-one-half years ago, surgeries, or chronic or serious illnesses.

Prior to the onset of her seizures, the patient was an honor roll student involved in extracurricular activities such as cheerleading, singing, and sports, and was elected prom queen. Her grades after the seizure onset have been in the B, C, and D ranges. She reports that currently she is spending her time working crossword puzzles, reading, cleaning the house, and skating. She stated that friends call her on the phone and visit occasionally; she implied that it is her friends and not herself who initiate the social contact.

Behavioral Observations

The patient is a black, left-handed, 19-year-old female of medium height and weight. Ms. C.'s testing appointment had to be rescheduled twice, the first time because the patient's mother forgot to bring her to the appointment, and the second time because the patient was unable to locate the testing lab and spent three hours wandering around the hospital grounds.

On arrival to the third testing appointment, the patient was observed to be attractively attired and well groomed. She was soft-spoken, tended to mumble, and appeared socially ill at ease and awkward. She spontaneously offered help to the examiner in handling test materials and appeared to be exerting her best effort on the tasks during the extended five-hour testing session. She was observed to be frustrated and surprised by her relatively poor confrontational naming performance and spontaneously commented, "I don't understand why I can't do this!" Her solving of tasks was noted to be much more rapid on nonverbal as opposed to verbal tasks. No overt evidence of delusions or other gross psychiatric disturbance was observed.

Tests Administered

See data summary sheet.

Test Results

Intellectual Scores

Ms. C. is currently functioning within the average range of general intellectual ability (Full Scale IQ = 103, 58th percentile). A slight and nonsignificant discrepancy was observed between overall Verbal and Performance IQs, with the Verbal IQ falling eight points below the Performance IQ (VIQ = 99; PIQ = 107).

Moderate scatter was noted across individual Verbal subtest scores (25th-91st percentiles); average scores were obtained on subtests tapping fund of general information, vocabulary range, select verbal abstract reasoning ability, and calculation ability, whereas a score within the average range was noted on a subtest involving digit span. It should be noted that considerable intrasubtest scatter was observed within the Information and Vocabulary subtests, and some word-finding difficulties and perseverations were noted in the patient's responses. In addition, although the patient's basic computational abilities appeared to be intact, she exhibited concreteness in her reasoning. For example, the fourth item on the Arithmetic subtest reads: "If a man buys six cents' worth of stamps and he gives the clerk ten cents, how much change should he get back?" The patient asked that the question be repeated three times and commented, "I don't understand. . .stamps cost 20 cents." After 40 seconds the patient finally provided the correct answer. The patient spontaneously reported, "I'm trying to get the words out of the way. The words get in the way."

Mild scatter was noted across individual Performance subtest scores with all scores within the average to high average ranges (37th-84th percentiles). The individual Performance subtest scores will be discussed in further detail in the section on perceptual organization skills.

Attention and Concentration Processes

The patient's brief passive attention skills and brief concentration for rote material were within the high average to superior range for her age. Specifically, the patient scored at the 91st percentile on the Digit Span subtest of the WAIS (F = 7; B = 7), and was able to rapidly and accurately count backwards from 20, recite the letters of the alphabet, and count by 3s to 40 (6, 4, and 22 seconds, respectively). Auditory rhythm discrimination skills were within the high average range as measured by the Seashore Rhythm Test (28/30). However, possible attentional difficulties (as well as possible comprehension and/or reasoning difficulties) were noted when the patient was required to mentally solve mathematical word problems (Arithmetic subtest of the WAIS = 25th percentile). Ms. C. frequently requested that the test questions be repeated, and her responses were provided tentatively.

Language Functioning

The patient's spontaneous speech was noteworthy for the previously mentioned soft-spokenness and mumbling, and occasional word-finding difficulties when attempting to provide names of well-known individuals ("I can see him in my mind. I can't think of his name.").

The patient's word generation skills were within the superior range for her age (56 words beginning with "f," "a," and "s" within three minutes); however, she demonstrated mild to moderate impairment on a formal confrontational naming test (Boston Naming Test). Specifically, she was only able to label 39 of 60 stimulus pictures; phonemic cues were useful in eliciting the correct name approximately 40% of the time.

Ms. C.'s ability to discriminate individual speech sounds was well within the average range for her age as measured by the Speech Sounds Perception Test (27/30). Receptive vocabulary level was within the low average range for her age (PPVT-R = 18th percentile), and consistent with her performance on a task involving definition of vocabulary items (Vocabulary subtest = 25th percentile). Language comprehension skills generally appeared to be intact, although the patient's performance on some tasks suggested the presence of selective difficulties in attending to and processing verbal material. Specifically, she repeatedly requested repetition of oral word problems on the Arithmetic subtest of the WAIS, and her immediate recall of paragraph details demonstrated some distortion of details.

Spelling and reading recognition skills are well within the average to superior range (WRAT Spelling = 66th percentile; Reading = 91st percentile).

Sensory Perceptual/Motor Exam

Ms. C. described herself as left-hand dominant. She denied any history of significant injury to her hands, arms, or shoulders. A finger agnosia exam was negative. On a task of finger tapping speed, the patient surprisingly scored substantially better with her nondominant hand (L = 40; R = 47.4); performance of the left hand was within the low average range, and performance of her right hand was within the high average range. In addition, on the placing of pegs in a pegboard, the patient performed more rapidly with her nondominant hand (L = 61 seconds; R = 55 seconds), although performance of both hands was well within the normal range.

Perceptual Organizational Skills

The patient's scores on perceptual organization tasks were variable. Scores well within the average range were obtained on visual perceptual tasks; she scored at the 63rd percentile on the Picture Completion subtest of the WAIS, and scored within the normal range on a task involving identification of obscured objects (Street Test = 9.5). In addition, scores on constructional tasks were well within the average to high average ranges; Ms. C. scored at the 75th and 84th percentiles respectively on the Block Design and Object Assembly subtests of the WAIS, and scored in the average range in the pencil and paper copying of a complex two-dimensional design (Rey-Osterrieth Complex Figure = 60th percentile, see Figure 4.2).

Some variability in performance on visual tracking and visual sequencing tasks was noted. The patient made two errors on the Rey Tangled Lines Test, and was observed to have some difficulty in finding specific numbers on Trails A, which lowered her score to the impaired range (40 seconds). She scored within the average range on Trails B (50 seconds). Her two lowest Performance subtest scores on the WAIS, although still well within the normal range, occurred

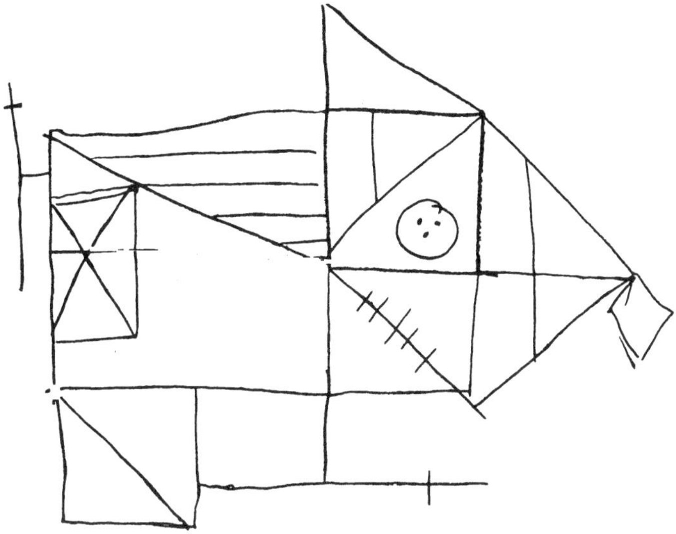

FIGURE 4.2. Case F.C. Rey-Osterrieth Complex Figure: copy. Reduced by 40%.

on the Picture Arrangement and Digit Symbol subtests (37th and 50th percentiles, respectively).

Verbal (Auditory) and Nonverbal (Visual) Learning and Memory

The patient's memory skills generally appear to be intact for both verbal and nonverbal material, although some difficulties in the initial learning/processing of verbal material and delayed recall of nonverbal information were suggested.

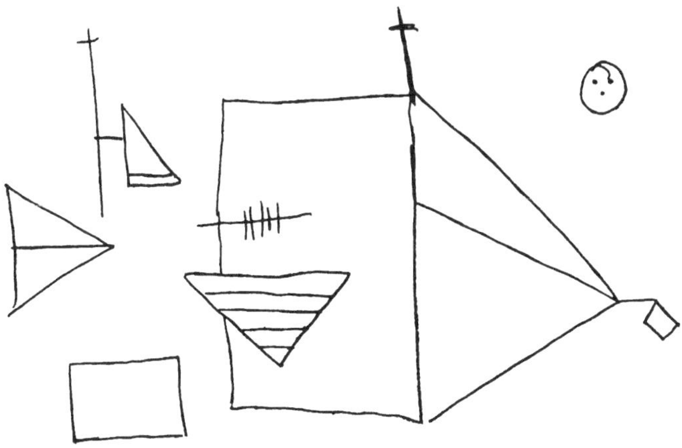

FIGURE 4.3. Case F.C. Rey-Osterrieth Complex Figure: delayed recall. Reduced by 40%.

The patient's overall ability to learn relatively easy as well as more difficult word pairs was in the average range for her age (WMS-AL = 68th percentile), however, on the initial learning trial the patient was unable to recall any of the four difficult word pairs. On the two subsequent trials the patient accurately recalled all four of the more difficult pairs as well as all of the six easier pairs. Following a 45-minute delay, the patient was able to recall 100% of the information originally learned. The patient's learning of a 15-item list of words (AVLT) was complete after five trials and well within the normal range (7-13-14-13-15). Following an interference task, only minimal information was lost (13/15), and following a 30-minute delay, the patient was able to recall all 15 of the words. The patient's immediate recall of paragraph details was within the high average range in terms of overall volume of recall (WMS-LM = 88th percentile); however, some mild confabulation/distortion of details was observed as well as occasional incorrect juxtaposition of information. Following a 45-minute delay, the patient was able to recall 80% of the information originally learned, a retention rate well within the normal range.

The patient's immediate recall reproduction of relatively simple geometric figures was within the average range for her age (WMS-VR = 64th percentile), and following a 45-minute delay, the patient was able to recall 100% of the information originally learned. Conversely, the patient's three-minute delayed recall of a complex two-dimensional figure showed good recall of specific details, but she was completely unable to recall the overall structural framework (Rey-Osterrieth = <10th percentile; Figure 4.3). This performance appeared to be related to a rather poor organizational strategy used in the original copying of the figure.

Conceptual Shifting and Response Inhibition

The patient completed all six categories on the Wisconsin Card Sorting Test but exhibited significantly more perseverative responses and errors than expected for her age and education (perseverative responses = 24; perseverative errors = 21); she showed some initial confusion after the first strategy shift but readily improved her performance on subsequent strategy shifts. The patient performed well within the average range on the Stroop Test, a task involving the screening out of distracting stimuli (A = 37 seconds; B = 54 seconds; C = 87 seconds).

Achievement Scores

<u>WRAT</u>
Reading: 91st percentile; 11.1 grade equivalent
Spelling: 66th percentile; 9.5 grade equivalent
Arithmetic: 25th percentile; 6.6 grade equivalent

Formal achievement testing suggested that the patient's sight reading skills are generally within expectation for her educational level, although spelling and mathematical skills are relatively depressed.

Personality Functioning

Personality assessment with the Rorschach Inkblot Test was suggestive of the presence of considerable stress and distress that appear to be in reaction to situational and environmental factors. Specifically, the patient appears to feel helpless, powerless, and at the mercy of forces outside her control. Her responses suggest that she is experiencing more stress than she has resources with which to cope, and as a result she has developed significant depressive affect, lapses in judgment, and some deterioration of thought processes. In addition, she appears to be withdrawing from others and becoming introversive, and may be having difficulty accurately interpreting the actions of others. Test responses also suggest that the patient may be underachieving at the present time and is experiencing feelings of low self-esteem and inadequacy. The presence of several special scores (INCOM = 3; DR = 1) suggest the possibility of psychotic thought processes.

Summary and Impressions

Neuropsychological findings point to the presence of selective deficits in a relatively well-functioning individual. We were particularly heartened by the presence of relatively intact cognitive skills given that the patient had experienced an episode of status epilepticus just a few weeks prior to the testing.

Intellectual scores indicate that the patient is functioning within the average range of general intellectual ability (Full Scale IQ = 103). Neuropsychological test scores document the presence of mild to moderate impairment in some language skills, with general sparing of perceptual organization skills; this pattern of scores would implicate dysfunction of the dominant hemisphere. Specifically, mild to moderate impairment was noted on a confrontational naming task, receptive vocabulary range was attenuated, spelling and mathematical ability were depressed, and some distortion was noted in the initial processing of verbal information on learning and computation tasks.

In addition to the selective language deficits, the patient demonstrated perseverative behavior on a categorization task, appeared to have some difficulty in visual scanning and tracking, and was unable to reproduce the overall gestalt of a line drawing on delayed recall.

Also of note, results of motor testing surprisingly revealed better performance with the nondominant hand as compared to the dominant hand. These motor findings, in the absence of peripheral nervous system explanations for the decreased performance of the left hand, would be suggestive of anterior right hemisphere dysfunction in addition to the documented left anterior temporal lobe EEG disturbance. The motor findings are consistent with the reported transient left-sided paralysis that accompanied the original seizure onset. Given that the patient is left-hand dominant, the possibility arises that she is right hemisphere dominant for language, or that she possesses bilateral language representation.

Personality testing revealed significant depression and suggested that the patient is experiencing considerable stress related to situational factors that is exceeding her coping resources. Also of note, tendencies toward disordered and idiosyncratic thought processes were noted, which indicate that the patient is experiencing some compromise in rational thinking interictally as well as during the observed episodes of frank delusions. The patient should be evaluated by a psychiatrist as to the appropriateness of antipsychotic medication. In addition, her suicidal tendencies should be carefully monitored. Supportive psychotherapeutic treatment, possibly including membership in an epilepsy support group, may be very beneficial to the patient.

We are somewhat puzzled by the patient's apparent disorientation and poor problem-solving skills on the date of her second missed testing appointment when she spent several hours wandering the hospital grounds. This behavior is in contrast to the relatively intact functioning noted one week later when the present test scores were obtained. Apparently the patient either experiences wide fluctuations in cognitive integrity, was still experiencing effects from her status episode at the time of the failed appointment, or suffered a seizure associated with amnestic "wandering."

NEUROPSYCHOLOGY TEST SCORE SUMMARY SHEET

Patient: F.C. Age: 19 Sex: F Handedness: L

I. Intelligence WAIS Age-Corrected Scores

VERBAL			PERFORMANCE		
Information	8	(25 %ile)	Picture Completion	11	(63 %ile)
Digit Span	14	(91 %ile)	Picture Arrangement	9	(37 %ile)
Vocabulary	8	(25 %ile)	Block Design	12	(75 %ile)
Arithmetic	8	(25 %ile)	Object Assembly	13	(84 %ile)
Comprehension	9	(37 %ile)	Digit Symbol	10	(50 %ile)
Similarities	11	(63 %ile)			
VERBAL IQ =	99	(47 %ile)	PERFORMANCE IQ =	107	(68 %ile)

FULL SCALE IQ = 103 (58 %ile)

II. Attention/Concentration
Digit Span: 7 forward + 7 backwards = 14 Total (91 %ile)
Mental Control, WMS: 9 (78 %ile)
Trails A: 40" (<1 %ile), Trails B: 50" (57 %ile)
Seashore Rhythm Test: 28/30

III. Language
Boston Naming Test: 39 /60
Controlled Word Association: F (21) + A (15) + S (20) + Age Corr.= 56 (>95 %ile)
PPVT-R: Standard Score = 139, 18 %ile
Speech Sounds Perception: 27/30

IV. Perceptual/Organizational
Rey-Osterrieth Complex Figure Copy: 33 /36 (60 %ile)
Street Test: 9.5/13
Rey Tangled Lines: 2 errors

V. Memory

VERBAL		NONVERBAL	
WMS Logical Memory	13 (88%ile)	WMS Visual Repro.:	12 (64%ile)
45 min. delay:	10.5	45 min. delay:	12
Percent retention:	80	Percent retention:	100

WMS Associate Learning
I Easy 6, 6, 6
I Hard 0, 4, 4
I Score: 17 (68%ile)
45 min. delay: 6 easy, 4 hard 100% retention

Rey-Osterrieth Fig: 33 (60 %ile)
3 min. delay: 10 (<10 %ile)

Rey Auditory Verbal Learning Test (15 items):
T1: 7 T2: 13 T3: 14 T4: 13 T5: 15 Recall after Interference: 13
30-min. Delayed Recall: 15

VI. Motor Exam	Dominant Hand	%ile	Nondom. Hand	%ile
Finger Tapping:	40	23	47.4	89
Grooved Pegbd.:	61"	34	55"	73

VII. Sensory
Finger Gnosis: intact

VIII. Frontal Systems
Stroop A: 37", Stroop B: 54", Stroop C: 87"
Wisconsin Card Sort: Categories: 6, Perseverative Responses: 24, Perseverative Errors: 21
Rey Tangled Lines: 2 errors

IX. Achievement		Grade Equivalent	Percentile Rank
WRAT:	Reading	11.1	91
	Spelling	9.5	66
	Arithmetic	6.6	25

X. Personality
Rorschach Inkblot Test

Commentary on Epilepsy Cases

When assessing the seizure patient, the clinician must gather specific information regarding seizure characteristics, in addition to querying basic information regarding medical, psychiatric, educational, and occupational history as was detailed in the introduction to this book. Data need to be obtained regarding seizure type(s), frequency, length of seizure disorder, familial history of seizures, and date of most recent seizure. As described in the introduction to this chapter, neuropsychological performance varies depending on seizure characteristics, and interpretation of neuropsychological scores needs to be conducted within the context of thorough knowledge of the patient's seizure history. Knowledge regarding the most recent ictal event is important because transient lowering of cognitive functioning can occur immediately following a seizure, particularly with generalized major motor seizures. If testing is conducted during this post-ictal period, test scores will be spuriously lowered.

Cases 1 and 3 illustrate the type of cognitive difficulties seen in patients with left temporal lobe seizures, namely verbal learning and recall deficits, lowered Verbal IQ, and subtle language impairments including declines in word finding, word generation, vocabulary range, and verbal comprehension/processing. As a general rule, the cognitive deficits in right temporal lobe seizure patients tend to be elusive and less obvious than those observed in left temporal seizure patients, but frequently a lowering of Performance IQ and decreased visual perceptual organization and nonverbal learning and recall abilities is observed.

Case 2 reveals the cognitive devastation that can occur with a long-standing severe seizure disorder. The reader will notice that the neuropsychological battery administered to the patient was abbreviated. Patients with IQs within the borderline to retarded range typically perform very poorly on neuropsychological tests, and thus it is usually not very productive to administer lengthy batteries. Neuropsychological tests were typically developed and standardized on patients with average premorbid IQs, and the tests generally do not discriminate well at low intellectual levels.

Psychiatric symptoms are a common finding in the epileptic population. Case 3 highlights the development of cognitive and psychotic symptoms in a left-handed female patient with left temporal lobe seizure onset. Female sinistrals with left temporal lobe seizure foci appear to be the most predisposed to exhibit psychosis. Case 1 provides an example of the type of episodic dyscontrol found in some seizure patients. Some authors suspect that these rage reactions may represent subclinical seizure activity in limbic areas (Rickler, 1982).

5
Brain Tumors, Cysts, and Abscesses

Space-occupying lesions in the central nervous system include tumors, cysts, and abscesses. The term "brain tumor" refers to a new growth (neoplasm) of cells in the brain that resembles other cell masses in the body but is arranged atypically and has no physiological usefulness. A brain cyst refers to a walled sack or pouch that contains fluid, semifluid, or solid material. A brain abscess is a collection of pus caused by disintegration of brain tissue that develops secondary to infections elsewhere in the head or body. Bacteria multiplies within the cerebral white matter, producing ischemia and thrombosis, which cause necrosis of brain tissue.

Literature on the neuropsychological correlates of brain cysts and abcsesses is sparse. This chapter is therefore devoted to neuropsychological findings in brain tumors. We have, however, presented a case of a brain cyst to provide an example of the type of cognitive profile that may be found in this population.

The following summary of brain tumor types is drawn from Adams and Victor (1985), Lezak (1983), Kolb and Whishaw (1985), and Walsh (1978), and we refer the reader to these sources for more thorough information.

Cerebral tumors develop from the supportive cells of the brain (e.g., glial cells) or from the brain coverings, rather than from the brain neurons themselves. The tumors are classified as malignant or benign based on whether or not they infiltrate the brain itself. Malignant tumors arise from the supportive brain cells, invade the surrounding brain tissues, and can rarely be removed entirely. Benign tumors typically grow from the meninges or coverings of the brain, do not invade actual brain tissue, and usually can be totally excised. Malignancy is classified on a four-point scale (Grades 1, 2, 3, and 4), with the higher grades referring to more highly malignant and fast growing lesions.

Brain tumors, whether benign or malignant, are categorized into three general types according to their site of origin. *Gliomas* develop from the glial cells in the brain and account for approximately 45% of all brain tumors. The three major types of gliomas are astrocytomas, glioblastomas, and medulloblastomas. Astrocytomas are the most commonly occurring gliomas (40%) and are typically found in adults over age 30. They are relatively slow growing and are generally viewed as not highly malignant. Due to the slow growth pattern, prognosis is usually fairly good after treatment, with some reports of 20 years of survival postoperatively. Glioblastomas, in contrast, are considered highly malignant, are fast growing, and account for approximately 30% of all gliomas. They are more prevalent among male adults over age 35. Prognosis is poor, with survival rates averaging about one year post surgery. Medulloblastomas occur in 11% of diagnosed gliomas, and are typically located in the cerebellum of children. These tumors are considered very malignant, and postoperative life expectancy usually ranges from one to two years.

A second major type of cerebral tumor is the *meningioma*, occurring in 12% to 15% of all brain tumors. Meningiomas arise from, and are usually confined to, the meninges of the brain. They are encapsulated and do not invade brain tissue, and they typically are located along the outer surfaces of the cerebral hemispheres. If removed completely, they usually do not reappear.

The third type of brain tumor is the *metastatic*, or secondary, tumor, the second most commonly occurring brain tumor (20–25%). This classification of neoplasm refers to tumor cells that originate at tumor sites located outside of the cranium and are carried to the brain via the bloodstream, where they grow independently. It is not uncommon for multiple brain metastases to occur, thus rendering treatment problematic and prognosis poor.

The general symptoms of cerebral tumor include seizures, mental disturbance, headache, vomiting, and dizziness. In addition, the presence of a growing mass in the brain leads to brain swelling, or edema, and raised pressure within the cranium, resulting in drowsiness, inertia, and diminished mental capacity. Brain function is specifically compromised by tumor through destruction of brain tissue by invasion or replacement, increased intracranial pressure, seizures, and alterations of endocrine functions.

There is no one pattern of neuropsychological findings found in tumor cases because the amount of neuropsychological impairment is determined by location, size, and rate of growth of the tumor, tumor type, and length of time the tumor has been present, as well as the presence of seizures, raised intracranial pressure, edema, and unfortunately, often the effects of treatment. Walsh (1978) concludes:

> While most space occupying lesions will produce a set of general symptoms, each particular case will have specific features which depend on the interruption of connections between different parts of the brain. Thus, a small lesion in a strategic situation may have disastrous early effects because it interferes with vital centres or cuts a large number of interconnections between different areas of the brain, while a large lesion in another area may be almost silent for a relatively long period. (p. 85)

The most recent, large-scale study of the effects of brain tumor on neuropsychological functioning was conducted by Hom and Reitan (1984). They administered the Halstead-Reitan neuropsychological battery and the Wechsler-Bellevue Scale (Form I), to a total of 92 cerebral tumor patients classified as having either rapid or slow growing tumors, and right or left hemisphere tumor location. Patients with the more malignant, rapidly growing tumors (glioblastomas, astrocytomas grade 3–4) consistently showed more intellectual and neuropsychological impairment than the patients with slowly progressive tumors (astrocytomas grade 1–2). However, on purely intellectual measures, the differences were generally slight and failed to reach statistical significance. For example, Full Scale IQ, Verbal IQ, and Performance IQ ranged between 90 and 94 for both groups (average range). Although statistically significant differences were reported between the two groups on the neuropsychological measures, performance of both groups was well within the impaired range when compared with normative data (Reitan, 1985; Bornstein, 1985). Unfortunately, the neuropsychological differences between groups were confounded in that the mean age of the rapidly growing tumor group was 16 years greater than that of the slow growing tumor group (53.40 versus 36.96). Hom and Reitan argue that the age differences are characteristic of the two types of tumors and that it would be misleading to attempt to equate the groups with regard to age. However, it seems fair to postulate that if the effects of age had been partialed out, the group differences may have been significantly reduced, suggesting that the differences are to some large degree due to the effect of superimposing a disease process on an older brain, rather than due to the disease process per se.

Comparison of patients with tumors in the right versus left hemispheres revealed statistically significant differences on mean IQs and selected neuropsychological measures. Normal IQ scores were obtained by patients with right cerebral lesions, although Performance IQs were slightly lower. Conversely, patients with left hemisphere lesions tended to obtain slightly lower scores on Full Scale and Verbal IQ scores (i.e., low average range), with average scores on Performance skills. Among individual subtest scores, Block Design and Object Assembly performances were lower in the right hemisphere-lesioned groups, and Vocabulary, Similarities, Arithmetic, Digit Span, Comprehension, and Information were substantially lower in the left hemisphere-lesioned groups. Both left- and right-lesioned patients demonstrated deficits on all neuropsychological measures, with the right-lesioned patients scoring particularly more poorly on the Tactual Performance Test, Trails A and B, and finger tapping with the left hand. Left hemisphere-lesioned patients scored more poorly on the Category test and on finger tapping with the right hand.

In an earlier study by the same authors (Hom & Reitan, 1982), 50 patients with neoplastic lesions were compared with patients with cerebrovascular lesions (n = 50) and head trauma (n = 50) on sensory perceptual and motor tasks (Tactual Performance Test, Finger Tapping, Grip Strength, Finger Agnosia, Finger Number Writing, Tactile Form Recognition, and Tactile, Auditory and Visual Imperception). Of interest, patients with right hemisphere lesions demonstrated more contralateral impairment than did left hemisphere-damaged patients. In addition, the right hemisphere-damaged patients showed a greater incidence of ipsilateral impairment than their left hemisphere-damaged counterparts. Performance of patients with cerebrovascular lesions was most impaired, and scores of patients with head trauma were least impaired, with tumor patient performance falling in the middle. Again age was a confound, with the head trauma patients averaging 20 years younger than the tumor and CVA groups.

Another investigation addressing the neuropsychological correlates of tumor patients was reported by Hochberg and Slotnick (1980), who examined cognitive performance in 12 adult astrocytoma patients one year post surgery and radiation therapy who had not returned to work or active social functioning. The Halstead-Reitan battery was administered, as well as other measures including the WAIS and WRAT-Arithmetic subtest. Intellectual scores were within the average range, but some signs of diffuse brain dysfunction appeared in all patients. Specifically, depressed performance was observed in all patients on the Category test and the localization section of the TPT, and over half the patients performed poorly on Trails B and the WRAT-Arithmetic subtest. Signs of focal dysfunction were also present on motor and tactile tasks, with all but two patients showing impairment contralateral to the lesion. Two of the patients exhibited marked diffuse intellectual impairment despite the absence of tumor reoccurrence. Hochberg and Slotnick indicate that the cause of the cognitive difficulties in their patients was not obvious, given that the patients did not exhibit hydrocephalus, increased intracranial pressure, or metabolic alterations. They implicate radiation therapy as an etiologic factor in the mental declines observed in their patients.

The Aphasia Screening Test portion of the Halstead-Reitan battery was not administered in the above studies and aside from the Verbal subtests of the Wechsler Scales, no information is available regarding language functioning in these patients. Coughlin and Warrington (1978) studied language functions in a large sample of patients, nearly 90% of whom had intracranial neoplasms. The left hemisphere-lesioned patients (n = 57) performed poorly on tasks measuring complex language comprehension (e.g., modified Token Test), vocabulary definition (Vocabulary subtest), receptive vocabulary (modified Peabody Picture Vocabulary Test), and word retrieval. Patients with temporal lobe lesions showed more severe disturbances of word retrieval and receptive vocabulary than patients with left hemisphere extratemporal tumors. Patients with right hemisphere tumors (n = 43) also scored relatively poorly on the language comprehension and receptive vocabulary tasks. The authors concluded that the deficient performance in the latter patients probably reflected higher level cognitive deficits rather than true linguistic impairment.

Memory abilities were also not addressed in the above neuropsychological studies. The neurological literature suggests that tumors located around the floor and sides of the third ventricle that impinge on the surrounding gray matter structures are frequently accompanied by profound amnesia involving remote and recent memory. For example, Williams and Pennybacker (1954) found evidence of memory impairment on mental status testing in 75% of 32 cases with third ventricle tumors. Older patients were more likely to demonstrate the memory loss than younger patients. For example, in patients aged 20 or younger, half showed a moderate memory loss and half showed no memory compromise. However, in patients aged 41 to 60, three fourths demonstrated a severe memory loss. Lobosky, Vangilder, and Damasio (1984) reported severe memory impairment associated with third ventricle colloid cysts, and they hypothesize the memory loss could be due to dysfunction of the mammillary body-thalamus connections, septum, or medial temporal regions (due to disturbance in the septum or thalamus).

Aside from these studies, little other recent literature addresses the neuropsychological findings characteristic of adult tumor patients. More information is available on the residual intellectual impairment in patients who had successfully treated brain tumors in childhood, although thorough neuropsychological data are lacking. The documented continuing intellectual difficulties may be the result of disruption of brain maturation and development by the tumor, or the effects of the radiologic and/or chemotherapeutic treatment. A consistent finding has been that the earlier the development and diagnosis of the condition (less than 5 years old), the more intellectual impairment is evidenced on formal testing ($\bar{x}$ IQ within the borderline range) (Bamford, 1976; Chin & Maruyama, 1984; Eiser, 1981; Ellenberg, McComb, Siegal, & Stowe, in press; Danoff, Cowchock, Marquette, Mulgrew, & Kramer, 1982). Children with diagnosis and treatment of the condition between the ages of 6 and 10 show minimal intellectual depression ($\bar{x}$ IQ in the low 90s), and treatment and diagnosis after age 10 was less likely to be associated with intellectual decline (Ellenberg et al., in press; Chin & Maruyama, 1984; Eiser, 1981). Some investigators have indicated that extension of the tumor into the hypothalamus and/or thalamus and brainstem is associated with the most intellectual deficit (Danoff et al., 1982); however, other authors report that hemispheric tumors were associated with more cognitive devastation than third and fourth ventricle tumors (Ellenberg et al., in press). No differential effect of tumor type on IQ has been reported (Eiser, 1981). In addition, the presence of mental retardation has not been directly associated with hydrocephalus or with amount of brain irradiated (Danoff et al., 1982).

The effects of the radiation and chemotherapeutic treatment of tumors on cognitive functioning is a growing area of interest. As noted previously, Hochberg and Slotnick (1980) suggest that radiation therapy was probably the major etiologic agent in the continuing cognitive difficulty noted in their adult brain tumor patients. In addition, Martins, Johnston, Henry, Stoffel, and Di Chiro (1977) reported that there is a small risk that standard therapeutic doses of radiation may result in actual necrosis of irradiated brain tissue nine months to two years after treatment, causing cognitive compromise. Diminished intellectual ability has also been a consistent finding in patients who underwent radiation therapy as children (Bamford et al., 1978; Danoff et al., 1982; Duffner, Cohen, & Thomas, 1983), although the exact relationship between the radiation and cognitive difficulties is not clear. Ellenberg and colleagues (in press) indicate that whole brain radiation, especially in young children, is associated with greater disruption of memory, attention, visuo-perceptual speed, and motor speed. Duffner and co-workers (1983) implicate radiation and chemotherapy in combination as adversely affecting intellectual functions, but others contest the role of chemotherapy in cognitive impairment (Ellenberg et al., in press; Hochberg & Slotnick, 1980).

In summary, the neuropsychological literature suggests that brain tumor patients have evidence of subtle diffuse cognitive impairment, particularly in more complex, novel problem-solving tasks, probably due to the effects of increased intracranial pressure, irradiation of the brain, and seizures. Focal signs are also typically present, such as impairment in language, visual perceptual organization skills, memory, and motor dexterity and tactile sensation, which are related to the tumor location. Overall intellectual scores are frequently preserved. The observed cognitive deficits can be expected to be more pronounced for rapidly growing tumors as compared to more slowly growing tumors. Adults with histories of successfully treated brain tumors in childhood will tend to show more marked intellectual impairment the earlier in life they were diagnosed and treated.

References

Adams, R.D., & Victor, M. (1985). *Principles of neurology* (3rd edition). New York: McGraw-Hill.

Bamford, F.N., Morris-Jones, P., Pearson, D., Ribeiro, G.G., Shalet, S.M., & Beardwell, C.G. (1976). Residual disabilities in children treated for intracranial space-occupying lesions. *Cancer, 37,* 1149–1151.

Bornstein, R.A. (1985). Normative data on selected neuropsychologic measures from a nonclinical sample. *Journal of Clinical Psychology, 41,* 651–659.

Chin, H.W., & Maruyama, Y. (1984). Age at treatment and long-term performance results in medulloblastoma. *Cancer, 53,* 1952–1958.

Coughlan, A.K., & Warrington, E.K. (1978). Word-comprehension and word-retrieval in patients with localized cerebral lesions. *Brain, 101,* 163–185.

Danoff, B.F., Cowchock, F.S., Marquette, C., Mulgrew, L., & Kramer, S. (1982). Assessment of the long-term effects of primary radiation therapy for brain tumors in children. *Cancer, 49,* 1580–1586.

Dorland, S. (1974). *Illustrated medical dictionary* (25th ed.). Philadelphia: W.B. Saunders.

Duffner, P.K., Cohen, M.E., & Thomas, P. (1983). Late effects of treatment on the intelligence of children with posterior fossa tumors. *Cancer, 51,* 233–237.

Eiser, C. (1981). Psychological sequelae of brain tumours in childhood: A retrospective study. *British Journal of Clinical Psychology, 20,* 35–38.

Ellenberg, L., McComb, J.G., Siegal, S.E., & Stowe, S. (in press). Factors affecting cognitive outcome in pediatric brain tumor patients. *Pediatrics.*

Hochberg, F.H., & Slotnick, B. Neuropsychologic impairment in astrocytoma survivors. *Neurology, 30,* 172–177.

Hom, J., & Reitan, R.M. (1982). Effect of lateralized cerebral damage upon contralateral and ipsilateral sensorimotor performances. *Journal of Clinical Neuropsychology, 4,* 249–268.

Hom, J., & Reitan, R.M. (1984) Neuropsychological correlates of rapidly versus slowly growing intrinsic cerebral neoplasms. *Journal of Clinical Neuropsychology, 6,* 309–324.

Kolb, B., & Whishaw, J.Q. (1985). *Fundamentals of human neuropsychology* (2nd ed.). New York: W.H. Freeman.

Lezak, M. (1983). *Neuropsychological assessment* (2nd ed.). New York: Oxford University Press.

Lobosky, J.M., Vangilder, J.C., & Damasio, A.R. (1984). Behavioural manifestations of third ventricular colloid cysts. *Journal of Neurology, Neurosurgery, and Psychiatry, 47,* 1075–1080.

Martins, A.N., Johnston, J.S., Henry, J.M., Stoffel, T.J., & Di Chiro, G. (1977). Delayed radiation necrosis of the brain. *Journal of Neurosurgery, 47*, 336–345.

Reitan, R.M., & Wolfson, D. (1985). *The Halstead-Reitan Neuropsychological Test Battery: Theory and clinical interpretation (pp. 97–100)*. Tuscon: Neuropsychology Press.

Walsh, K.W. (1978). *Neuropsychology: A clinical approach*. New York: Churchill Livingstone.

Williams, M., & Pennybacker, J. (1954). Memory disturbances in third ventricle tumor. *Journal of Neurology, Neurosurgery, and Psychiatry, 17*, 115–123.

Case 1: Third Ventricle Tumor

Reason for Referral and Background Information

Ms. W.B. was referred for neuropsychological testing to assess the extent of brain dysfunction following removal of a third ventricle tumor one month ago and subsequent radiation treatment. Specifically, this patient was referred to document current short-term and long-term memory deficits, as well as any other cognitive impairments.

Presenting Situation and Background Information

This 38-year-old, right-handed female was hospitalized two months ago with complaints of disorientation and decreased memory. Four days prior to admission she became disoriented while driving to church. On the day of admission she left work to pick up her children from school and never arrived at the school grounds. One hour later she arrived at her mother's house and was unable to account for her whereabouts during the previous hour. In addition, one-and-one-half weeks before admission the patient had complained of generalized dull aching bifrontal headaches, which occurred primarily in the morning. The headaches were not associated with nausea or vomiting.

A CT scan revealed a large markedly enhancing lesion in the region of the foramen of Monroe. The patient subsequently underwent a right frontoparietal craniotomy for subtotal resection of the third ventricular mass. Analysis of the tumor suggested metastatic breast carcinoma. One-and-one-half weeks after surgery the patient developed a right parietal subdural hydroma and required draining of the collection of cerebral spinal fluid.

During her postoperative hospitalization the patient exhibited poor short-term memory, disorientation, and lack of spontaneity in her speaking. Subsequently the patient and her family have reported short-term and remote memory impairment. The patient also experienced confusion, low energy, and incontinence during the period of the 10 whole brain radiation treatments that ended four days prior to the first testing session. Specific information regarding the radiation treatment was unavailable.

The patient's medical history is remarkable for a mastectomy two-and-one-half years ago for breast carcinoma. She and her family deny any history of alcohol or drug abuse, head injury, birth or developmental abnormalities, seizure disorder, chronic illnesses, surgeries or hospitalizations aside from the mastectomy, or psychiatric symptoms or treatment. Currently the patient is prescribed tamoxifen.

The patient is a high school graduate with two years of junior college business and secretarial training. She has no history of learning disabilities. She has been employed as a secretary for the past 10 years.

Behavioral Observations

Ms. B. presented as a pleasant, friendly, 38-year-old, black woman who was generally cooperative throughout the evaluation. The patient was tested in three sessions over a three-week period. She reported at the third session that some remote memories were returning to her, but when asked to recall specific events during each decade of her life (e.g., where she attended school and lived as a child), she was rather vague. Her recall of more remote memories appeared to be better preserved than memories from the most recent decade. Specifically, she was often confused regarding events of the past five years and frequently confabulated information. Particularly notable was her lack of recall for significant negative incidents such as her parents' divorce, her husband's extramarital affair during her second pregnancy, and the fact that she had been divorced from her husband prior to her mastectomy three years ago. Ms. B. insisted in the first interview that she had been separated from her husband just a few weeks before, although in fact she had been divorced for nearly four years.

The patient appeared to become fatigued with the testing, particularly during the more extended sessions. Frequently she would laugh inappropriately when she was unable to recall information from her past. For example, when corrected by her mother regarding the time of her divorce from her husband, she merely laughed and appeared unconcerned. She also demonstrated lack of insight into the extent of her current disability; she requires close supervision by her mother yet indicated that she planned to assume care for her two daughters, aged 10 and 12, and that she wanted to return to work full-time as a secretary in a law office.

Tests Administered

See data summary sheet.

Test Results

Intellectual Scores

Ms. B. is functioning within the low average range of general intellectual ability (Full Scale IQ = 83, 13th percentile). A slight but nonsignificant discrepancy was observed between Verbal and Performance IQs, with the Performance IQ falling seven points below the Verbal IQ (VIQ = 87; PIQ = 80).

In relation to Verbal subtests, Ms. B.'s performance varied from high average (Vocabulary = 75th percentile) to borderline (Similarities = 5th percentile). Most difficulty was noted on a task of abstract reasoning ability (Similarities). The patient's score on the Vocabulary subtest is probably indicative of high average premorbid verbal ability. Less intersubtest scatter was evident among the Performance subtest scores, which varied from the borderline range (Object Assembly = 5th percentile) to the average/low average range (Picture Completion and Picture Arrangement = 25th percentile). Fatigue appeared to be a factor in the performance of several subtests, particularly the Object Assembly task.

Attention and Concentration Processes

Ms. B. demonstrated somewhat variable performance across attention and concentration tasks. Although her score on the Digit Span subtest of the WAIS-R was within the average range (25th percentile), distractibility was observed during her performance of the Arithmetic subtest of the WAIS-R (9th percentile). The patient frequently failed to recall stimulus questions even after they were repeated. She indicated that prior to the development of the tumor she had been proficient at math-related tasks. Also, impaired performance was found on a timed task of attention and visual tracking ability (Trail Making = <1st percentile).

Language Functioning

Ms. B.'s basic language skills appear to be intact. She made no language errors on the Aphasia Screening Test, and scored within the normal range on a formal confrontational naming test (Boston Naming Test = 51/60) and on a verbal fluency test (FAS = 25th-29th percentile). Vocabulary range was at the high average level (WAIS-R Vocabulary = 75th percentile).

Motor Exam

The patient describes herself as right-handed. She stated that there are no left-handed individuals in her family. Scores on a finger tapping task were well within the normal range for both hands (R = 49.8; L = 49), although the expected dominant-hand advantage was not observed. The patient and her family denied any history of injuries to the patient's hands, arms, or shoulders.

Perceptual Organizational Skills

Performance was variable on perceptual organization tasks. Scores within the average to low average range were obtained on visual perceptual tasks (Picture Completion = 25th percentile; Hooper Visual Organization Test = 22.5/30; Line Orientation = 22nd percentile). On visual sequencing and tracking tasks, the patient's performance varied from average to impaired. The patient scored within the average/low average range on the Picture Arrangement subtest (25th

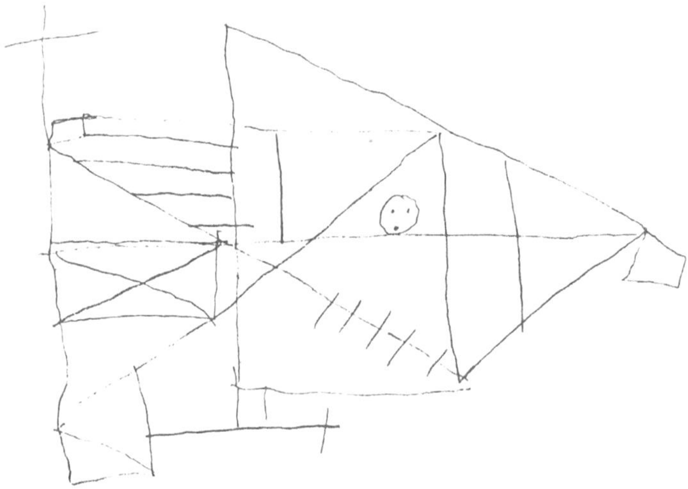

FIGURE 5.1. Case W.B. Rey-Osterrieth Complex Figure: copy. Reduced by 55%.

percentile), within the low average range on the Digit Symbol subtest (16th percentile), and within the impaired range on Trails A and B (57 and 167 seconds, respectively).

Performance across constructional tasks revealed some disturbance; the patient scored below the 10th percentile in her pencil and paper copy of a complex two-dimensional line drawing (Rey-Osterrieth, see Figure 5.1) and at the fifth and ninth percentiles respectively on the Object Assembly and Block Design subtests of the WAIS-R. Of note, Ms. B.'s pencil and paper copying revealed disturbance primarily on the left side of the figure. On the puzzle-solving task (Object Assembly), the patient was unable to deduce the identity of the second and fourth puzzles (human profile and elephant) or to correctly assemble any of the pieces of these test items.

Verbal (Auditory) and Nonverbal (Visual) Learning and Memory

Significant impairment of the patient's verbal learning and recall was evident throughout the testing. Her immediate recall of paragraph details was at the first percentile (WMS-Logical Memory). She was only able to repeat one-and-one-half details from the first story and no information from the second story, even though it was read twice. Following a 30-minute delay she did not recall having been read the stories. In addition, she failed to learn any of the easy or more difficult rote word pairs on the WMS-Associate Learning task (< 1st percentile). On the Rey Auditory Verbal Learning Test, she scored well below the norm, learning a maximum of six out of 15 words, recalling one word after an interference task and zero words after a five-minute delay. She was only able to recognize six of the items when presented in paragraph format, and committed nine false-positive errors. The patient performed at the first percentile on a "divided" attention task involving retaining consonant trigrams over a distraction (Consonant Trigrams).

Ms. B.'s immediate recall reproduction of relatively simple geometric figures was within the impaired range (WMS-VR-2nd percentile). When she was required to reproduce the Rey-Osterrieth Complex Figure and WMS-Visual Reproduction designs on three-minute and 30-minute delays respectively, she could not recall any of the information. Even when the framework of the Rey-Osterrieth figure was provided as a cue, she could not recall any details. Interpretation of the nonverbal visual memory performance was somewhat problematic due to the patient's poor constructional ability.

Performance on the Information subtest of the WAIS-R provided data regarding the patient's remote memory functioning. She was unable to name four men who have been president of the Untied States since 1950; she was only able to cite the current president. She was able to adequately describe who Martin Luther King, Jr., was.

Abstraction, Conceptual Tracking, and Response Inhibition

Ms. B. was able to complete only two of the six categories on the Wisconsin Card Sorting Test, a task involving conceptual tracking and categorization skills. This performance falls within the impaired range (< 1st percentile). The patient was noted to make several perseverative and "other" responses (i.e., no obvious strategies employed to sort the cards). At the conclusion of the testing, the patient indicated that she used sorting strategies involving color and symbols but was unable to deduce the strategy of sorting by number.

The patient required considerably more time than the average for her age to complete the color interference section of the Stroop Test (C = 260 seconds), a task involving the maintaining of a course of action in the face of distracting stimuli. Speed of word reading and color naming was intact (A = 42 seconds; B = 75 seconds).

Verbal abstraction skills were also depressed. The patient obtained a borderline score on the Similarities subtest of the WAIS-R (5th percentile), and could not successfully define proverbs (WAIS-R Comprehension).

Summary and Impressions

Results of intellectual testing indicate that the patient is currently functioning within the low average range of general intellectual ability (Full Scale IQ = 83).

The neuropsychological test findings reveal the presence of a severe impairment in the ability to learn and retain new verbal and nonverbal material. The patient also displayed difficulties in attention, and some of her problems in new learning could be explained by this. However, her intact digit span performance coupled with other characteristics of her memory failure provide support for a distinct memory disorder. For example, questioning of the patient regarding personal historical information revealed a significant remote memory deficit, particularly for the most recent years. In addition to the presence of a temporal gradient characterizing a retrograde amnesia, her profile was marked by frequent confabulations. The patient's amnestic disorder is similar to the diencephalic amnesia observed in Korsakoff's patients who have sustained damage to the mammillary bodies and other memory structures adjacent to the third ventricle. The patient's tumor, surgery, and/or radiation treatment appear to have compromised these same structures. The limited neuropsychological literature on third ventricle tumors documents a very high frequency of severe memory impairment in these patients.

Test results also provide evidence of "frontal systems" dysfunction characterized by deficient categorization and abstraction, and poor performance on alternation tasks and tasks involving mental flexibility and response inhibition. The patient's inappropriate laughter and apparent unconcern during the interview further suggest the possibility of disruption of frontal systems. Due to the connections between the frontal lobe and structures adjacent to the third ventricle, it is not surprising that impairment in frontal system skills was suggested. In addition, direct damage to the right frontal area was sustained during the tumor resection.

Additionally, performance on constructional tasks was significantly depressed. The patient's paper and pencil constructional skills reveal left-sided distortion. The disturbance in constructional skills and mild left-sided neglect is probably associated with the surgical resection approach (right frontoparietal) and/or damage due to the postsurgical right parietal subdural hydroma. The patient's basic language skills, motor functioning, and visual perceptual skills appeared to be intact.

The observed cognitive deficits are consistent with the documented structural lesions, but it is also possible that the radiation treatment has been etiologic in the neuropsychological impairments.

Retesting in six months to one year would be useful in documenting any changes in cognitive functioning. The patient is likely to experience a longstanding memory disorder that will require her to receive ongoing financial assistance as well as support in organizing and implementing daily tasks. Also of concern is the fact that the patient is a single parent with custody of two adolescent daughters. Provisions will need to be made to insure adequate supervision and care of the daughters given that the patient's insight and judgment are currently compromised.

NEUROPSYCHOLOGY TEST SCORE SUMMARY SHEET

Patient: W.B. Age: 38 Sex: F Handedness: R

I. Intelligence WAIS-R Age-Corrected Scores

VERBAL			PERFORMANCE		
Information	7	(16 %ile)	Picture Completion	8	(25 %ile)
Digit Span	8	(25 %ile)	Picture Arrangement	8	(25 %ile)
Vocabulary	12	(75 %ile)	Block Design	6	(9 %ile)
Arithmetic	6	(9 %ile)	Object Assembly	5	(5 %ile)
Comprehension	9	(37 %ile)	Digit Symbol	7	(16 %ile)
Similarities	5	(5 %ile)			

VERBAL IQ = 87 (19 %ile) PERFORMANCE IQ = 80 (9 %ile)
FULL SCALE IQ = 83 (13 %ile)

II. Attention/Concentration
Digit Span: 6 forward + 4 backwards = 10 Total (25 %ile)
Trails A: 57 sec. (<1 %ile), Trails B: 167 sec. (<1 %ile)

III. Language
Boston Naming Test: 51/60
Controlled Word Association: F (10) + A (6) + S (8) + Age Corr.= 30 (25-29 %ile)
Aphasia Screening Exam: intact

IV. Perceptual/Organizational
Rey-Osterrieth Complex Figure Copy: 26 /36 (<10 %ile)
Hooper Visual Organization Test: 22.5 /30
Judgement of Line Orientation: 20/30 (22 %ile)

V. Memory

VERBAL		NONVERBAL	
WMS Logical Memory	.75 (1 %ile)	WMS Visual Repro.:	5.5 (2 %ile)
30 min. delay:	0	30 min. delay:	0
Percent retention:	0	Percent retention:	0

WMS Associate Learning	Easy 0 , 0 , 0	Rey-Osterrieth Fig:	26 (<10 %ile)
	Hard 0 , 0 , 0	3 min. delay:	0
	Score: 0 (<1 %ile)		

Rey Auditory Verbal Learning Test (15 items):
T1: 4 T2: 6 T3: 4 T4: 5 T5: 5 Recall after Interference: 1
5-min. Delayed Recall: 0
Recognition: 6 Hits, 9 False Identifications

VI. Motor Exam

	Dominant Hand	%ile	Nondom. Hand	%ile
Finger Tapping:	49.8	83	49	93

VII. Frontal Systems
Stroop A: 42", Stroop B: 75", Stroop C: 260"
Wisconsin Card Sort: Categories: 2
Auditory Consonant Trigrams: 35/60

Case W.B.

WMS- Logical Memory:

Immediate recall:

Story A: "It (story) went in and out...Annette Thompson, a scrub woman from the city...nothing else."

Story B: "It went in and out."
Second presentation: "It (story) left."

WAIS-R Comprehension Proverbs:

Strike while the iron is hot: "For shaping or molding something, hit it while it's hot."

Shallow brooks are noisy: "Because of the shallowness, it's noisy, hitting the rocks and what have you."

One swallow doesn't make a summer: "If you see one swallow (laughs), I don't know."

WAIS-R Similarities:

Coat-suit: "One complements the other; coat goes with a suit."

Boat-automobile: "Both operated by motors."

Button-zipper: "Both on some garment."

North-west: "They're alike in no way that I know of."

Egg-seed: "An egg is like a seed in a sense."

Table-chair: "You need a chair to go with a table."

Case 2: Right Parietal Osteoma[1]

Reason for Referral

Ms. H.D. was referred for comprehensive neuropsychological testing to evaluate her current level of cognitive functioning following two surgeries for osteoma with subsequent seizure disorder. Assessment of personality functioning was also requested.

Presenting Situation and Background Information

Ms. H.D. is a 49-year-old, right-handed female who underwent surgery for two benign right cerebral osteomas 22 and 18 years ago. The first growth was found in the right parietal area and the second in the right temporal area. She experienced paralysis of the left side after the first surgery, which was nearly resolved within one-and-one-half years. Eight years ago the patient experienced onset of seizures; she suffered three generalized major motor seizures that were followed by left-sided weakness. She subsequently developed an intractable partial complex seizure disorder. EEGs obtained eight years ago were judged to be within normal limits and a CT scan revealed no recurrence of the tumors. Dilantin was prescribed but multiple side effects were noted. Currently the patient is prescribed Mysoline 250 mg. tid, Cimetidine 300 mg. tid, and Ativan 2 mg. bid.

The patient reports experiencing seizures approximately three to four times per month, although EEGs have consistently been judged to be normal. Her seizures are initiated by an aura of confusion that may last up to 20 minutes. During these episodes the patient does not recognize the voices of her husband or children, and her speech becomes slurred. She then becomes unresponsive and stares, and may continue to engage in activities. She is usually tired the day before a seizure and sleeps for four to five hours after a seizure. She generally experiences some residual confusion upon awakening. Approximately two to three years ago, the patient began experiencing episodes involving several minutes of "confusion" that occur once every two to three days. Occasionally she will experience a full day of confusion during which she forgets family members' names and does not recognize their faces, and gets lost driving to familiar places.

The patient indicated that her concentration abilities have declined since the onset of her seizure disorder. In addition, her calculation abilities have deteriorated and she reports difficulty in determining where numbers should be entered on accounting sheets. She notes that she now has difficulty correctly reversing crochet patterns when executing crochet projects. In writing letters for her hobby of geneologic research, she discovered that she was writing street numbers backward. She denied the presence of depression but admitted to guilt, in terms of "what did I do to deserve" the illnesses, and concern about the financial

[1]An osteoma is defined as a tumor composed of bone tissue (Dorland, 1974, p. 1106).

burden placed on her family. She experienced suicidal ideation eight years ago when she was informed that she had a seizure disorder but denied any current suicidal ideation.

The patient's medical history is positive for peptic ulcer, a rectus sheath hematoma, and bilateral oophorohysterectomy two years ago with incidental appendectomy. Subsequent to the surgery the patient suffered a pulmonary embolism. She has reportedly suffered from chronic diarrhea for the past one-and-one-half years that has resulted in a 65-pound weight loss and caused her to resign her position as a grocery store manager nine months ago. She indicated that her sleep is normal and that she eats "like a horse" but has continued to lose weight. Despite extensive medical evaluation, no cause for the diarrhea has been found, and in fact the diarrhea temporarily remitted following admission for GI evaluation. The patient also reports "uncontrollable vomiting" when upset. The possibility of Briquet's syndrome or somatoform disorder has been postulated. The patient's medical history is negative for head injury, birth or developmental abnormalities, or psychiatric treatment.

The patient obtained an A.A. degree in accounting from a junior college. She described herself as an "A" student, and was able to complete in three semesters a program that normally requires five semesters. She has been employed in the grocery business since age 15 and, for the last four months of her employment, was a store manager. She has been married 34 years to a man who is also epileptic. She has 2 sons, aged 26 and 30, and a daughter, aged 33. She reports that she does not drink and discontinued smoking eight months ago.

Behavioral Observations

Ms. D. is an extremely thin, Caucasian, right-handed female. She was casually dressed and wore her very long hair in a braid. Affect was appropriate, and mood was mildly dysphoric. Speech was generally unremarkable. Test behavior was cooperative and compliant; the patient expressed interest in her performance and frequently asked to be told the correct answers to problems. She frequently verbalized instructions to herself during the completion of problems. The patient's most recent partial complex seizure reportedly occurred approximately one week ago.

Tests Administered

See data summary sheet.

Test Results

Intellectual Functioning

Ms. D. is currently functioning within the low average range of overall intelligence (Full Scale IQ = 89). Verbal and Performance IQ scores did not differ significantly (VIQ = 91; PIQ = 89). A mild degree of intersubtest scatter was noted, with age-corrected scaled scores ranging from average (Vocabulary, Picture Completion, Comprehension, Object Assembly, Similarities, Information, Arithmetic, and Digit Symbol) to low average (Digit Span, Picture Arrangement, and Block Design).

Mental Control

The patient's brief passive attention skills, as measured by digit span (F = 5; B = 4), were within the low average range for her age. She was able to accurately recite the alphabet and count backward from 20 (5 and 13 seconds, respectively) but made two errors in counting by 3s to 40 (27 seconds). The patient performed within the borderline and low average range respectively on two timed visuomotor tasks requiring drawing lines between numbers, or alternating between numbers and letters, in sequential order (Trailmaking A = 41 seconds; B = 97 seconds).

Sensory Perceptual and Motor Skills

Ms. D. denied any history of injury to hands, arms, or shoulders.

She committed twice as many left-sided sensory perceptual errors as right-sided errors on the Halstead-Reitan Sensory Perceptual Exam (R = 4; L = 9). Half of the errors on the left side were under conditions of simultaneous stimulation; four were suppressions of the left hand and one was an error of astereognosis. One astereognosis error for the right hand was also noted with simultaneous stimulation.

The patient is right-hand dominant and displayed the expected right-hand advantage on motor tasks. Her dominant-hand performance on finger tapping was within the average range, but impaired tapping speed was present with the left hand (R = 37.4; L = 22). On a task requiring the placing of pegs in a pegboard, the patient performed within the borderline range with her right hand but demonstrated particularly impaired performance with her left hand (R = 75 seconds; L = 92 seconds). Grip strength was significantly depressed bilaterally, but again the left hand performance was particularly impaired (R = 18 kg., L = 6 kg.).

Language Ability

The patient's spontaneous speech was unremarkable, and she was able to comprehend spoken language without difficulty. Her range of vocabulary, as assessed by the WAIS-R Vocabulary subtest, was well within the average range (63rd percentile). Her ability to name pictured objects on the Boston Naming Test was normal (56/60). Word generation skills were also within the average range; the patient was able to generate 28 words beginning with the letters "f," "a," and "s" within three minutes. The patient made one error on an aphasia screening exam, misspelling triangle as "tryingle."

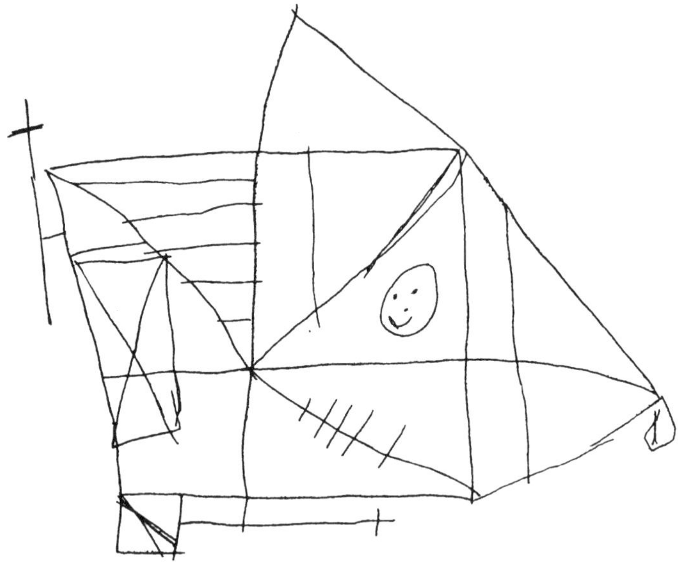

FIGURE 5.2. Case H.D. Rey-Osterrieth Complex Figure: copy. Reduced by 50%.

Verbal Learning and Memory

The patient's immediate auditory memory span was within the low average range for her age (Digit Span = 16th percentile). Her immediate recall of new word associations and short story paragraphs on the WMS was within the average range for her age on the Associate Learning and Logical Memory subtests of the WMS (64th and 39th percentiles, respectively). Her performance on a 15-item word list learning task was within the average to high average range (AVLT); by the fifth learning trial she was able to recall 13 of the items.

A 30-minute delayed recall of the details of story paragraphs and the word associations was also within the average range (86% and 100% retention, respec-

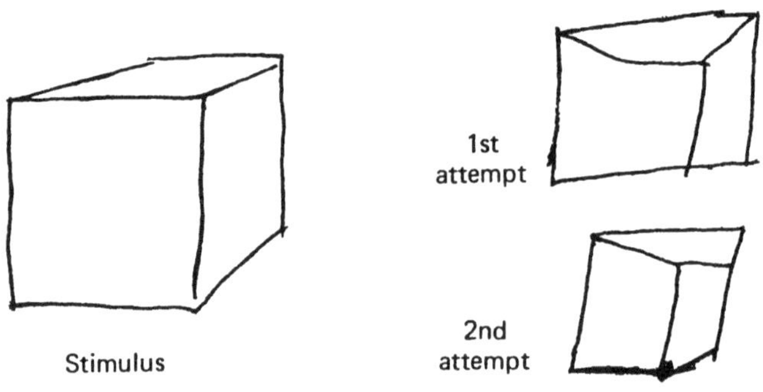

FIGURE 5.3. Case H.D. Three-dimensional cube: copy (2 attempts). Reduced by 15%.

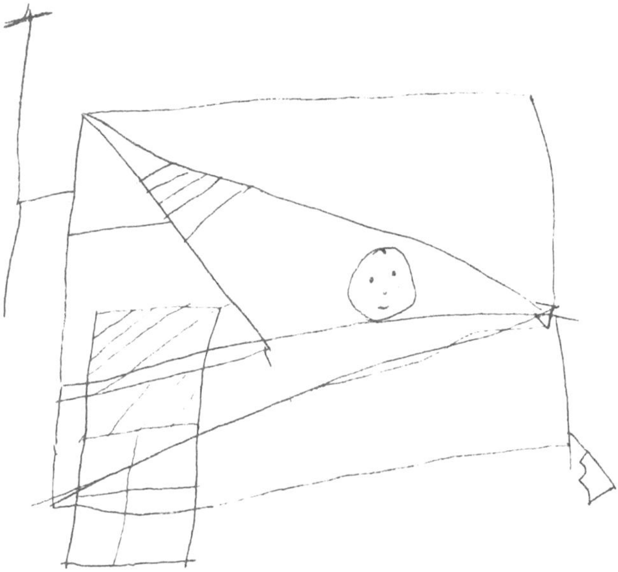

FIGURE 5.4. Case H.D. Rey-Osterrieth Complex Figure: delayed recall. Reduced by 35%.

tively). After an interference trial, the patient was able to recall 12 words on the word list learning task, a performance well within the normal range. After a 30-minute delay, she recalled nine of the 15 words, a performance within the low average range, and correctly recognized all items when presented in paragraph format, with no false identifications.

Visual Perception/Construction/Memory

Ms. D. did not report any difficulties in primary visual acuity. Her performance on WAIS-R subtests that required attention to fine visual details, such as Picture Completion and Picture Arrangement, was within the average to low average range (63rd and 16th percentiles, respectively). Average to low average scores were also obtained on visuo-spatial constructive tasks requiring block arrangement and puzzle-solving (Block Design = 16th percentile, Object Assembly = 37th percentile). On the other hand, the patient's pencil and paper copy of a complex two-dimensional line drawing was within the low average borderline range and demonstrated omissions and distortions (Rey-Osterrieth, see Figure 5.2). In addition, her drawing of a three-dimensional cube was inaccurate (Figure 5.3).

The patient's immediate recall of simple line drawings was within the average range for her age on the WMS-Visual Reproductions subtest (34th percentile) and she was able to retain the information at a normal rate over a 30-minute delay (two of three designs recalled). Her delayed recall of the Rey-Osterrieth figure following a three-minute delay was impaired and revealed significant distortions (< 10th percentile) (Figure 5.4).

Frontal Systems Tests

Ms. D.'s performance on the Wisconsin Card Sorting Test was within the superior range for her age and education level; she was able to complete 10 categories and provided 112 correct responses with minimal perseverative errors. Her performance on the Consonant Trigrams was within the average to low average range (42/60).

Brief Personality Evaluation

The patient's MMPI protocol was valid and revealed a profile in which the primary complaints are somatic, with secondary complaints of depression and anxiety (1"23'780-4/956 L-FK/). Persons with this profile tend to experience abdominal pains, stomach complaints, weight disturbance, dizziness, head pain, insomnia, irritability, nervousness, weakness, and worrying. Ms. D. endorsed five of 11 critical items pertaining to depression and distress, and six of 10 items relating to somatic concerns.

On the Sentence Completion task, themes of the importance of family closeness and a dislike of lying and dishonesty emerged. There was also regret expressed regarding her illness, and hope and optimism regarding recovery.

Summary and Impressions

Ms. D. is a right-handed, 49-year-old former grocery store manager who has a history of seizures dating from eight years ago, and two intracranial surgeries 18 and 22 years ago for right cerebral osteomas. In addition, the patient has lost 65 pounds in the last one-and-one-half years due to chronic diarrhea.

The current pattern of neuropsychological test results revealed overall average to low average intelligence. Most areas of measured cognitive function were intact, although selective areas of deficit were noted. Specifically, motor function tasks were generally depressed bilaterally, with particularly low scores obtained with the nondominant left hand. In addition, a relatively high number of sensory perceptual suppressions were found for the left hand. Pencil and paper constructional abilities were within the borderline range, and delayed recall of complex nonverbal visual material was impaired, although simpler nonverbal material was adequately retained over time. These results are suggestive of a cerebral dysfunction in the nondominant hemisphere, consistent with the location of the tumors. Specifically, errors in tactile discrimination with the left hand and deficits on constructional tasks might be anticipated with a right parietal lesion, and difficulties in nonverbal visual memory are common with right temporal lobe disturbance. The depressed motor functioning would suggest extension of dysfunction to posterior frontal lobe areas.

In addition to the documented declines on functions associated with the nondominant hemisphere, some mild disruption of attentional abilities was also evidenced.

The only difficulties of a verbal nature noted on testing involved spelling. The patient denied any history of spelling learning disability, and the clinical significance of the single gross spelling error present on current testing is unclear. Given the history of excellent grades in junior college, current low average intellectual scores may reflect a slight decline from premorbid levels.

In terms of psychological functioning, Ms. D. displayed an MMPI pattern that is seen in patients who are highly concerned with their physiologic state and have developed a depression related to somatic concerns. Such individuals are typically not receptive to intrapsychic or dynamic interpretation of their symptoms. Treatment of the depression through medication and supportive psychotherapy might be beneficial.

Addendum: The patient was subsequently placed on an antidepressant (nortriptyline) and experienced improvement in her energy level, decrease in somatic complaints, and virtual disappearance of the diarrhea.

NEUROPSYCHOLOGY TEST SCORE SUMMARY SHEET

Patient: H.D. Age: 49 Sex: F Handedness: R

I. Intelligence WAIS-R Age-Corrected Scores

VERBAL			PERFORMANCE		
Information	8	(25 %ile)	Picture Completion	11	(63 %ile)
Digit Span	7	(16 %ile)	Picture Arrangement	7	(16 %ile)
Vocabulary	11	(63 %ile)	Block Design	7	(16 %ile)
Arithmetic	8	(25 %ile)	Object Assembly	9	(37 %ile)
Comprehension	10	(50 %ile)	Digit Symbol	8	(25 %ile)
Similarities	9	(37 %ile)			
VERBAL IQ =	91	(27 %ile)	PERFORMANCE IQ =	89	(23 %ile)

FULL SCALE IQ = 89 (23 %ile)

II. Attention/Concentration
Digit Span: 5 forward + 4 backwards = 9 Total (16 %ile)
Mental Control, WMS: 5 (20 %ile)
Trails A: 41" (7 %ile), Trails B: 97" (14 %ile)

III. Language
Boston Naming Test: 56/60
Controlled Word Association: F (10) + A (7) + S (11) + Age Corr.=
34 (35-39 %ile)
Aphasia Screening Exam: 1 spelling error

IV. Perceptual/Organizational
Rey-Osterrieth Complex Figure Copy: 29 /36 (10 %ile)

V. Memory

VERBAL		NONVERBAL	
WMS Logical Memory	9 (64 %ile)	WMS Visual Repro.:	7 (34 %ile)
30 min. delay:	7.75	30 min. delay:	5
Percent retention:	86	Percent retention:	83
WMS Associate Learning I Easy	6 , 6 , 6	Rey-Osterrieth Fig:	29 (10 %ile)
Hard	1 , 2 , 1	3 min. delay:	10.5 (<10 %ile)
Score:	13 (39 %ile)		

Delay: 6 easy, 1 hard 100% retention

Rey Auditory Verbal Learning Test (15 items):
T1: 6 T2: 8 T3: 11 T4: 12 T5: 13 Recall after Interference: 12
30-min. Delayed Recall: 9
Recognition: 15 Hits, 0 False Identifications

VI. Motor Exam

	Dominant Hand	%ile	Nondom. Hand	%ile
Finger Tapping:	37.4	33	22	1
Grooved Pegbd.:	75"	6	92"	1
Grip Strength:	18	2	6	<1

VII. Sensory
Halstead-Reitan Sensory Perceptual Exam
Simultaneous Stimulation - R = 4, L = 9

VIII. Frontal Systems
Wisconsin Card Sort: Categories: 10
Auditory Consonant Trigrams: 42 /60

IX. Personality
MMPI: 1"23'780-4/956 L-FK/
Sentence Completion Test

Case 3: Bilateral Frontal Cysts

Reason for Referral and Background Information

Mr. C.G. was referred for neuropsychological testing to evaluate and document the presence of cognitive deficits associated with an extensive bilateral frontal lobe epidermoid cyst.

Mr. G. is a 31-year-old, right-handed Caucasian male who presented at the emergency room with a generalized tonic-clonic seizure associated with nausea, vomiting, and incontinence. A CT scan revealed a large cystic bifrontal mass. An EEG documented abnormal mild slowing of background rhythm with no epileptiform activity. Two months later the patient experienced onset of severe headaches and underwent elective resection of the cyst. The cyst was found to extend into the cella and occupied the majority of the frontal fossa and part of the middle fossa with extension posteriorly to the thalamus. Neuropsychological testing was completed six weeks prior to surgery.

Mr. G. has a long history of neurologic-related problems dating from infancy. His birth was apparently unremarkable, but when he was two weeks old he developed pertussis and required a two-week hospitalization. He was readmitted when he became "stuporous" and was noted to turn "blue" when he coughed. He is thought to have suffered anoxic encephalopathy secondary to the pertussis encephalitis. The patient was slow to walk and talk (two and three years, respectively) and exhibited marked behavioral abnormalities including "extreme" hyperactivity, tics and odd mannerisms (facial grimacing, throat-clearing), inappropriate social behavior and preference for mechanical objects and gadgets, and occasional suicidal ideation. He was alternately diagnosed with Gilles de la Tourette syndrome, hyperactive organic behavior disorder, and "childhood schizophrenic reaction" and was prescribed Thorazine, Mellaril, and Ritalin at various times.

He was described as a "slow learner" with "motor visual handicap" and was placed in classrooms for the emotionally handicapped. IQ testing at age 5 revealed a Full Scale IQ of 80, a Verbal IQ of 92, and a Performance IQ of 71. Verbal ability was reported to be intact, but paper and pencil constructional skills were depressed. Marked intersubtest scatter was present with impaired scores noted on constructional (Block Design, Object Assembly) and visual motor tracking tasks (Coding). Neurologic exams and EEG recordings were unremarkable. Retesting at age 10 documented a Full Scale IQ of 85, Verbal IQ of 91, and Performance IQ of 80. Significant scatter was again present with impaired scores noted in constructions (Object Assembly, Block Design), rapid grapho-motor tracking (Coding), digit span, verbal abstraction (Similarities), and knowledge of social norms and judgment (Comprehension). At age 11 the hyperactivity worsened, and the patient began to experience headaches. An EEG obtained at that time showed mild left anterior temporal spiking.

Mr. G. was able to complete high school with tutoring. At age 19 he began to experience absence seizures and in recent years has exhibited occasional generalized tonic-clonic seizures that have been well controlled with Dilantin. Five years ago the patient obtained psychiatric treatment for "uncontrollable outbursts of temper"; for example, he became angry at his mother and "squeezed" her, fracturing some of her ribs. Some improvement in impulse control was reported. During this same time he sought medical treatment for periodic dizziness. An EEG obtained at that time showed mild slowing of background rhythm but no epileptiform activity. The patient reports a history of LSD, PCP, and marijuana abuse at that time.

One year ago the patient began experiencing frequent dizzy spells without loss of consciousness or vertigo. An EEG recorded at that time was read as normal. He continued to experience periodic dizziness and six months ago reportedly suffered a tonic-clonic seizure, although he did not seek medical treatment. A second grand mal seizure occurred the day of admission.

Mr. G.'s medical history is also noteworthy for several eye surgeries for strabismus and exotropia in the right eye and a hernia repair. He is the third of four siblings. Family history is noteworthy for a younger sister who was born three months premature and is partially blind. She developed a partial complex seizure disorder at age 25. The patient's younger and older sisters were described as exhibiting significant psychiatric disturbance as children. The patient's mother is an alcoholic. The patient is currently prescribed Dilantin, 300mg., qhs.

The patient reports that he has no friends either currently or in the past, and he has only been able to temporarily hold employment as a janitor, truck driver, and gas station attendant. He has resided primarily with his parents but currently is living in a hotel. Mr. G.'s mother states that she has to remind her son to maintain personal hygiene and must assist and direct him in general self-care activities, including applying for public assistance and preparing to attend appointments. The patient is currently receiving general relief assistance, and reportedly has difficulty budgeting his money. He reports that social welfare agencies and missions provide him with most of his food. Although Mr. G. recognizes his difficulties in organizing his life, he resents others treating him "like a child." He reported that he would like to be more self-sufficient in managing his life. He describes his mother as being very supportive and actively involved in structuring his life. His mother stated a desire to become less involved, and her son agreed to consider other options.

Behavioral Observations

Mr. G. appeared as a somewhat disheveled, friendly, 31-year-old, Caucasian male who expressed considerable enthusiasm for the assessment process. He was frequently jocular, laughing loudly at his jokes, commenting freely in a childlike manner, and using expressions like "right on," and "far out." He frequently verbalized to himself to "hurry up" and "come on, brain," and when he missed an item, he would often chastise himself with comments like "I'm as ignorant as they come."

Mr. G. was early for his appointments and very cooperative throughout the evaluation. He apologized for his appearance. Following completion of two tests of motor functioning (finger tapping, grip strength), there was a noticeable tremor in his left hand. One eye often wandered to the side (most often his right eye).

Tests Administered

See data summary sheet.

Test Scores

Intellectual Scores

Mr. G. is currently functioning within the average range of general intellectual ability (Full Scale IQ = 90, 25th percentile). A mild but nonsignificant discrepancy was observed between overall Verbal and Performance IQs, with the Performance IQ falling seven points below the Verbal IQ (VIQ = 94; PIQ = 87).

On the Verbal subtests, Mr. G.'s performance was consistently within the average range (25th-63rd percentiles). More notable scatter was observed among the Performance subtest scores, which varied from the borderline range (Digit Symbol) to the average range (Picture Completion). It should be noted that during the administration of the Block Design subtest, Mr. G. appeared to have difficulty attending to the task and frequently introjected inappropriate comments that interfered with the speed of his performance and lowered his score to the 16th percentile. Mr. G. also failed to organize his responses in a methodical manner and demonstrated poor planning ability on this test.

Overall, Mr. G.'s intellectual profile is consistent with that obtained in childhood using a similar measure of intelligence.

Attention and Concentration Processes

On tests of attention and concentration, Mr. G. performed within the borderline to average range for his age. He obtained a forward digit span of five and a backward span of up to six, performances at the 25th percentile. On the Consonant Trigrams test, which measures the ability to engage in "divided attention," Mr. G. performed within the borderline range for his age (5th percentile).

Language Functioning

Mr. G.'s spontaneous speech was often jocular and tangential. His basic language skills appear to be grossly intact. He scored within the normal range on a formal confrontational naming test (Boston Naming Test = 53/60) and on a word generation test (FAS = 55th–59th percentile).

Motor Exam

The patient denied any history of significant injury to his hands, arms, or shoulders. Variable performance was noted on motor testing. Although the patient described himself as right-handed, he actually performed slightly better with his left hand on a finger tapping task (R = 58; L = 62); scores for both hands were

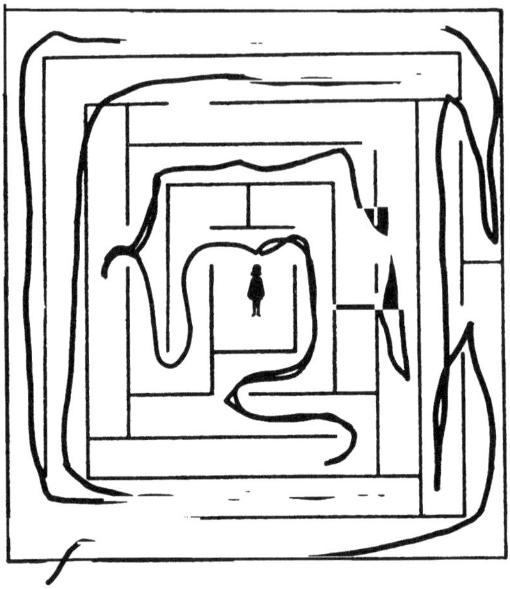

FIGURE 5.5. Case C.G. WISC-R Mazes Figure 7: 7 errors, 52 seconds. Reduced by 25%.

well above the normal range. Evaluation of the patient's grip strength also failed to reveal the expected dominant-hand advantage (R = 29; L = 30), and performance was within the impaired range bilaterally. Mr. G. reported that subjectively his left hand feels stronger than his right.

Perceptual Organizational Skills

Mr. G.'s performance on perceptual organization tasks was variable. Scores within the average range were obtained on visual perceptual tasks (Picture Completion = 37th percentile; Hooper Visual Organization Test = 27/30). However, on tasks involving visual sequencing and tracking, performance ranged from average to impaired. Specifically, the patient scored within the average range on the Rey Tangled Lines Test (no errors) and the Picture Arrangement subtest (25th percentile), but he scored within the borderline range on the Digit Symbol subtest (5th percentile) and within the impaired range on Trails A and B (45 and 193 seconds, respectively). In addition, Mr. G.'s performance on the Mazes subtest of the WISC-R demonstrated a significant problem in planning and anticipating outcome; he tended to repeatedly enter "blind alleys" (Fig. 5.5).

The patient's constructional ability was within the average to borderline range (Block Design = 16th percentile; Object Assembly = 25th percentile; Rey-Osterrieth = 10th percentile). His scores appeared to be depressed by poor organization strategies rather than deficient constructional skills.

Verbal (Auditory) and Nonverbal (Visual) Learning and Memory

Mr. G.'s performance on verbal and nonverbal learning and recall tasks was generally intact, although some variability was present in delayed recall of nonverbal visual material. He scored well within the normal range on the AVLT. He was able to recall 13 words by the fifth learning trial, and 13 and 14 words respectively after an interference task and a 30-minute delay. On the Logical Memory subtest of the Wechsler Memory Scale, he scored at the 70th percentile on immediate recall, and he was able to recall 90% of the information learned on 30-minute delayed recall. Scores on the WMS-Associate Learning subtest were also within the average range (34th percentile), and delayed recall of the word pairs was within the normal range (6 "easy" pairs, 1 "hard" pair).

Mr. G.'s immediate recall reproduction of simple geometric figures was at the 74th percentile (WMS-Visual Reproduction), and after a 30-minute delay, he was able to recall 58% of the information originally learned (2 of 4 designs), a retention rate below the normal range. However, his recall of a complex two-dimensional line drawing following a three-minute delay was well within the average range (Rey-Osterrieth = 30th percentile).

Abstraction and Mental Flexibility

Mr. G. was only able to complete four categories (7th percentile) on the Wisconsin Card Sorting Test, a task involving conceptual tracking and categorization skills. Despite being told that he was sorting incorrectly, Mr. G. continued to make perseverative errors (27) and failed to maintain set two times.

When asked to interpret proverbs, the patient provided highly concrete answers and appeared not to recognize that the statements were proverbs (WAIS-R Comprehension).

Achievement Scores

<u>WRAT-R</u>
Reading: 11th grade equivalent; 27th percentile
Spelling: 3rd grade equivalent; .9 percentile
Arithmetic: 7th grade equivalent; 9th percentile

Achievement test scores indicate that Mr. G.'s sight reading skills are relatively intact but that his ability to spell is impaired. His performance of mathematical calculations is also somewhat depressed.

Summary and Impressions

Intellectual scores indicate that the patient is currently functioning within the average range of general intellectual ability (Full Scale IQ = 90). A mild but nonsignificant discrepancy was observed between his Verbal and Performance IQs (VIQ = 94; PIQ = 87). Mr. G.'s intellectual profile is consistent with that obtained in childhood using a similar measure.

Neuropsychological test scores revealed impairment on some tasks sensitive to frontal lobe dysfunction as well as some depression of academic skills (e.g., spelling, mathematics). Specifically, Mr. G. performed poorly on tasks requiring conceptual tracking and categorization, sequencing and alternation, "divided attention," maze-solving, motor strength, and planning and organizational ability. However, given the massive size of the frontal lobe cyst, we are surprised that the patient scored well on other tasks measuring frontal systems integrity; namely, word generation, motor dexterity, and screening out of visual distractors. It should be noted that the patient's behavioral presentation and history also provided evidence of frontal lobe dysfunction; for example, his personal hygiene was relatively poor, he made jocular and rather childlike comments, he has trouble budgeting his money, and he has difficulty applying for public assistance services and meeting appointments and requires his mother's assistance.

In contrast, performance on other measures of higher level cognitive functioning was intact. This was evidenced by the patient's normal fund of information, average intellectual scores, and intact language, visual perceptual, memory, and motor skills. The norm of motor dexterity and language skills would suggest that the frontal lobe cysts are not likely to be of recent origin, but rather developed relatively slowly and gradually, which allowed for some brain reorganization and compensation.

While the deficits in "frontal lobe" skills would be anticipated given the bifrontal cysts, it is also possible that some of the observed cognitive and behavioral difficulties may also be sequelae of the history of anoxic encephalopathy, seizures, Tourette's syndrome, childhood hyperactivity, learning disabilities, drug abuse, and possible childhood schizophrenia. The documented poor performance in spelling and arithmetic would not be unexpected given the history of learning disability and tutoring in high school.

The pattern of cognitive difficulties manifested by the patient would indicate that he will function best in a work environment in which he is given specific direction and structure. Due to his problems in organizing and planning ahead, the patient also requires support in his daily functioning. It is recommended that Mr. G. be referred to the social work department for vocational counseling. Mr G. is motivated to obtain a job within his range of ability and to receive direction regarding the attainment of improved life-skill functioning.

Reevaluation of neuropsychological functioning following surgery is recommended to assess possible changes in cognitive status.

NEUROPSYCHOLOGY TEST SCORE SUMMARY SHEET

Patient: C.G. Age: 31 Sex: M Handedness: R

I. Intelligence WAIS-R Age-Corrected Scores

VERBAL			PERFORMANCE		
Information	11	(63 %ile)	Picture Completion	9	(37 %ile)
Digit Span	8	(25 %ile)	Picture Arrangement	8	(25 %ile)
Vocabulary	10	(50 %ile)	Block Design	7	(16 %ile)
Arithmetic	9	(37 %ile)	Object Assembly	8	(25 %ile)
Comprehension	9	(37 %ile)	Digit Symbol	5	(5 %ile)
Similarities	10	(50 %ile)			
VERBAL IQ =	94	(34 %ile)	PERFORMANCE IQ =	87	(19 %ile)

FULL SCALE IQ = 90 (25 %ile)

II. Attention/Concentration
Digit Span: 5 forward + 6 backwards = 11 Total (25 %ile)
Trails A: 45" (<1 %ile), Trails B: 193" (<1 %ile)

III. Language
Boston Naming Test: 53 /60
Controlled Word Association: F (14) + A (10) + S (11) + Age Corr. = 39 (55-59 %ile)

IV. Perceptual/Organizational
Rey-Osterrieth Complex Figure Copy: 29/36 (10 %ile)
Hooper Visual Organization Test: 27 /30
Rey Tangled Lines: intact
WISC-R Mazes: 13, SS = 2

V. Memory

VERBAL		NONVERBAL	
WMS Logical Memory	9.5 (70%ile)	WMS Visual Repro.:	12 (74%ile)
30 min. delay:	8.5	30 min. delay:	7
Percent retention:	90	Percent retention:	58

WMS Associate Learning I Easy 6 , 6 , 6   I Hard 1 , 1 , 3   I Score: 14 (34 %ile)
30 min. delay: 6 easy, 1 hard 78 % retention

Rey-Osterrieth Fig: 29 (10 %ile)
3 min. delay: 18.5 (30 %ile)

Rey Auditory Verbal Learning Test (15 items):
T1: 6 T2:8 T3:9 T4:11 T5: 13 Recall after Interference: 13
30-min. Delayed Recall: 14

VI. Motor Exam

	Dominant Hand	%ile	Nondom. Hand	%ile
Finger Tapping:	58	93	62	99
Grip Strength:	29	1	30	2

VII. Frontal Systems
Wisconsin Card Sort: Categories: 4 , Perseverative err: 27
Auditory Consonant Trigrams: 40 /60 Rey Tangled Lines: 0 err.

VIII. Achievement

WRAT-R:	Grade Equivalent	Percentile Rank
Reading	11	27
Spelling	3	.9
Arithmetic	7	9

WAIS-R Comprehension Proverbs:

Strike while the iron is hot: "Referring to metal iron. It's more malleable when soft. It can become a liquid state if it gets hot enough."

Shallow brooks are noisy: "Because the water is shallow...tends to tumble over rocks...white noise, pink noise, random sound."

Commentary on Brain Tumor Cases

All three cases reveal the unique focal cognitive deficits that can be present with brain mass lesions in various locations, despite normal intellectual scores. Patient 1 exhibits the severe amnesia and frontal systems dysfunction that may be found with damage to mammillary bodies, thalamus, and/or other subcortical structures adjacent to the third ventricle. Patient 2 demonstrates the constructional, nonverbal memory, and left-hand motor and tactile deficits often associated with right hemisphere tumors. Patient 3 shows the relatively discrete and subtle cognitive abnormalities that may accompany frontal lobe disruption and that nonetheless have profound implications for a patient's level of function within society.

In Patient 1 we see the acute deterioration associated with fast growing tumors of recent origin. Patient 3 provides an example of the substantial brain reorganization and compensation that is frequently present with long-standing, albeit massive, brain lesions.

These three patients illustrate the various associated features of brain masses and their treatment that impact cognition in addition to the effects of the actual brain mass. Patients 2 and 3 experienced seizures as sequelae of the brain lesions. Patients 1 and 2 received radiation treatment, and Patient 1 suffered direct insult to the right fronto-parietal area during tumor resection and subsequent subdural hydroma.

6
Long-Term Alcohol Abuse

There is little doubt about the neurotoxic effects of alcohol on the human nervous system, and multiple (though sometimes mild) neuropsychological deficits have been documented in long-term, chronic alcohol abusers. The purpose of this chapter is to acquaint the reader with the variety of deficits common to long-term alcohol abusers and the assessment measures that may best be utilized to tease out sometimes subtle deficits. We will not review in detail the interesting but differing views on various models that have been purported to explain the nature of these deficits (e.g., the "premature aging" hypothesis, the "right hemisphere" hypothesis), but the interested reader is referred to Brandt and Butters (1986), Loberg (1986), and Parsons and Farr (1981) for a more comprehensive discussion of these models.

Many individuals view the profound amnesic presentation of the patient with Korsakoff's disease as typifying the neuropsychological sequelae following long-term alcohol abuse, and indeed, such impairment does occur in a small number of chronic alcoholics. However, specific patterns of neuropsychological deficits may characterize patients in the early to middle phases of alcohol abuse who have not developed the Korsakoff's amnestic disorder or even the more global alcohol dementia, both of which will be discussed later in this chapter.

Neuropsychological Sequelae of the Early and Middle Phases of Alcohol Abuse

Clinical research on alcoholic patients is sometimes difficult to interpret given the varied subject populations used and the length of sobriety/detoxification prior to testing. For instance, variables such as age, duration and degree of alcohol abuse, in-patient versus out-patient status, past psychiatric history, number of blackouts, history of head injury, premorbid medical variables, and duration of detoxification at the time of testing may greatly affect test results and yield artifactual differences among studies. Additionally, the clinician administering a neuropsychological test battery to a chronic alcohol abuser must take these factors into account when making clinical interpretations of the findings, such as in the case of a patient with not only a chronic history of alcohol abuse but also with one or more head injuries, as is frequently found in this population.

At the time of acute intoxication, the heavy alcohol abuser will generally present with a picture characteristic of an individual in an acute confusional state, with decreased attention and deficits in most cognitive spheres assessed. Thus, it is important that the individual *not* be tested in the acute withdrawal phase because notable, but not necessarily lasting, cognitive deficits will usually be seen. Ryan and Butters (1980) reported that the greatest improvement in cognitive functioning takes places in the first week of abstinence but that continuing improvement still occurs and plateaus at three to six weeks post cessation of drinking. Many studies have required at least two weeks of abstinence before testing; however, some have required as much as four weeks. In our clinical work, we recommend a minimum of three weeks of abstinence before a patient undergoes neuropsychological testing.

Chronic alcoholics typically demonstrate a variety of cognitive difficulties, including mild deficits in visuo-spatial, perceptual, and graphomotor tasks (Butters, Cermak, Montgomery, & Adenolfi, 1977; Goldstein, 1976), learning and memory, and tasks assessing "executive functions" such as abstraction, planning, and complex problem-solving tasks (Oscar-Berman, 1973; Cutting, 1979). Despite these findings affecting specific cognitive domains, overall intellectual functioning appears largely uncompromised. For instance, in a study by Butters (1981) comparing chronic alcoholics (with Korsakoff's disease) with matched controls on the WAIS, no significant differences were found on overall IQ scores (although Digit Symbol subtest scores were significantly lower in the alcohol group). Others (e.g., Parsons, Tarter, & Edelberg, 1972), however, have noted mildly lowered Performance IQ scores relative to the Verbal scores in chronic alcohol abusers, and this will be discussed more fully below.

Deficits in visuo-spatial tasks have been the most consistently documented deficits shown by long-term alcohol abusers. For instance, Goldstein (1976) notes the dramatic perceptual/analytic abnormalities in the chronic alcoholic on tasks of field dependence/independence. Tarter (1976) and others report that alcoholics exhibit deficits on visuo-spatial tasks such as Block Design, the Tactual Performance Test, Rod and Frame Test, and Embedded Figures Test. As early as the 1940s, it was noted (Teicher & Singer, 1946) that alcoholics as a group obtained higher Verbal IQ scores than Performance IQ scores, though the differences admittedly were slight and usually did not exceed 10 points. These consistent findings have led some (e.g., Jones & Parsons, 1972) to suggest a "right hemisphere hypothesis," implying a selective vulnerability of the right hemisphere to the effects of alcohol. However, more recent research has questioned this hypothesis, and other competing and tenable hypotheses have been offered. One problem with this theory is the difficulty explaining why alcohol would be more toxic to one hemisphere than the other. Others (e.g., Parsons & Leber, 1981) have used these findings to suggest a "premature aging" hypothesis because the alcoholic exhibits some cognitive deficits comparable to the pattern seen in normal aging (such as depressed performance on visuo-spatial and speeded tasks).

Deficits in "frontal systems" tasks (i.e., those tasks dependent upon intact frontal lobe/subcortical connecting structures) have also been consistently noted in this group, and have even led some (e.g., Tarter, 1975) to suggest a selective fronto-limbic-diencephalic dysfunction. Support for this hypothesis comes from studies documenting consistently poorer performance in chronic alcoholics on tasks such as the Halstead Category Test (Fitzhugh, Fitzhugh, & Reitan, 1965; Jones & Parsons, 1971), and the Wisconsin Card Sorting Test (e.g., Tarter, 1973). Additional support for this hypothesis is obtained from the findings of cortical atrophy in frontal parietal regions on CT scans in a majority of chronic alcoholics (Lezak, 1983).

Until recently, most studies reported relatively normal memory functioning in chronic alcoholics who did not display a Wernicke-Korsakoff's syndrome or alcohol dementia. This may largely be attributable to the lack of sensitive assessment instruments used in the past, such as the global "MQ" score from the Wechsler Memory Scale (unmodified) that contains no measure of delayed (secondary) memory and equates overlearned information with more recent memory. In fact, Brandt and Butters (1986) quote Parsons and Prigatano as concluding that "there is no evidence of lasting impairment of memory in detoxified alcoholic men" (p. 464). However, more recent studies specifically designed to assess more subtle memory impairment in chronic alcoholics have documented mild deficits. Ryan, Butters, Montgomery, Adinolfi, and Didario (1980) tested 18 chronic alcoholics (with at least a 10-year history of alcohol abuse), 18 matched nonalcoholics, and seven chronic alcoholic patients with Korsakoff's disease (KD). The results revealed notable memory deficits, not only for the Korsakoff's patients but also for the subjects with chronic alcohol abuse without the full amnestic syndrome. On the three memory tasks in the battery, the chronic alcohol abusers (without Korsakoff's disease) performed more poorly than the matched normal controls but better than the fully amnestic KD patients. Thus, careful neuropsychological assessments that include tests sensitive to memory dysfunction (e.g., immediate and delayed recall tasks, serial-list learning tasks, paired-associated learning tasks) are very important to include in the assessment of this group and are likely to elicit mild to moderate memory dysfunction.

A final area of commonly reported difficulty on neuropsychological tests is on measures of speed of performance and the solution of novel, complex tasks. These individuals have been shown to perform poorly on such tasks as the Trail Making Test and, as already mentioned, the Digit Symbol test, a composite measure involving speed, learning, and the ability to rapidly devise a strategy to solve a novel problem (cf. Goldman, 1983).

Thus, careful neuropsychological assessment will reveal deficits in many cognitive domains, including perceptual organizational abilities, learning and memory, "executive functions" such as complex problem solving, abstract reasoning, and planning, as well as on speeded tasks. We now proceed to a more severe and debilitating disorder occurring in some chronic alcohol abusers, the amnestic disorder of Korsakoff's disease.

Korsakoff's Disease

Korsakoff's disease (KD) occurs when an individual has not only had a course of chronic alcohol abuse, but also sustained a nutritional deficiency resulting in damage to thalamic and hypothalamic structures. It is also reported that KD patients suffer neuronal loss in the nucleus basalis of Meynert similar to that found in patients with Alzheimer's disease (Arendt, Bigl, Arendt, & Tennstedt, 1983; see Butters, 1985).

The most striking feature of the chronic alcoholic who has developed Korsakoff's disease is the severe anterograde memory deficit they possess. Testing will immediately disclose a prominent amnestic syndrome in the presence of relatively normal overall intellectual skills, in which the patient cannot learn any new information. These patients will often have no recall on subsequent testing sessions (even minutes, hours, days, or weeks apart) of ever having been tested before. It is not uncommon for their primary doctor, with whom they have come in contact on a frequent (even daily) basis, to seem to them a stranger who requires a new introduction upon each visit. Though "primary memory" is intact, resulting in relatively normal digit span scores, "secondary" memory or delayed recall is usually essentially nonexistant. Thus, though a patient may be able to recall four or more of 15 words presented across five trials (often demonstrating a primacy or recency effect), he or she will be unable to recall any of the items following a distractor, and the introduction of many intrusion responses (i.e., words that were never on the original 15-item list) is common. Although fewer patients with KD actually confabulate or create elaborate stories to fill the vacuum of their amnesia than is commonly thought, the tendency to confabulate is present in a sizeable percentage of these patients and is usually confined to the first year following onset of the disease (Brandt & Butters, 1986).

Another hallmark of the Korsakoff syndrome is the temporal gradient characterizing the retrograde amnesia. That is, these patients can recall more accurately events and faces from the distant past (but still not as well as matched normal controls) than they can events and faces more recent to the onset of their amnesia. This has been demonstrated in several studies, such as by Seltzer and Benson (1974) who showed that patients with KD could recall well-known events more accurately from the 1930s and 40s than from the 1960s and 70s. In a series of studies, Albert, Butters, and colleagues (e.g., Albert, Butters, & Levin, 1979) used a "Remote Memory Battery" to assess memories spanning the decades from the 1920s to the 70s. The three tests in this battery included a "Famous Faces" test (pictures of famous people such as Charlie Chaplin and Richard Nixon), a "recall" test (a series of questions about famous people and events), and a "recognition" test (a series of questions about famous people and events with three choices for each item). They found the now well-known "temporal gradient" on both "easy" and "hard" items, indicating that people and events from the more remote decades (1920 to 1949) were recalled far more accurately than more recent events (1950 to 1979). In a series of studies, Squire and colleagues (e.g., Cohen & Squire, 1981) have demonstrated similar findings using a "TV test" consisting of names of television programs from various decades that aired for one season or less.

In addition to these prominent deficits, the patient with Korsakoff's disease will also typically present with deficits characterizing the non-Korsakoff chronic alcoholic patient, such as visuo-spatial impairment, "executive systems" dysfunction, and poor performance on timed, speeded tasks, especially those that require the development of rapid problem solving and visuo-motor tracking, such as the Digit Symbol subtest from the WAIS-R.

Thus, the psychologist assessing a patient suspected of having Korsakoff's disease would expect to find a relatively "pure" amnesia, characterized by an *inability* to learn new information except that which can be held for a few moments in the patient's immediate memory span as well as a temporal gradient indicating better recall for more remote events and people. In our battery for these patients, we recommend not only the essential core battery of neuropsychologic tests, but also prescribe adding a measure of remote memory, such as the "Remote Memory Battery" developed by Albert, Butters, and colleagues.

Alcohol Dementia

The final disorder on what some (e.g., Brandt & Butters, 1986) have termed the "continuum of alcohol abuse" is the alcohol dementia (Lishman, 1981). The patient with alcohol dementia has had a long and chronic history of alcohol abuse culminating in definite decline in overall intellectual/cognitive abilities from premorbid abilities, as well as moderate to severe deficits in many other cognitive domains. It is a condition that is not well researched, perhaps because the striking amnesia in the patients with KD has attracted so much clinical attention (Lishman, 1981) and because the tendency, until recently, has been not to distinguish among various dementia syndromes. The patient with an alcohol dementia may or may not also have sustained KD along the way. We do not know of any systematic and comprehensive research specifically examining the specific cognitive deficits versus preserved abilities in this disorder. Until the research is undertaken on this neglected syndrome, we can only speculate as to the prototypic mental status abnormalities in this syndrome. The first two cases presented below, we believe, represent cases of alcohol dementia encountered in our clinical work thus far and may serve as examples representing this intriguing syndrome.

Summary

It is clear from the above discussion that subtle to more serious neuropsychological deficits are present in long-term alcohol abusers, with the most serious effects found in the first six weeks post cessation of drinking. Following this acute period, residual compromise may be found in long-term alcohol abusers, most commonly in: (1) visuo-spatial constructional and analytic tasks; (2) tasks dependent upon intact "frontal systems," such as planning, organizing, complex, rapid problem solving, and abstract thinking; and (3) learning and memory tests. The patient who has sustained Korsakoff's disease will usually present with a prominent anterograde amnesia within the context of relatively preserved intelligence and overall cognitive functioning. The patient with an alcohol dementia will exhibit serious memory disturbance and intellectual decline along with notable compromise in multiple other cognitive domains. Finally, the neuropsychologist must take into account past history of head injury, nutritional deficiencies, and other variables in the interpretation of test results in this group.

References

Albert, M.S., Butters, N., & Levin, J. (1979). Temporal gradients in the retrograde amnesia of patients with alcoholic Korsakoff's disease. *Archives of Neurology, 36,* 211-216.

Arendt, T., Bigl, V., Arendt, A., & Tennstedt, A. (1983). Loss of neurons in the nucleus basalis of Meynert in Alzheimer's Disease, paralysis agitans and Korsakoff's Disease. *Acta Neuropatholigica, 61,* 101-108.

Brandt, J., & Butters, N. (1986). The alcoholic Wernicke-Korsakoff syndrome and its relationship to long-term alcohol abuse. In I. Grant & K. Adams (Eds.), *Neuropsychological assessment of neuropsychiatric disorders* (pp. 441-477). New York: Oxford University Press.

Butters, N. (1981). Amnestic disorders. In K. Heilman & E. Valenstein (Eds.), *Clinical neuropsychology* (pp. 439-474). New York: Oxford University Press.

Butters, N. (1985). Alcoholic Korsakoff's syndrome: Some unresolved issues concerning etiology, neuropathology, and cognitive deficits. *Journal of Clinical and Experimental Neuropsychology, 7,* 181-210.

Butters, N., Cermak, L.S., Montgomery, K., & Adenolfi, A. (1977). Some comparisons of the memory and visuoperceptive deficits of chronic alcoholics and patients with Korsakoff's disease. *Alcoholism: Clinical and Experimental Research, 1,* 73-76.

Cohen, N.J., & Squire, L.R. (1981). Retrograde amnesia and remote memory impairment. *Neuropsychologia, 19,* 337-356.

Cutting, J. (1979). Differential impairment of memory in Korsakoff's syndrome. *Cortex, 15,* 501-516.

Fitzhugh, L., Fitzhugh, K., & Reitan, R. (1965). Adaptive abilities and intellectual functioning of hospitalized alcoholics: Further considerations. *Quarterly Journal of Studies on Alcohol, 26,* 402-411.

Goldman, M.S. (1983). Cognitive impairment in chronic alcoholics: Some cause for optimism. *American Psychologist, 38,* 1045-1054.

Goldstein, G. (1976). Perceptual and cognitive deficits in alcoholics. In G. Goldstein & C. Neuringer (Eds.), *Empirical studies of alcoholism* (pp. 115-151). Cambridge, MA: Ballinger.

Jones, B., & Parsons, O. (1971). Impaired abstracting ability in chronic alcoholics. *Archives of General Psychiatry, 24,* 71-75.

Jones, B., & Parsons, O.A. (1972). Specific vs. generalized deficits of abstracting ability in chronic alcoholics. *Archives of General Psychiatry, 26,* 380-384.

Lezak, M. (1983). *Neuropsychological assessment* (2nd ed.) New York: Oxford Univer-

Lishman, W.A. (1981). Cerebral disorder in alcoholism: Syndromes of impairment. *Brain, 104,* 1-20.
Loberg, T. (1986). Neuropsychological findings in the early and middle phases of alcoholism. In I. Grant & K. Adams (Eds.), *Neuropsychological assessment of neuropsychiatric disorders* (pp. 415-440). New York: Oxford University Press.
Nelson, L.D., Satz, P., & Mitrushina, M.N. (1988). Validation of a test to measure personality and affective change in a brain-injured population: Preliminary results. *Journal of Clinical and Experimental Neuropsychology, 10,* 59 (abstract).
Oscar-Berman, M. (1973). Hypothesis testing and focusing behavior during concept formation by amnestic Korsakoff patients. *Neuropsychologia, 11,* 191-198.
Parsons, O.A., & Farr, S.D. (1981) The neuropsychology of alcohol and drug use. In S.B. Filskov & T.J. Boll (Eds.), *Handbook of clinical neuropsychology* (pp. 320-365). New York: John Wiley and Sons.
Parsons, O.A., & Leber, W.R. (1981). The relationship between cognitive dysfunction and brain damage in alcoholics: Causal, interactive or epiphenomenal? *Alcoholism: Clinical Experimental Research, 5,* 326-343.
Parsons, O.A., Tarter, R.E., & Edelberg, R. (1972). Altered motor control in chronic alcoholics. *Journal of Abnormal Psychology, 72,* 308-314.
Ryan, C., & Butters, N. (1980). Further evidence for a continuum-of-impairment encompassing male alcoholic Korsakoff patients and chronic alcoholic men. *Alcoholism: Clinical and Experimental Research, 4,* 190-197.
Ryan, C., Butters, N., Montgomery, K., Adinolfi, Al., & Didario, B. (1980). Memory deficits in chronic alcoholics: Continuities between the "intact" alcoholic and the alcoholic Korsakoff patient. In H. Begleiter (Ed.), *Biological effects of alcohol* (pp. 701-717). New York: Plenum Press.
Seltzer, B., & Benson, D.F. (1974). The temporal pattern of retrograde amnesia in Korsakoff's disease. *Neurology, 24,* 527-530.
Tarter, R.E. (1973). An analysis of cognitive deficits in chronic alcoholics. *Journal of Nervous and Mental Disease, 157,* 138-147.
Tarter, R.E. (1975). Brain damage associated with chronic alcoholics. *Disorders of the Nervous System, 36,* 185-187.
Tarter, R.E. (1976). Neuropsychological investigations of alcoholism. In G. Goldstein & C. Neuringer (Eds.), *Empirical studies of alcoholism* (pp. 231-256). Cambridge, MA: Ballinger Publishing Company.
Teicher, M., & Singer, E. (1946). A report on the use of the Wechsler-Bellevue scales in an overseas general population. *American Journal of Psychiatry, 103,* 91-93.

Case 1: Chronic Alcohol Abuse

Reason for Referral and Presenting Situation

Mr. T.C. is a 61-year-old, right-handed, black male with a high-school education who was referred for neuropsychological evaluation after staff observation of possible memory deficits. A complete assessment was requested to delineate the nature of the patient's cognitive impairment. Mr. C. was recently admitted to the hospital from a nursing home because he had been threatening to strike another patient. Mr. C. had been placed in a nursing home originally when his family refused to continue to care for him and, because of cognitive decline, he could not care for himself at home. Past history is significant for almost lifelong chronic alcohol abuse, though the patient reportedly has not ingested alcohol for five months. He has been employed in several semi-skilled jobs over the years. There is no known history of head trauma or other neurologic injury, or history of past psychiatric disturbance. A CT scan performed on admission revealed only very mild cortical atrophy, and an EEG was normal. Neurologic exam revealed only mild peripheral neuropathy. The patient is currently on no medications.

Behavioral Observations

Mr. C. appeared as a gregarious and friendly man who conversed in a tangential manner about his varied experiences over the years. It was frequently necessary to interrupt him and structure the conversation in order to complete the testing. Otherwise, he was fully cooperative during the evaluation, and the results are believed to reflect an accurate portrayal of Mr. C.'s current level of cognitive functioning.

Tests Administered

See data summary sheet.

Test Results

Gross Cognitive Functioning

Mr. C. obtained a score of 23/30 on the Mini-Mental State Exam, indicating borderline impairment of cognitive functioning. He was unable to name the current season, did not know the name of the hospital, made four errors on consecutive serial 7 subtractions, and recalled only two of three words following a short delay.

Intelligence

Intellectual assessment reveals a Verbal IQ of 93, a Performance IQ of 80, and a Full Scale of 87, placing the patient in the low average range of intellectual ability. The disparity between Verbal and Performance IQ scores was marginally significant. Mr. C. performed best on tasks measuring his knowledge of vocabulary definitions (Vocabulary), social judgment and understanding of common social conventions (Comprehension), and selective attention (Digit Span). In contrast, he scored less well on many of the visuo-spatial tasks and performed very poorly on a subtest measuring his ability to abstract commonalities between objects (Similarities). These results may reflect mild decrement in intellectual functioning relative to his probable premorbid level of functioning, primarily in the nonverbal domain.

Attention and Concentration

Performance in this domain was variable. Mr. C. was able to repeat seven digits forward and four backward (Digit Span), an average performance. He performed in the average range on tasks requiring him to count backwards from 20, recite the alphabet, and count forward by 3s (WMS–Mental Control). However, as mentioned above, he made several errors in consecutive serial 7 subtractions. In addition, on tests of visual tracking and cognitive flexibility (Trail-Making Test, Parts A and B), the patient performed poorly. He scored in the impaired range on the Trail Making Test, Part A, and was not able to correctly complete Part B. On this latter portion, he became quite confused, and after almost 3½ minutes seemed to have lost the instructional set and could not sequentially alternate from number to letter. His performance on the Stroop Test was within normal limits. Together, these results reveal variable performance with intact brief passive and sustained attention, and impairment on tasks measuring visual scanning, tracking, calculations, and set shifting abilities.

Language

Mr. C.'s spontaneous speech was fluent and meaningful, and he was quite hyperverbal throughout the evaluation. The rate and rhythm of his speech was within normal limits. The results of a confrontational naming task indicate mildly impaired performance (Boston Naming Test = 43/60). His word list generation (FAS) was in the high average range, and gross assessment of comprehension, reading, and writing to dictation was all intact. Thus, language assessment is essentially within normal limits except for a mild deficit in confrontational naming abilities.

Visuo-Spatial Abilities

Mr. C. performed in the impaired range (< 10th percentile) in his copy of a complex two-dimensional figure (Rey-Osterrieth). Additionally, though his overall strategy was fairly good, he was very concrete in his approach, retracing with the second color of pencil what he had already drawn with the first colored pencil. Though he performed in the low average range on another visuo-spatial task requiring him to construct a matrix of blocks to match a design (Block Design), he performed in the average range on a task requiring him to put puzzle pieces together to form a familiar object (Object Assembly). Thus, there is possible evidence of a very mild visuo-spatial deficit relative to verbal intellectual scores.

Motor

Motor examination using the Finger Tapping Test revealed normal performance bilaterally (R = 46.8; L = 40.4), although a slightly greater than expected (14%) dominant-hand advantage was present.

Learning and Memory

Mr. C. performed in the average range in his immediate recall of logical prose (WMS–Logical Memory), similar to conversational speech. However, following a 30-minute delay, he was unable to recall any of the elements of the two stories and, in fact, confabulated two rather elaborate stories that contained elements that were in neither of the originally presented stories. When given a paired-word associate learning task (WMS–Associate Learning), he was able to learn all six of the easy word pairs by the first learning trial, though he could only learn one of the four more difficult pairs by the second learning trial and recalled none on the third learning trial. He was only able to learn five of 10 words presented him on a serial list learning task (Shopping List Test) by the fourth learning trial, and his recall strategy was poor, revealing recency and primacy effects on most recall trials. Following a 15-minute delay, he was able to recall four of the 10 words. On a recognition portion of this test, he correctly identified nine of the 10 items that were on the list, with only one false-positive identification.

The patient performed in the low average range on his immediate recall of simple line drawings (WMS–Visual Reproduction), and he could recall only 50% of the information following a 30-minute delay, a performance below expected levels. Thus, tests of learning and memory reveal consistently poor performance for both verbal and nonverbal material, and his recognition of the material appears better than free recall.

Tasks of Set Shifting and Concept Learning

Significantly, the patient was unable to complete even one of the categories on the Wisconsin Card Sorting Test and made many perseverative errors. Additionally, the patient was very concrete on a test of abstract thinking (Similarities subtest of the WAIS-R). Together, these results indicate deficits on tasks of set shifting/concept learning and abstract thinking.

Summary and Conclusions

Selective impairment of higher cognitive functioning was observed in an individual with low average intelligence. Most notable impairment was observed on tests measuring memory functions, especially for complex verbal material following a delay and on tasks of abstraction, concept learning, and shifting of set. In addition, a possible naming disturbance was found. It is significant to note that he does not appear to be fully amnestic as he is able to recall limited amounts of previously presented information following a delay and his recognition appears better preserved than recall. Thus, his pattern is not characteristic of a Korsakoff's syndrome. He also evidenced depressed performance on visuo-spatial tasks. These results are quite consistent with the effects of chronic alcohol abuse and indeed, raise the possibility of a mild alcohol-related dementia.

The patient's verbally abusive behavior and attempt to strike out while in the nursing home may in fact be a consequence of deficits in frontal lobe functioning, secondary to the alcohol abuse. Therapeutic interventions that are concrete and simple will be most helpful for this patient. Verbal instructions given him should be written. Nonverbal memory is also deficient, and he may have difficulty learning his way around novel environments. His impulsivity and tendency to be inappropriately aggressive should be monitored.

Together, testing results are believed to be of a chronic, static nature, though mild improvement may take place over the next several months to one year if the patient continues to abstain from alcohol.

NEUROPSYCHOLOGY TEST SCORE SUMMARY SHEET

Patient: T.C.   Age: 61   Sex: M   Handedness: R

I. Gross Cognitive Functioning
Mini-Mental State Exam: 23/30

II. Intelligence WAIS-R Age-Corrected Scores

VERBAL			PERFORMANCE		
Information	9	(37 %ile)	Picture Completion	6	(9 %ile)
Digit Span	10	(50 %ile)	Picture Arrangement	7	(16 %ile)
Vocabulary	11	(63 %ile)	Block Design	6	(9 %ile)
Arithmetic	8	(25 %ile)	Object Assembly	9	(37 %ile)
Comprehension	12	(75 %ile)	Digit Symbol	6	(9 %ile)
Similarities	2	(4 %ile)			
VERBAL IQ =	93	(32 %ile)	PERFORMANCE IQ =	80	(9 %ile)

FULL SCALE IQ = 87 (19 %ile)

III. Attention/Concentration
Digit Span: 7 forward + 4 backwards = 11 Total (50 %ile)
Mental Control, WMS: 5 (29 %ile)
Trails A: 94 " (<1 %ile), Trails B: 200" (<1 %ile)

IV. Language
Boston Naming Test: 43/60
Controlled Word Association: F (13) + A (11) + S (18) + Age Corr.= 49 (85-89 %ile)

V. Perceptual/Organizational
Rey-Osterrieth Complex Figure Copy: 28.5 /36 (<10 %ile)

VI. Memory

VERBAL		NONVERBAL	
WMS Logical Memory	5.5 (26%ile)	WMS Visual Repro.:	2 (14 %ile)
30 min. delay:	0	30 min. delay:	1
		Percent retention:	50

WMS Associate Learning
I Easy 6 , 3 , 6
I Hard 0 , 1 , 0
I Score: 8.5 (22 %ile)

Shopping List Test (10 items):
T1: 3 T2: 6 T3: 5 T4: 6 T5: 5   5-min. Delayed Recall: 4
Recognition: 9 Hits, 1 False Identifications

VII. Motor Exam

	Dominant Hand	%ile	Nondom. Hand	%ile
Finger Tapping:	46.8	79	40.4	57

VIII. Frontal Systems
Stroop A: 49", Stroop B: 89", Stroop C: 165"
Wisconsin Card Sorting Test: 0 Categories

Case 2: Documented Intellectual Decline Following Chronic Alcohol Abuse: A Probable Alcohol Dementia

Presenting Situation and Reason for Referral

Mr. M.F. presents as a 60-year-old, right-handed, black male with a ninth-grade education who has worked as a truck driver and cook for most of his life. He was referred for neuropsychological assessment to rule out an amnestic syndrome secondary to several decades of chronic alcohol abuse. For the past five years, the patient has resided in a nursing home because of memory difficulties and an inability to control his drinking on his own. His length of alcohol abuse spans some four decades, though he has reportedly not drunk alcohol since entering the nursing home five years ago. Past medical history is noncontributory, though he does have a history of one prior psychiatric admission five years ago when initially placed in the nursing home because of alcohol abuse and memory problems. At that time, he was given brief psychological testing, including an intelligence test (WAIS). Laboratory findings (including CT and EEG) were essentially within normal limits except for mild cortical atrophy on CT scan. The patient reports no prior history of neurologic injury and currently is taking no medications.

Behavioral Observations

Mr. F. appeared as a reasonably pleasant but quiet individual who participated in the testing in a compliant manner. His affect appeared blunted and mood was euthymic with no complaints of depression. There was no evidence of psychomotor retardation. The patient seemed generally indifferent to his performance on the testing, and when he encountered difficulties on the tests, he seemed mildly aware of these difficulties but not concerned by them. The test results are believed to be an accurate estimate of the patient's current level of cognitive functioning.

Tests Administered

See data summary sheet.

Test Results

Gross Cognitive Functioning

Mr. F. obtained a score of 20/30 on the Mini-Mental State Exam, indicating mild impairment of gross cognitive functioning. He made errors on five of 10 orientation items, and two of five serial 7 subtractions. In addition, he recalled only one of three words following a short delay and incorrectly reproduced two intersecting pentagons.

Intelligence

On the WAIS-R, Mr. F. obtained a Verbal IQ of 82, a Performance IQ of 80, and a Full Scale IQ of 80, placing him in the low average range of intellectual functioning overall. Within the verbal domain, the patient consistently performed within the low average to average range on every subtest except for a very poor performance (0 raw score points) on a test of abstract thinking and ability to conceptualize the relationship between two related items (Similarities subtest). Within the nonverbal domain, the patient performed in the low average range on all tests except for an average performance on a test assessing the patient's attention to visual details (Picture Completion).

We are fortunate to have test data on this patient from five years ago, using the non-revised WAIS. It must be noted that there is an expected eight-point discrepancy between WAIS and WAIS-R Full Scale IQ scores, favoring the WAIS. Comparison of this patient's performance reveals a 21-point decline from the WAIS to WAIS-R Full Scale IQ scores. If the eight-point discrepancy is taken into account, the decline appears to actually be 13 points overall, indicating a marginally significant decline in overall intellectual/cognitive abilities over the last five years.

Attention and Concentration

Mr. F. was able to repeat six digits forward and three backwards (Digit Span), placing him in the low average range. He performed rapidly and without error on a mental control task requiring such rote skills as counting backwards from 20, reciting the alphabet, and counting forward by 3s (WMS–Mental Control). However, when given a visual scanning and tracking task, the patient performed below the first percentile (Trails A) and he was unable to perform the more complex portion of the task (Trails B), which requires cognitive flexibility and alternation. Thus, no deficits were noted in simple selective attention abilities, but speed of performance was notably slow on a task of visual scanning and tracking, and the patient was entirely unable to complete a divided attention task (Trails B) involving alternation between tasks.

Language

Mr. F.'s spontaneous speech was fluent and meaningful. Gross assessment of comprehension and repetition were intact, though a mildly depressed score was present on a confrontational naming task (Boston Naming Test). However, this score must be interpreted with caution given the patient's limited educational background. In contrast, word list generation (FAS) was in the superior range. Thus, no clear language abnormalities were evident except for a possible mild naming deficit, although, again, it is possible that his performance was artifactually lowered due to his lowered education level and lack of familiarity with some of the pictured items.

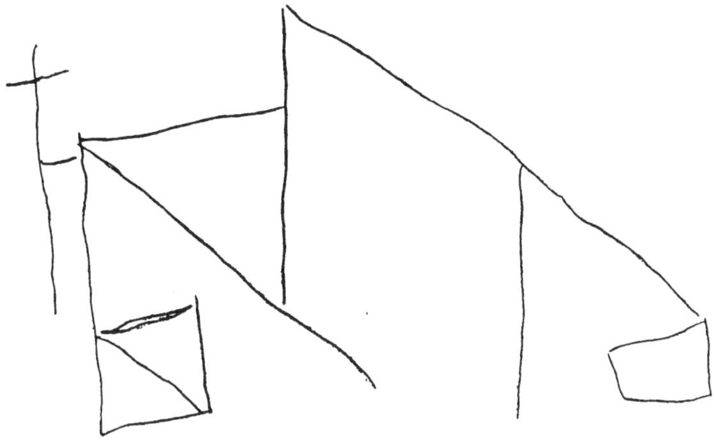

FIGURE 6.1. Case M.F. Rey-Osterrieth Complex Figure: copy. Reduced by 50%.

Visuo-Spatial

Mr. F. performed well below the 10th percentile in his copy reproduction of a complex two-dimensional figure (Rey-Osterrieth, see Fig. 6.1) and his construction was notably incomplete. He scored in the low average range (9th percentile) in his construction of red and white blocks to match a design (Block Design), and in the low average range in his construction of puzzle pieces to form a familiar object (Object Assembly). Thus, low average to impaired performance was evident on visuo-spatial construction tasks.

Learning and Memory

The patient performed in the second percentile in his immediate recall of conversational prose passages (WMS–Logical Memory), and following a 30-minute delay, he was unable to recall any of the material originally learned. When presented with related and unrelated word pairs (WMS–Associate Learning), he was able to learn all six of the easy word pairs by the third learning trial but was never able to learn any of the four unrelated word pairs over the three presentations. On a serial list learning task of 15 unrelated words (AVLT) presented over five trials, the patient did not evidence a learning curve, recalling only five of the 15 words by the fifth trial. Following an interference trial, the patient could recall all five words earlier learned, but after a 15-minute delay, he could recall only one of the words and provided four intrusion responses. Assessment of recognition memory revealed clear deficits; he gave 12 correct identifications in conjunction with eight false-positive responses. This implies clear deficits in both encoding, storage, and retrieval mechanisms.

Assessment of nonverbal memory also reveals deficits, though this is difficult to conclusively conclude given the patient's constructional deficit described

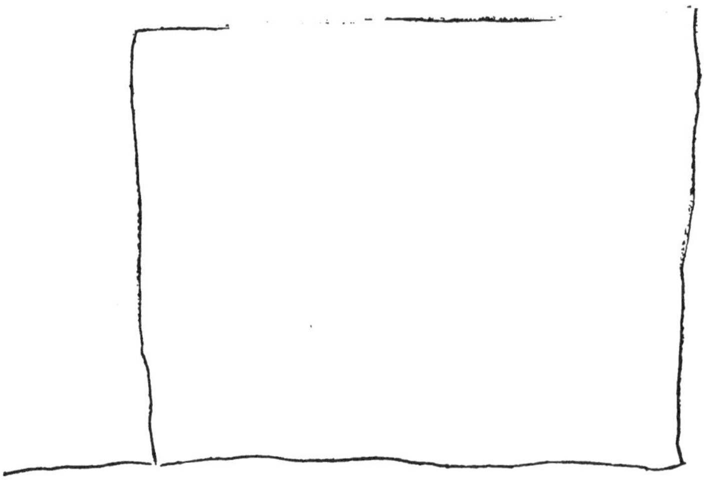

FIGURE 6.2. Case M.F. Rey-Osterrieth Complex Figure: delayed recall. Reduced by 20%.

above. He performed in the low average range in his immediate recall reproduction of simple line drawings (WMS–Visual Reproduction), and following a 30-minute delay, he could recall none of the information presented him earlier. Also, following a 3-minute delay, the patient was virtually unable to reproduce any elements, besides the borders, of a complex figure he was asked to copy earlier (Figure 6.2). These results reveal impairment in both initial encoding and storage and retrieval mechanisms of both verbal and nonverbal material.

"Frontal Systems" Tasks

On the Wisconsin Card Sorting Test, the patient solved no categories. The test was stopped after the first 64 cards because he became increasingly frustrated when unable to obtain correct responses—though again, interpretation of this performance must be made with caution given his age and limited education level. Of note, the patient obtained 0 raw score points on a test of abstract thinking (Similarities), revealing very concrete answers. Thus, deficits were evident on at least two tasks administered in this domain.

Personality

Personality assessment using the MMPI reveals a slightly depressed individual who is confused by the abnormalities in his thinking process. He presents also with an increase in somatic concerns. At present, it is likely that Mr. F. is mildly depressed, in addition to having the cognitive difficulties described above.

SUMMARY

Interpretation of neuropsychological test scores was rendered somewhat problematic due to the patient's low education level. Mr. F. presents as a 60-year-old, black male with low average IQ and with notable cognitive deficits in a variety of spheres. Memory evaluation reveals an inability to learn new information, confirming an anterograde amnestic process. In addition to the memory disturbance is a documented decline in overall intellectual ability from testing five years ago, in conjunction with deficits in visuo-spatial skills, abstraction ability and other "frontal systems" measures, and confrontational naming. Together, these results would appear to support the presence of a mild dementia syndrome, most probably secondary to his history of alcohol abuse. As part of this alcohol dementia, the presence of an underlying Korsakoff's disorder is also indicated.

Other factors must also be considered. The patient appears mildly depressed, and a medication evaluation is recommended. Could his depression account for the deficits described above? Results of assessment by clinical interview, MMPI, and Hamilton Depression Score (4) would argue against a severe depression. Most probably the patient is suffering from a mild depressive-adjustment reaction to his overall cognitive disturbance. Thus, depression is not a likely explanation for the overall cognitive loss and deficits noted on current testing.

Could his loss in overall intellectual abilities be from a different type of dementia syndrome? The data are not wholly consistent with a prototypic pattern typical of Alzheimer's disease, given the disproportionate memory impairment relative to intact word list generation and only a possible mild confrontational naming disturbance. Other etiologies of his dementia syndrome are not readily suggested, though of course others must be considered and ruled out by follow-up neurologic examination.

Taken together, these results appear consistent with overall cognitive loss secondary to decades of alcohol abuse in a man who once demonstrably functioned in the average range of intelligence, and are consistent with a mild alcohol dementia. On a practical level, he will continue to require supervised care because of his severe memory, visuo-spatial, and frontal systems deficits.

NEUROPSYCHOLOGY TEST SCORE SUMMARY SHEET

Patient: M.F. Age: 60 Sex: M Handedness: R

I. Gross Cognitive Functioning
Mini-Mental State Exam: 20/30

II. Intelligence WAIS-R Age-Corrected Scores

VERBAL			PERFORMANCE		
Information	8	(25 %ile)	Picture Completion	8	(25 %ile)
Digit Span	7	(16 %ile)	Picture Arrangement	6	(9 %ile)
Vocabulary	8	(25 %ile)	Block Design	6	(9 %ile)
Arithmetic	8	(25 %ile)	Object Assembly	7	(16 %ile)
Comprehension	9	(37 %ile)	Digit Symbol	6	(9 %ile)
Similarities	3	(1 %ile)			
VERBAL IQ =	82	(12 %ile)	PERFORMANCE IQ =	80	(9 %ile)

FULL SCALE IQ = 80 (9 %ile)

III. Attention/Concentration
Digit Span: 6 forward + 3 backwards = 9 Total (16 %ile)
Mental Control, WMS: 9 (88-89 %ile)
Trails A: 86" (<1 %ile), Trails B: 148" (4 %ile) with errors

IV. Language
Boston Naming Test: 48/60
Controlled Word Association: F (17) + A (11) + S (20) + Age Corr.= 57 (95 %ile)

V. Perceptual/Organizational
Rey-Osterrieth Complex Figure Copy: 9 /36 (<10 %ile)

VI. Memory

VERBAL		NONVERBAL	
WMS Logical Memory	1.5 (2%ile)	WMS Visual Repro.:	2 (14 %ile)
30 min. delay:	0	30 min. delay:	0

WMS Associate Learning
I Easy 2 , 4 , 6
I Hard 0 , 0 , 0
I Score: 6 (10 %ile)

Rey Auditory Verbal Learning Test (15 items):
T1: 5 T2: 4 T3: 5 T4: 6 T5: 5 Recall after Interference 5 15-min. Delayed Recall 1
Recognition: 12 Hits, 8 False Identifications

VII. Frontal Systems
Wisconsin Card Sorting Test: 0 Categories

VIII. Personality
MMPI: 8*5"21'9037-64/F"L-K/
Hamilton Depression Score: 4

Case 3: Korsakoff's Syndrome

SIGNIFICANT HISTORY

Mr. K.B. is a 50-year-old, right-handed, Caucasian male of slender frame who was referred for neuropsychological evaluation to rule out an amnestic disorder. Recently, the patient's wife called the neurology clinic and expressed concern over her husband's recent memory deficits, citing incidents in which her husband has turned on stove gas burners and forgotten about them. The patient admitted to a "poor memory" but added, "I never had a good memory."

Mr. B.'s history is noteworthy for a 35-year history of heavy alcohol abuse, involving ingestion of approximately 12 beers per day. According to Ms. B., he has not had any alcohol for the past 12 months. At that time (one year ago) he was seen in the emergency room because of repeated episodes of vomiting. He returned to the emergency room a week later with complaints of confusion, incoherent speech, and gait disturbance. He was admitted with a diagnosis of Wernicke's encephalopathy.

Mr. B.'s medical history is notable for a 20-year history of hypertension. He had a left carotid body tumor removed two years ago, followed by damage to the ninth cranial nerve and intermittent left eyelid drooping. His family history is remarkable for alcohol abuse in his father, mother, and uncle. The patient's father died in his 60s with hypertension and heart disease.

The patient was born in France, where he lived until his 19th birthday when he and his family immigrated to America. Though the patient is a native speaker of French, he quickly became conversant in English and even served as a translator during his tour of service in the U.S. Army. Mr. B. has two years of college education and was employed as a stock clerk since his military discharge. The patient has been unemployed for the past year because he has been unable to work in light of his memory difficulties.

BEHAVIORAL OBSERVATIONS

Mr. B. was enthusiastically cooperative during the four-hour testing session. He stated that the tasks were interesting and novel to him. The patient's speech was fluent and remarkable for a French accent. His mood and affect were appropriate to the testing situation. During a conjoint interview, Mr. B.'s wife appeared supportive and concerned about her husband's welfare, and was cooperative in relating information about her husband's biographic history. Overall, the results are believed to be an accurate reflection of the patient's current level of cognitive functioning.

TESTS ADMINISTERED

See data summary sheet.

Test Results

Gross Cognitive Functioning

Mr. B.'s performance on the Mini-Mental State Exam yielded a score of 26/30. He accurately recalled only one of three words following a short delay and made two errors in a series of five consecutive serial 7 subtraction tasks. These results suggest intact gross cognitive functioning.

Attention and Concentration

The patient's performance on tasks measuring attention and concentration was variable, ranging from average to impaired levels of functioning. He was able to accurately repeat six digits forward and four backwards (Digit Span), a performance falling at the 25th percentile. On the Arithmetic subtest of the WAIS-R, a subtest heavily tapping attentional abilities, the patient also performed at the 25th percentile. However, on the Mental Control portion of the Wechsler Memory Scale, a measure sensitive to attentional processes, the patient performed below the first percentile. His performance was adversely affected by delayed response times and multiple errors, particularly on a task requiring him to count forward by 3s.

Intelligence

Intellectual assessment using the WAIS-R yields a Verbal IQ of 94, a Performance IQ of 91, and a Full Scale IQ of 92, placing him in the average range of intellectual ability. Based upon his educational and vocational history, these findings are generally consistent with expected levels of functioning and are not believed to represent significant decline from estimated premorbid levels. On the nonverbal portion of the WAIS-R, the patient's performance was marked by wide scatter among the subtests. Mr. B.'s performance on tasks measuring visuo-spatial ability and rapid graphomotor tracking showed greatest compromise compared to performance on other nonverbal measures. The patient's performance on a more pure measure of visuo-spatial ability and speed of performance (Block Design) was marked by distortions in many of his constructions. On two of the five trials, he failed to maintain the 2×2 or 3×3 matrix necessary to complete the task. Verbal abilities were all within the average range, with slightly better performance evident on tasks assessing long-held cultural information and fund of vocabulary.

In sum, Mr. B.'s current level of intellectual functioning falls in the average range and most likely does not represent an appreciable decline from expected premorbid levels. Specific measures of nonverbal intellectual functioning were adversely affected by the patient's difficulties in visuo-spatial processing.

Language

Mr. B.'s spontaneous speech was fluent and unremarkable except for a mild French accent. On formal screening, he was able to repeat a sentence, follow a three-step command, write a spontaneous sentence, and read simple material. On a test of confrontational naming (Boston Naming Test), however, the patient performed in the low average to borderline range (BNT = 47/60), though his score could have been lowered by his not being a native English speaker. The patient's score on a task of verbal fluency (FAS) fell below the fourth percentile (FAS = 13). Despite his impoverished performance on this task of word list generation, the words given were reflective of an average fund of vocabulary, such as "sociology," "scholar," and "Fahrenheit."

These results suggest a disturbance in language functioning characterized by a possible mild word-finding disturbance and decreased word list generation. An important factor to consider in relation to this performance is that Mr. B. is not a native speaker of English. However, that he was an interpreter in the military and that he performed well on an English vocabulary measure argue against this as accounting in large part for the deficits described above.

Perceptual Organizational Abilities

On a task that taps visual perception and alertness to visual details (Picture Completion subtest), the patient performed in the superior range (91st percentile). He scored in the average range (50th percentile) on a task of logical visual sequencing (Picture Arrangement). On a visuo-constructional task (Object Assembly subtest), Mr. B. performed in the average range (37th percentile). His performance on another measure of visuo-constructive ability (Block Design) placed him in the borderline range (5th percentile) and was marked by his failure to maintain the 2 × 2 or 3 × 3 matrix on two of five trials. Mr. B.'s copy of a complex two-dimensional figure was in the average range (Rey-Osterrieth = 25th percentile). Thus, variable performance was evident in this domain, with performance ranging from superior to borderline levels.

Verbal and Nonverbal Learning and Memory

On the AVLT, a test tapping verbal/auditory memory processes, the patient was able to recall only five of the 15 items by the fifth learning trial and no learning curve was noted. Following an interference task, the patient was unable to recall any of the previously learned items, although he was able to recognize five of the 15 items with no false positives from a paragraph read to him. Mr. B.'s memory for logical prose was examined by having him recall paragraphs read to him (WMS–Logical Memory). His performance fell at the third percentile for immediate recall of the verbal information. Following a 30-minute delay, Mr. B. was unable to recall any of the previously learned verbal material. On the Boston

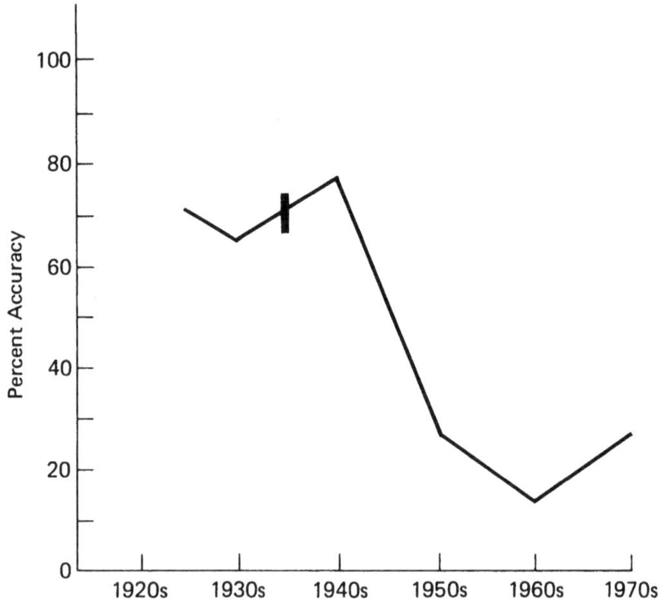

FIGURE 6.3. Case K.B. Boston Remote Battery–Recognition Test. Heavy line indicates patient's date of birth.

Remote Memory Battery, a task tapping remote memory across decades, the patient's performance yielded a substantial temporal gradient on several of the subtests, and his performance overall was depressed compared to a normative population (Figure 6.3). It should be noted that a recognition format was utilized for the Famous Faces and Recall subtests because of the patient's naming deficit.

Mr. B.'s performance on an immediate recall nonverbal memory measure fell in the low average range (WMS–Visual Reproduction, 9th percentile). Following a 30-minute delay, he was unable to recall any of the previously learned information. On the multiple-choice format of a nonverbal memory measure (Benton Visual Form Recognition Test), the patient was able to accurately recognize five of the 16 designs, a performance at chance levels (there are four multiple choices for each of the 16 designs). The patient performed in the impaired range in his recall following a 3-minute delay of the Rey-Osterrieth Complex figure.

In summary, these results indicate marked impairment for immediate and delayed recall of both verbal and nonverbal material, with more remote memories better preserved than more recent material.

Motor

Mr. B.'s motor abilities were assessed using the Finger Tapping Test. The patient's performance in this task is within normal limits bilaterally compared to

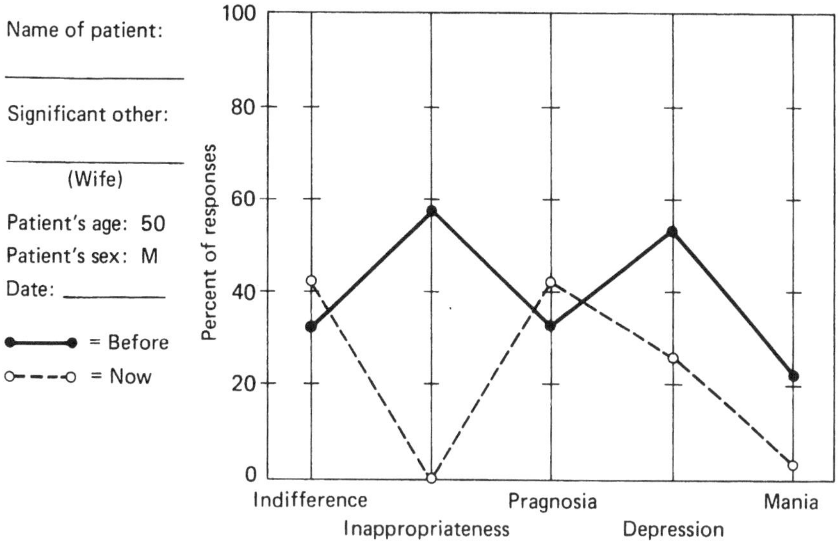

FIGURE 6.4. Case K.B. Neuropsychology Behavior and Affect Profile. The term *pragnosia* was coined to describe a deficit in linguistic pragmatic ability. Copyright 1985 by Satz, Van Gorp, Lewis, and Van Lancker. All rights reserved. Reprinted by permission.

persons in his age group (R = 40.8; L = 34.6), and the dominant to nondominant superiority is consistent with expected limits.

Personality

The patient's present and past personality functioning was assessed using the UCLA Neuropsychology Behavior and Affect Profile (Nelson, Satz, & Mitrushina, 1988) (Figure 6.4), which was completed by his wife. Scales measuring depression, mania, and inappropriateness reflect the most notable changes, with scores on all three scales *lower* now than before his illness. Thus, it seems that Mr. B. has become less depressed and energetic since his illness, with a greater appropriateness in his behavior as assessed by his wife. Perhaps these changes are related to the patient's abstinence from alcohol for the past 12 months.

Summary and Impressions

Neuropsychological test findings are consistent with an alcoholic Korsakoff's syndrome. Results indicate marked impairment for immediate and delayed recall of verbal and nonverbal information, and his recognition memory abilities are also depressed compared to persons in his age group. Testing of the patient's remote memory reveals a temporal gradient with distant memories appearing more spared than recent memories. Overall, the neuropsychological picture is characterized by a marked anterograde and retrograde amnesia, the latter characterized by a temporal gradient.

These findings are not consistent with an alcohol dementia. Intellectual functioning appears largely intact (average range), and although his visuo-spatial deficits are variable, most are generally within expected levels for his intellectual level.

We are perplexed regarding the marked decrement in verbal fluency and milder yet significant deficits in confrontational naming, especially in view of his intact vocabulary performance. Perhaps his not being a native English speaker can account for some of these deficits. Frontal systems involvement is frequently suggested in the alcoholic syndrome and could be causal in the depressed verbal fluency, but this would not account for the naming deficit. It is also possible that these language results represent the effects of the left carotid body tumor, though this is unknown at this time. Additionally, given the patient's 20-year history of hypertension, a vascular etiology contributing to his deficits must also be considered.

On a practical level, we are concerned about Mr. B.'s ability to care for himself in light of his memory disturbance, and we believe he would function best in a structured environment where he would have assistance with activities of daily living.

There may be some additional recovery of cognitive functioning if Mr. B. continues to abstain from alcohol, though most probably, most of the recovery he will achieve following cessation of drinking has already occurred.

Reassessment in six to 12 months may be helpful in clarifying whether any recovery or further decline in cognitive functioning occurs.

NEUROPSYCHOLOGY TEST SCORE SUMMARY SHEET

Patient: K.B. Age: 50 Sex: M Handedness: R

I. Gross Cognitive Functioning
Mini-Mental State Exam: 26/30

II. Intelligence WAIS-R Age-Corrected Scores

VERBAL			PERFORMANCE		
Information	11	(63 %ile)	Picture Completion	14	(91 %ile)
Digit Span	8	(25 %ile)	Picture Arrangement	10	(50 %ile)
Vocabulary	12	(75 %ile)	Block Design	5	(5 %ile)
Arithmetic	8	(25 %ile)	Object Assembly	9	(37 %ile)
Comprehension	8	(25 %ile)	Digit Symbol	6	(9 %ile)
Similarities	11	(63 %ile)			
VERBAL IQ =	94	(34 %ile)	PERFORMANCE IQ =	91	(27 %ile)

FULL SCALE IQ = 92 (30 %ile)

III. Attention/Concentration
Digit Span: 6 forward + 4 backwards = 10 Total (25 %ile)
Mental Control, WMS: 2 (1 %ile)

IV. Language
Boston Naming Test: 47/60
Controlled Word Association: F (4) + A (2) + S (7) + Age Corr.= 17 (<4 %ile)

V. Perceptual/Organizational
Rey-Osterrieth Complex Figure Copy: 30.5 /36 (25 %ile)

VI. Memory

VERBAL		NONVERBAL	
WMS Logical Memory	3.25 (3 %ile)	WMS Visual Repro.:	4 (9 %ile)
30 min. delay:	0	30 min. delay:	0
		Rey-Osterrieth Fig:	30.5 (20 %ile)
		3 min. delay:	8 (<1 %ile)

Rey Auditory Verbal Learning Test (15 items):
T1:4 T2:5 T3:5 T4:4 T5:5 Recall after Interference: 0
Recognition: 5 Hits, 0 False Identifications

Benton Visual Form Recognition Test: 5/16 with 5 PE, 5 MR, 1 MD

Boston Remote Memory Battery: see text

VII. Motor Exam

	Dominant Hand	%ile	Nondom. Hand	%ile
Finger Tapping:	40.8	37	34.6	20

VII. Personality
Neuropsychology Behavior and Affect Profile: see text

Commentary on Alcohol-Abuse Cases

Together, these cases represent common findings in a collection of chronic alcohol abusers. Case 1 represents the prototypic findings in chronic alcohol abusers in the middle to latter stages of chronic alcoholism: the dramatic deficits in nonverbal, perceptual/organizational, and memory abilities oftentimes seen in this group.

Case 2 was intriguing in demonstrating a dementia syndrome with a documented decrease from a prior level of functioning. Though it is possible that his dementia could have resulted from other etiologies (such as multi-infarct dementia), there were no risk factors or other medical/neurologic abnormalities apparent on physical examination or lab studies to immediately suggest an alternate etiology. Therefore, though neuroradiographic studies would be appropriate to rule out another etiology (such as stroke or tumor), the most likely etiology is a dementia secondary to chronic alcohol abuse. A diagnosis of Alzheimer's disease is certainly possible, though the relative sparing of language functions makes this somewhat less likely. It is unknown why some chronic alcoholics are more vulnerable to eventual global cognitive decline whereas others, despite roughly similar histories of alcohol abuse, retain more modest deficits. Also unclear is why some alcoholics who admittedly undergo nutritional deficiencies sustain KD, and others, who may well undergo similar deficiencies, do not. More research remains to be done.

Finally, Case 3 illustrates well the prototypic pattern of deficits seen in KD. Though Mr. B. retained overall intact intellectual functioning, his severe anterograde memory disturbance illustrates the disproportionate memory impairment in patients with KD. The temporal gradient evident on Albert's Remote Memory Battery also is typical of that found in KD patients.

Thus, the three patients presented in this chapter may be considered "prototypic" of those in the middle and latter stages of alcohol abuse. We might have selected more representative cases by selecting those with multiple processes, such as (as is perhaps most common) those with one or more head injuries, and those with a concurrent psychiatric history (e.g., schizophrenia or severe depression). Though these reflect "real cases" that commonly are seen with long histories of alcohol abuse, we felt that it would not be clear to the reader what the effects of the alcohol abuse might be and what could be attributable to the effects of the co-condition, such as head injury or schizophrenia. Thus, our cases are perhaps less representative of a broad cross-section of alcoholics at large, but they illustrate well the deficits than can result from alcohol abuse itself.

7
Adult Presentation of Learning Disorders

There is a growing body of evidence indicating that childhood learning disorders tend to persist through adolescence and adulthood (Dykman, Peters, & Ackerman, 1973; Gottesman, Belmont, & Kaminer, 1975; Kline, 1972; Muehl and Forell, 1973; Rourke, Young, Strang, & Russell, 1986; Sarazin & Spreen, 1986). Accordingly, there is little support for the maturation hypothesis, which posits that children tend to outgrow learning problems manifested in childhood. Disorders of learning are referred in the literature by a multiplicity of terms such as learning disability, Attention Deficit Disorder (ADD), Minimal Brain Dysfunction (MBD), and dyslexia. Unfortunately, individuals with often quite disparate learning-related disorders are grouped together. Most researchers and clinicians agree that there is a strong need to retire the general term of "learning disabilities" that is often used to describe a heterogeneous group of individuals manifesting distinct disorders. Rather, more attention should be directed toward identifying the specific attributes of the individual's learning problem.

The American Psychiatric Association's Diagnostic and Statistical Manual III–Revised (DSM-III-R) refers to learning disabilities as Specific Developmental Disorders characterized by "inadequate development of specific academic, language, speech, and motor skills and that are not due to demonstrable physical or neurologic disorders, a Pervasive Developmental Disorder, Mental Retardation, or deficient educational opportunities" (DSM-III-R, 1987, pp. 39–42). Within the subclass of specific Developmental Disorders are Developmental Arithmetic Disorder, Developmental Expressive Writing Disorder, Developmental Reading Disorder (e.g., dyslexia), Developmental Articulation Disorder, Developmental Expressive Language Disorder, Developmental Receptive Language Disorder, and Developmental Coordination Disorder. Attention-deficit Hyperactivity Disorders are also tied to learning problems and are grouped under the subclass of Disruptive Behavior Disorders, defined as "developmentally inappropriate degrees of inattention, impulsiveness, and hyperactivity." The age at onset of each disorder is usually below seven years. Thus, the diagnosis of learning disability in adulthood relies on a retrospective assessment in childhood.

Although distinct terms for specific learning disabilities are available, the literature often refers to subgroups interchangeably. This introduction will cover the research findings relating to individuals with various types of learning disabilities.

Differential Diagnosis

In adults it is important to differentiate between acquired brain damage and developmental disability usually present since the perinatal period. To help make this determination, it is useful for the clinician to conduct an in-depth interview and ascertain historical information regarding the patient and his or her family. If the symptoms are tied largely to acquired brain damage, one may find a history of head injury, stroke, drug or alcohol abuse, seizures, cerebral infection, chemical exposure, or other types of acquired brain dysfunction. It is quite possible for an acquired lesion to coexist with a preexisting learning disability, but the pattern of neuropsychological functioning will usually clue the clinician regarding this event because brain-injured patients typically present with more severe deficits than the learning disabled (see below).

If the adult manifestation of learning deficits rests on enduring traits from childhood, reports of childhood learning disability are expected. The clinician should ascertain information regarding the patient's childhood history, including pre- and perinatal events. The clinician should also identify possible history of academic problems involving math, reading, writing, or language. Also, there may be reports of clumsiness and problems with coordination and balance. Signs of attention deficit disorder (ADD) with hyperactivity including impulsivity, inattention, and hyperactive behavior may have been present. Children with ADD and accompanying hyperactivity are often described as having a short attention span and difficulty staying on task, and are distractible, careless, restless, and disorganized. History of prescription of a stimulant medication, such as Ritalin, in childhood may clue the clinician to an hyperactive state that may have accompanied ADD. Onset of the childhood disorder is usually by age 3 but often is not diagnosed until the child enters the school system. ADD is often associated with nonlocalized "soft" neurologic signs, visual motor dysfunction, and EEG abnormalities. The disorder is more prevalent among males than females (4:1 ratio) and has a familial basis. The etiology is not well understood, although it has been tied to central nervous system dysfunction.

Another important differential is between learning disorders and personality disorders. The adult with a residual learning disorder may present with increased emotional problems (Eisenberg, 1966; Gaddes, 1976; Gates, 1968; Herjanic & Penick, 1972; Kline, 1972) and is sometimes diagnosed with Borderline Personality Disorder or an affective disorder, without consideration of a residual learning disorder.

Adult Presentation

Follow-up studies of children with learning disabilities have addressed occupational and emotional outcome, social adjustment, academic achievement, socioeconomic status, and specific cognitive deficits. Unfortunately, the conclusions are limited in that there are few systematic studies on this topic (for a review, see Horn, O'Donnell, & Vitulano, 1983; Schonhaut & Satz, 1983). The available literature, however, strongly indicates that at least a subset of the individuals who are learning disabled during childhood remain so through adulthood (Andrulis & Alio, 1976; Birely & Manley, 1980; Frauenheim, 1978; Kahn, 1980; Rourke et al., 1986; Sarazin & Spreen, 1986; Spreen & Haaf, 1986). In general, learning disability is not always outgrown over time but rather may lead to problems in fulfilling educational and vocational goals. Even when they do not pose a threat to adult success, childhood learning disorders are infrequently fully overcome (Schonhaut & Satz, 1983). Overall, the prognosis is not a positive one as Spreen (1982) points out:

> Most children who are referred to a clinic for a learning or reading disability do not catch up. In fact, their disability is likely to become worse over time. In addition, remedial instruction has in general not been shown to improve the prognosis for these children. (p. 483)

Sarazin and Spreen (1986) conducted one of the more carefully controlled studies on the long-term follow-up of learning-disabled children to measure the adult consequences. They studied the neuropsychological performance of 175 subjects diagnosed with learning disability, brain damage, and minimal brain damage in childhood. Performance was assessed between the ages of 8 and 12 and again between 9 and 17 years later using essentially the same battery of standardized tests, including the Wechsler Intelligence Scale and the Wide Range Achievement Test. Their results convincingly supported the persistence of learning deficits from childhood to young adulthood.

Although academic problems usually endure (Dykman et al., 1973; Gottesman et al., 1975; Kline, 1972; Muehl & Forell, 1973; Rourke & Orr, 1977; Rourke et al., 1986; Rutter, Tizard, Yule, Graham, & Whitmore, 1976; Satz, Taylor, Friel & Fletcher, 1978; Trites & Fiedorowicz, 1976), they are often attenuated by subject-moderator variables such as socioeconomic status and intellectual level. Individuals with above average intellectual levels generally are more successful in terms of finishing school and/or in attaining satisfying employment. An 18- to 35-year follow-up investigation of dyslexic, average, and superior readers conducted by Rawson (1968) highlights this point. Subjects were first seen between the ages of 6 to 8 years and were later interviewed between 26 and 40 years of age. Her sample consisted of exceedingly bright children (Mean Binet IQ = 130) from upper-class and upper-middle-class families. The results indicate a good prognosis in that 18 of the 20 dyslexics graduated from college with no significant differences between dyslexics and nondyslexics on years of education or adult socioeconomic status. This study differs from other research relying on data from reading or other learning-disabled individuals with average to low average intellect and middle-class socioeconomic status, which generally show a less favorable outcome. The literature indicates that children with learning disorders generally tend to drop out of school (Herjanic & Penick, 1972; Kline, 1972; Satz et al., 1978) and are apt to end up in lower socioeconomic occupations (Eisenberg, 1966).

General Cognitive Pattern of Learning Disorders in Adults

The overall cognitive profile for learning disorders in adults is similar to that seen in children (McCue, Shelley, & Goldstein, 1986; Buchanan & Wolf, 1986; Horn et al., 1983). In general, adults with learning disorders present with at least average intelligence, lower academic achievement scores relative to IQ and grade expectations, and selected cognitive deficits (McCue et al., 1986; O'Donnell, Kurtz, & Ramanaiah, 1983). They may also present with a lower Verbal IQ relative to Performance IQ. The neuropsychological deficits tend to be mild; learning-disabled individuals are usually less impaired than brain-damaged individuals but more so than normals (O'Donnell et al., 1983; Sarazin & Spreen, 1986). Academic problems are usually not limited to one subject area (Dykman et al., 1973; Rourke & Orr, 1977; Rutter et al., 1976; Satz et al., 1978; Spreen & Haaf, 1986; Trites & Fiederowicz, 1976).

Learning disabilities are not a homogeneous population (Benton & Pearl, 1978) but rather consist of various subtypes. Much of the research conducted in childhood learning disorders in recent years has focused on the identification of subtypes (Bakker, 1979; Boder, 1970; Denckla, 1977; Doehring & Hoshko, 1977; Fisk & Rourke, 1979; Lyon & Watson, 1981; Marshall & Newcombe, 1973; Mattis, French, & Rapin, 1975; Rourke & Orr, 1977; Satz & Morris, 1981).

An important issue is whether learning disability subtypes identified in childhood persist into adulthood. In a longitudinal study addressing this issue, Spreen and Haaf (1986) evaluated test performance of two groups of learning-disabled children and a matched control group in childhood, and again in adulthood. The subjects were administered a battery of neuropsychological and achievement tests—including the Wechsler Intelligence Scale, the Wide Range Achievement Test, the Peabody Individual Achievement Test, Sentence Repetition, Word Fluency, Purdue Pegboard, and the Halstead Category Test—initially at a mean age of 10 years and again at a mean age of 24 years. The results were cluster analyzed to assess for the persistence of subtypes into the adult years. Findings indicated that subjects could be grouped into generally impaired, specifically reading impaired, and specifically arithmetic impaired subtypes. Overall, visuospatial, reading, and arithmetic impairments that surfaced in childhood were likely to continue into adulthood. However, linguistic problems that were found in childhood were unlikely to persist into adulthood. In general, tracing individuals from childhood into their adult years revealed a moderate degree of persistence in terms of their subtypes.

Another study reported by McCue, Goldstein, Shelly, and Katz (1986) also attempted to determine if patterns of learning disability subtypes identified in children would be present in adulthood. Their results corroborate those of Spreen and Haaf (1986). Small groups of specific subtypes were identified: some groups did well at reading but poorly at arithmetic; others did poorly at reading but relatively better, though not normally, at arithmetic. Neuropsychological testing of the former group revealed difficulties in visuo-spatial, nonverbal problem-solving and complex psycho-motor tasks, while the latter group performed better on those tasks but more poorly on linguistic measures.

It should also be recognized that many learning-disabled individuals, particularly those with above average intellectual level, are able to develop and/or use cognitive strategies to help compensate for their deficits. The fact that some learning-disabled individuals are able to attain education levels and vocation status commensurate with normal learners provides some support that learning-disabled individuals are able to effectively use compensatory strategies.

Specific Neuropsychological Functioning

Learning-disabled individuals can be differentiated from brain-damaged and normal subjects in terms of their neuropsychological profiles. In general, the neuropsychological performance of learning-disabled individuals is less impaired than that of brain-damaged patients but more so than that of normal learners (O'Donnell et al., 1983; Sarazin & Spreen, 1986). O'Donnell and colleagues (1983) compared 60 learning-disabled adults, 20 brain-damaged adult victims of head trauma, and 30 normal college student volunteers in terms of their performance on the Halstead-Reitan Battery. Their results showed that all tests in the battery yielded significant differences between the normal and brain-damaged groups and between the learning-disabled and brain-damaged groups. They found that, despite roughly equivalent intellectual levels between the learning disabled and the normals, all of the Halstead-Reitan tests except the Tactual Performance Test–Memory component, the Finger Tapping Test, and the Trail Making Test (Part A) significantly differentiated the two groups.

On the other hand, a different pattern of findings was reported by McCue, Shelly, and Goldstein (1986). They provided neuropsychological performance data on intellectual and academic testing of 100 learning-disabled adults. Despite the fact that all subjects were in the low average range of intelligence, performance was below expectation on selected cognitive measures. They found mild impairment most frequently on the sample's performance on the Tactual Performance Test, Finger Tapping Test, Speech Perception, and Rhythm Test of the Halstead-Reitan Battery. The difference between these results and those reported above by O'Donnell and colleagues (1983) may reflect methodological differences between the two studies, including differences in sample selection.

Summary

The literature supports the view that learning disorders tend to persist into adulthood. The general cognitive profile for a learning-disabled adult is similar to that of a learning-disabled child. For example, the learning-disabled adult will frequently present with: at least average intellectual level, significantly lower academic achievement scores relative to IQ and grade expectation, and selected cognitive deficits. In light of such findings, neuropsychological evaluation of patients suspected of a learning disability should include administration of tests designed to measure academic achievement functioning, such as the Wide Range Achievement Test–Revised (WRAT-R) and the Peabody Picture Vocabulary Test–Revised (PPVT-R). These tests should be incorporated into the core battery of neuropsychological tests to assess whether the patient's academic achievement functioning is at a level consistent with intellectual functioning.

References

Andrulis, R.S., & Alio, J.P.(1976). Primary investigation into learning disabilities in adults. American Psychological Association. Paper presented at the Annual Convention in Washington, D.C.

American Psychiatric Association (1987). Diagnostic and Statistical Manual of Mental Disorders (3rd ed.-Revised). Washington, D.C.: Author.

Bakker, D.J. (1979). Hemispheric differences and reading strategies: Two Dyslexias? *Bulletin of the Orton Society, 29*, 84–100.

Benton, A.L., Pearl, D. (1978). *Dyslexia: An appraisal of current knowledge*. New York: Oxford University Press.

Birely, M., & Manley, E. (1980). The learning disabled student in a college environment: A report of State University's Program. *Journal of Learning Disabilities, 13*, 12–15.

Boder, E. (1970). Developmental dyslexia: A new diagnostic approach based on the identification of three subtypes. *Journal of School Health, 40*, 289–290.

Buchanan, M., & Wolf, J.S. (1986). A comprehensive study of learning disabled adults. *Journal of Learning Disabilities, 19*, 34–38.

Denckla, M.B. (1977). Minimal brain dysfunction and dyslexia: Beyond diagnosis by exclusion. In M.E. Blaw, I. Rapin, & M. Kinsbourne (Eds.), *Topics in child neurology*. New York: Spectrum Publications.

Doehring, D.G., & Hoshko, I.M. (1977). Classification of reading problems by the Q technique of factor analysis. *Cortex, 13*, 281–294.

Dykman, R.A., Peters, J.E., & Ackerman, P.T. (1973). Experimental approaches to the study of minimal brain dysfunction: A follow-up study. *Annals of the New York Academy of Science, 205*, 93–107.

Eisenberg, L. (1966). Reading retardation: I. Psychiatric and sociologic aspects. *Pediatrics, 37*, 352–365.

Fisk, J.L., & Rourke, B.P. (1979). Identification of subtypes of learning disabled children at three age levels: A neuropsychological, multivariate approach. *Journal of Clinical Neuropsychology, 1*, 289–310.

Frauenheim, J.G. (1978). Academic achievement characteristics of adult males who were diagnosed as dyslexic in childhood. *Journal of Learning Disabilities, 11*, 476–483.

Gaddes, W. (1976). Learning disabilities: Prevalence estimates and the need for definition. In R. Knights & D.J. Bakker (Eds.), *The neuropsychology of learning disorders: Theoretical approaches* (Proceedings of NATO Conference). Baltimore: University Park Press.

Gates, A.I. (1968). The role of personality maladjustment in reading disability. In G. Natches (Ed.), *Children with reading problems*. New York: Basic Books.

Gottesman, R., Belmont, I., & Kaminer, R. (1975). Admission and follow-up status of reading disabled children referred to a medical clinic. *Journal of Learning Disabilities, 8,* 642–650.

Herjanic, B., & Penick, E. (1972). Adult outcome of disabled child readers. *Journal of Special Education, 6,* 397–410.

Horn, W.F., O'Donnell, J.P., & Vitulano, L.A. (1983). Long-term follow-up of learning-disabled persons. *Journal of Learning Disabilities, 16,* 542–555.

Kahn, M.A. (1980). Learning problems of the secondary and junior college learning disabled student: Suggested remedies. *Journal of Learning Disabilities, 13,* 40–44.

Kline, C.L. (1972). The adolescents with learning problems: How long must they wait? *Journal of Learning Disabilities, 5,* 127–144.

Lyon, R., & Watson, B. (1981). Empirically derived subgroups of learning disabled readers: Diagnostic characteristics. *Journal of Learning Disabilities, 14,* 256–261.

Marshall, J.C., & Newcombe, F. (1973). Patterns of paralexia: A psycholinguistic approach. *Developmental Medicine and Child Neurology, 2,* 175–199.

Mattis, S., French, J., & Rapin, I. (1975). Dyslexia in children and young adults: Three independent neuropsychological syndromes. *Developmental Medicine and Child Neurology, 17,* 150–163.

McCue, M., Goldstein, G., Shelly, C., & Katz, L. (1986). Cognitive profiles of some subtypes of learning-disabled adults. *Archives of Clinical Neuropsychology, 1,* 13–23.

McCue, P.M., Shelly, C., & Goldstein, F. (1986). Intellectual, academic and neuropsychological performance levels in learning disabled adults. *Journal of Learning Disabilities, 19,* 233–236.

Muehl, S., & Forell, E.R. (1973). A follow-up study of disabled readers: Variables related to high school reading performance. *Reading Research Quarterly, 9,* 110–123.

O'Donnell, J.P., Kurtz, J., & Ramanaiah, N.V. (1983). Neuropsychological test findings for normal, learning-disabled, and brain-damaged young adults. *Journal of Consulting and Clinical Psychology, 51,* 726–729.

Rawson, M.B. (1968). *Developmental language disability: Adult accomplishments of dyslexic boys.* Baltimore, MD: The Johns Hopkins Press.

Rourke, B.P., & Orr, R.R. (1977). Prediction of the reading and spelling performances of normal and retarded readers: A four-year follow-up. *Journal of Abnormal Child Psychology, 5,* 9–20.

Rourke, B.P., Young, G.C., Strang, J.D., & Russell, D.L. (1986). Adult outcomes of central processing deficiencies in childhood. In I. Grant & K.M. Adams (Eds.), *Neuropsychological assessment of neuropsychiatric disorders* (pp. 244–267). New York: Oxford University Press.

Rutter, M., Tizard, J., Yule, W., Graham, P., & Whitmore, K. (1976). Research report: Isle of Wright studies, 1964–1974. *Psychological Medicine, 6,* 313–332.

Sarazin, F.F.A., & Spreen, O. (1986). Fifteen-year stability of some neuropsychological tests in learning-disabled subjects with and without neurological impairment. *Journal of Clinical and Experimental Neuropsychology, 8,* 190–200.

Satz, P., Morris, R. (1981). Learning disability subtypes: A review. In F. Pirrozollo & J. Wittrock (Eds.), *Neuropsychological and cognitive processes in reading* (pp. 109–141). New York: Academic Press.

Satz, P., Taylor, H.G., Friel, J., & Fletcher, J.M. (1978). Some developmental and predictive precursors of reading disabilities: A six-year follow-up. In A. Benton & D. Pearl (Eds.), *Dyslexia: An appraisal of current knowledge.* New York: Oxford University Press.

Schonhaut, S., & Satz, P. (1983). Prognosis for children with learning disabilities: A review of follow-up studies. In M. Rutter (Ed.), *Developmental neuropsychiatry* (pp. 542–563). New York: The Guilford Press.
Spreen, O. (1982). Adult outcome of reading disorders. In R.N. Malatesha & P.G. Aaron (Eds.), *Reading disorders: Varieties and treatments*. New York: Academic Press.
Spreen, O., & Haaf, R.G. (1986). Empirically derived learning disability subtypes: A replication attempt and longitudinal patterns over 15 years. *Journal of Learning Disabilities, 19*, 170–180.
Trites, R.L., & Fiedorowicz, C. (1976). Follow-up study of children with specific or primary reading disability. In R.M. Knight & D.J. Bakker (Eds.), *The neuropsychology of learning disorders: Theoretical approaches*. Baltimore, MD: University Park Press.
Wender, P.H., Reimherr, F.W., Wood, D., & Ward, M. (1985). A controlled study of methylphenidate in the treatment of Attention Deficit Disorder, Residual Type, in adults. *American Journal of Psychiatry, 142*, 547–552.

Case 1: Residual Signs of a Developmental Learning Disorder

Reason for Referral

Mr. R.F. referred himself for neuropsychological evaluation in an attempt to document a learning disability. Historical information presented below was supplied by the patient.

Presenting Situation and Background Information

Mr. F. is a 25-year-old, right-handed, Caucasian male with a bachelor's of science degree in public communications from a major university. He reported a history of learning difficulties since he began school with greatest difficulty in science, spelling, and reading. Mr. F. stated that he attended Montessori-type schools (e.g., open classroom, no tests, no grades) between the third and 12th grades. He graduated from a major university three years ago with a 2.6 grade-point average and reported that he frequently obtained tutoring to assist him in his coursework.

Since college graduation, Mr. F. has repeatedly applied for admission to several graduate schools without success. He is quite motivated and hopes to cultivate a career in the motion picture industry with script writing and perceives that a graduate education could help him to obtain such work. His rationale for referring himself for a neuropsychological evaluation was to obtain documentation that he has a learning disability so that he might be eligible for special services to gain entrance to graduate school, such as an untimed version of the Graduate Record Examination.

The patient denied any past head injuries, seizures, high fevers, convulsions, or other neurological or psychological illnesses. He also denied having a history of birth trauma or developmental delay. He reported having a "bad" memory in that he tends to forget things quite rapidly. He stated that he drinks occasionally (once a month) and does not use recreational drugs or medications. Family history is negative for learning disorders and left-handedness.

Behavioral Observations

Mr. F. is a thin young man who was very casually dressed for both of the testing sessions. He appeared younger than his stated age. He seemed very relaxed and attempted to give the appearance of being unconcerned about his test performance, although he appeared to exert good effort throughout the evaluation. The results are believed to represent the patient's best efforts.

Tests Administered

See data summary sheet.

Test Results

Intelligence

Mr. F. is currently functioning overall in the average range of intelligence with a Full Scale IQ of 103, a Verbal IQ of 107, and a Performance IQ of 101. On the verbal subtests, the patient performed in the high average to very superior range on all subtests except those measuring attention abilities (Digit Span and Arithmetic), which were in the low average range. In fact, his Vocabulary score, which taps word knowledge, was in the very superior range. His Verbal IQ can be estimated to be in the high average range if the subtests associated with attentional abilities are partialled out from his score. Performance subtests were generally in the average range. He performed best on a subtest measuring visual alertness to details (Picture Completion).

Attention

As noted above, the patient exhibited difficulty on tasks measuring attention abilities. His recitation of digits forward was in the normal range (6), but digits backwards was impaired (3). This suggests that he has difficulty holding digits briefly and mentally manipulating them for verbal output. He also showed difficulty in the mental manipulation of arithmetic problem-solving (Arithmetic subtest of the WAIS-R), although this may be attributed to problems with mathematics rather than primarily in attentional processing.

Language

The patient was fluent and articulate and showed no signs of aphasia on gross screening. No evidence of language deficits emerged on formal testing. His verbal productivity, as measured by the Verbal Fluency task, was above the 95th percentile. Mr. F.'s confrontational naming was also intact as measured by the Boston Naming Test (59/60). His writing was intact for both writing to dictation and copying sentences.

Sensory/Perceptual/Motor

No impairments were observed in either sensory/perceptual or motor functioning. There was no evidence of motor slowing; finger tapping performance was within normal limits (R = 50.4, L = 48.0) and the expected right-hand dominance was found. There was no evidence of finger agnosia or problems with right-left orientation for personal or extrapersonal space. His three-dimensional drawings were performed well, and his performance on the Beery VMI revealed intact visual-graphic skills (score = 23/24 correct). Mr. F. displayed intact organizational structure of a complex figure (Rey-Osterrieth copy = 36, 100%). He also performed above average on the Street test (11/13 correct), which is a visual gestalt task of perception.

Memory

Verbal

Mr. F. performed within the average range when he was asked to immediately recall short stories as assessed with the Logical Memory subtest of the WMS (40th percentile). He was also able to retain this material normally over a 90-minute interpolated delay (88% retention). In addition, his ability to learn a list of unrelated words (AVLT) was within the average range. Over the five trials that the 15-item word list was presented, Mr. F. recalled 5, 7, 9, 10, and 13 items respectively. Following a second (distractor) word list, he was able to recall 12 of the 13 previously learned items.

Nonverbal

No impairments were found on memory tests that involve less verbally direct material and that were presented visually. Mr. F. performed in the average range (69th percentile) on a three-minute delayed recall of the Rey-Osterrieth complex figure. He also scored within normal limits on both immediate and on 90-minute delayed recall on the Visual Reproduction subtest of the WMS.

Academic Achievement

The pattern of performance found on achievement testing using the PIAT and the WRAT suggests that Mr. F. is functioning significantly below expected levels in math and spelling based on his educational attainments and intellectual functioning. Mr. F. demonstrated significant problems on tests in which he was required to generate correct spelling (WRAT Spelling subtest) as well as choose correctly spelled words from a multiple-choice array (PIAT Spelling). It appears that the patient attempts to spell words based on their phonetic sounds. His reading, although slow and labored, was intact for comprehension and recognition.

Summary and Impressions

The test results are indicative of residual signs of a developmental learning disability. Mr. F. is currently showing some of the features commonly reported in the learning disabled; that is, marked difficulty in academic achievement areas despite average intellectual functioning. The patient is functioning significantly below expected levels on both math and spelling tests, given his educational attainments, intellectual functioning, and chronological age. He is currently performing at seventh- to ninth-grade levels in these two achievement areas, significantly below expected levels for one with a B.S. degree granted by a major university. Inadequate elementary and high-school education may have contributed, in part, to his poor performance on these standard achievement tests.

There are also signs of a residual childhood hyperactive disorder suggested by his problems with attention tasks. No other impairments in neuropsychological testing were observed. Perceptual, motor, memory, and language functions are all within a range that is compatible with his average intellectual functioning. Further, there is nothing in his history suggestive of a change in intellectual status. Intellectual scores are within the average range, although when the lowered scores on attention tasks are partialled out, at least high average verbal intellectual scores are suggested.

In sum, this is a young man who is showing residual signs of a childhood learning disability with primary deficits in math and spelling. There are also residual signs of a childhood attention disorder. Despite these problems, we feel that Mr. F. has sufficient native intelligence, motivation, and self-initiation to surmount most academic hurdles. History certainly documents this statement. His learning handicap has made it much more difficult, yet he is able to progress through many academic obstacles. We truly have never seen an individual with as much single-mindedness and motivation to overcome obvious developmental handicaps. If history serves as any forecast, this young man should succeed. We strongly recommend personal interviews for him for graduate school admission.

NEUROPSYCHOLOGY TEST SCORE SUMMARY SHEET

Patient: R.F. Age: 25 Sex: M Handedness: R

I. Intelligence WAIS-R Age-Corrected Scores

VERBAL			PERFORMANCE		
Information	13	(84 %ile)	Picture Completion	12	(75 %ile)
Digit Span	6	(9 %ile)	Picture Arrangement	11	(63 %ile)
Vocabulary	18	(99.6 %ile)	Block Design	10	(50 %ile)
Arithmetic	7	(16 %ile)	Object Assembly	9	(37 %ile)
Comprehension	12	(75 %ile)	Digit Symbol	10	(50 %ile)
Similarities	13	(84 %ile)			

VERBAL IQ = 107 (68 %ile) PERFORMANCE IQ = 101 (53 ile)
FULL SCALE IQ = 103 (58 %ile)

II. Attention/Concentration
Digit Span: 6 forward + 3 backwards = 9 Total (9 %ile)

III. Language
Boston Naming Test: 59/60
Controlled Word Association: F (19) + A (19) + S (20) + Age Corr.= 58 (>95 %ile)

IV. Perceptual/Organizational
Rey-Osterrieth Complex Figure Copy: 36/36 (100 %ile)
Street Test: 11 /13 Beery VMI: 23/24 Copy-A-Cube: intact

V. Memory

VERBAL		NONVERBAL	
WMS Logical Memory:	8.5 (40 %ile)	WMS Visual Repro.:	13 (77 %ile)
90 min. delay:	7.5	90 min. delay:	8
Percent retention:	88	Percent retention:	62
		Rey-Osterrieth Fig:	36 (100 %ile)
		3 min. delay:	25.5 (69 %ile)

Rey Auditory Verbal Learning Test (15 items):
T1: 5 T2: 7 T3: 9 T4: 10 T5: 13 Recall after Interference 12
Recognition: 14 Hits, 1 False Identification

VI. Motor Exam

	Dominant Hand	%ile	Nondom. Hand	%ile
Finger Tapping:	50.4	61	48.0	69

VII. Sensory
Finger Gnosis: intact R-L Differentiation: intact

VIII. Achievement

		Standard Score	Grade Equiv.	Percentile Rank
WRAT:	Spelling	93	7.5	32
PIAT:	Math	91	8.6	28
	Reading Rec.	103	12	57
	Reading Comp.	110	12	74
	Spelling	86	9	17

Case 2: Residual Signs of Attention Deficit Hyperactivity Disorder

Reason for Referral

Mr. M.N. is a 23-year-old, right-handed Caucasian male who was referred by his psychologist for evaluation of possible residual cognitive deficits associated with a childhood diagnosis of attention deficit disorder with hyperactivity.

Presenting Situation and Background Information

Mr. N. reported with symptoms of decreased ability to concentrate and motor restlessness that interfere with his ability to complete college courses. He currently is completing his second semester at a local city college. He obtained grades of Bs and Cs in general required courses, although the patient indicated that he "barely made it through the semester." He also stated that he did poorly in high school. In addition, the patient reported that he attended many high schools because he was expelled from several due to behavior problems. Mr. N. stated that he was diagnosed as having hyperactivity as a child and was treated with a medication, whose name he does not recall, for approximately one to two years from the ages of 8 to 10. The patient also reported that he was probably diagnosed as having dyslexia as a child, and he recalls being placed in special classes for the purpose of enhancing his reading skills. He stated that he now believes that his reading skills are above the average range for his age.

Birth history is significant for a cesarean section delivery. He reports no history of abnormal early development or of encephalitis, seizures, or significant head trauma. Mr. N. reported that from the ages of 12 to 19 he engaged in significant elicit drug use including PCP, Quaaludes, LSD, and marijuana, and denied drug use at present. Family history is negative for alcoholism, hyperactivity, learning disorders, and left-handedness.

Behavioral Observations

The patient is of short height and medium stature. Mr. N. was casually attired and wore a pierced earring in his left ear. The patient's behavioral presentation was noteworthy for obvious signs of restlessness, impatience, and distractibility. Two tests were discontinued because the patient indicated that he was tired and not doing his best and was "not into this." The patient tended to respond very rapidly to test questions without apparent forethought, and frequently he spontaneously corrected his answer after providing initial incorrect responses. Impulsivity and low frustration tolerance were noted when tasks became more difficult. An example of this type of behavior was noted upon completion of the last design of the Block Design subtest of the WAIS-R when Mr. N. impulsively scrambled his last design approximately halfway through the task stating, "I don't like this."

Tests Administered

See data summary sheet.

Test Results

Intellectual Scores

An abbreviated version of the WAIS-R (Satz-Mogel) was administered due to the patient's decreased concentration and restlessness. Mr. N. is currently functioning in the average range of general intellectual ability (Full Scale IQ = 98, 45th percentile). A minimal overall discrepancy was noted between his Verbal IQ (99) and his Performance IQ (96). Individual subtest scores need to be interpreted cautiously due to the abbreviated test administration format, but some trends emerged that deserve comment. Within the Verbal subtests, the patient's lowest scores (although still within the average range) were found on subtests tapping attention and concentration processes (Digit Span and Arithmetic subtests).

On the Performance subtests, Mr. N. scored most poorly on a subtest tapping alertness to visual details (Picture Completion = 9th percentile). In striking contrast, Mr. N. performed in the very superior range (99th percentile) on the Picture Arrangement subtest, which measures the ability to sequentially arrange pictures depicting stories.

Attention and Concentration Processes

Performance across attention and concentration tasks consistently tended to show compromise. The patient scored at the first percentile for his age on the Mental Control subtest of the WMS; specifically, he omitted the number 10 when counting backwards from 20, repeated the letters "u," and "v," when reciting the letters of the alphabet, and made an error when counting by 3s to 40. In addition, as noted previously, the patient's scores on subtests of the WAIS-R that tap attentional processes (e.g. Arithmetic and Digit Span) were lower than expected in relation to other verbal skills. On a letter-cancellation task requiring the patient to put a line through every "h" in an array of letters, the patient occasionally skipped over some of the target letters but caught these omissions at a later point. Mr. N. performed particularly poorly on the Consonant Trigrams Test, a complex attention task in which the patient is auditorily presented with three letters and then asked to recall the letters after counting backwards aloud from various numbers for 3, 9, or 18 seconds. The patient was unable to correctly recall any of the eight three-letter sequences presented, and the test was discontinued when the patient abruptly indicated disinterest in completing the remaining items.

Language Skills

Overall, there were no significant impairments on gross language functioning. The patient's performances on the Verbal subtests of the WAIS-R suggest that he has average to high average abilities in select verbal abstract-reasoning skills, vocabulary range, and fund of general information. Moreover, his scores on formal reading and spelling achievement tests were within the average to high average range (86th and 58th percentiles, respectively). The patient's performance on a word generation task was in the average range for his age (FAS = 40th–44th percentile).

Motor Exam

The patient denied any history of significant injury to his hands, arms, or shoulders. Motor testing revealed intact motor speed and skill bilaterally. On a task of finger tapping speed, the patient performed above average with each hand, and a slightly greater than expected dominant-hand advantage was observed (R = 58, L = 49). On a task requiring the patient to skillfully and rapidly place pegs in slots positioned at various angles (Grooved Pegboard Test), Mr. N. performed within the normal range despite dropping pegs, and the slight expected dominant-hand advantage was observed (R = 69 seconds, 1 error; L = 75 seconds, 2 errors).

Perceptual Organizational Skills

Performance on perceptual organization tasks was rather inconsistent and difficult to interpret; lower scores appeared to be related to impulsive and poorly organized response patterns. Scores on visual perceptual tasks were variable; the patient scored within the normal range on a task requiring the identification of obscured objects (Street Test), but scored within the low average range on tasks involving identification of missing details (Picture Completion = 9th percentile) and discrimination of embedded figures (Satz Embedded Figures Test). Also, a mild visuo-perceptual difficulty was noted on the Hooper Test. Some inconsistency was also observed in performance on visual-sequencing and visual tracking tasks; the patient performed within the very superior range on the Picture Arrangement subtest of the WAIS-R (99th percentile) and responded rapidly and accurately on Trails A but scored within the borderline range on Trails B. In addition to requiring more than the average amount of time to complete the latter task, the patient was also observed to make a sequencing error.

Scores on construction tasks were also variable and appeared to be negatively affected by the patient's marked impulsivity. Mr. M. scored within the average range on the Object Assembly and Block Design subtests of the WAIS-R (25th and 37th percentiles, respectively). The patient's Bender drawings were generally accurate, although crudely and rapidly rendered. His copy of a complex line drawing was poorly organized and overall performance was below the 10th percentile (Rey-Osterrieth).

Memory

Verbal

Performance on learning and recall tasks showed considerable fluctuation and inconsistency that appeared to be strongly related to attention and concentration deficits. The patient's ability to learn relatively easy as well as more difficult rote word pairs was in the borderline/impaired range for his age (WMS–Associate Learning = 3rd percentile). Specifically, Mr. N. was unable to learn any of the more difficult associations until the last learning trial in which he recalled two of the four pairs; although the patient rapidly learned the more simple associations, his performance on these items actually declined on the third trial despite the appearance of effortful performance. This pattern of performance strongly suggests the presence of attention difficulties. Mr. N.'s learning of a 15-item list of unrelated words (AVLT) showed a learning curve that was within the average range; again, however, evidence for deficient concentration was observed. The patient's recall of the stimulus items across the five learning trials was erratic (T1 = 7, T2 = 9, T3 = 6, T4 = 12, T5 = 11), and following an interference task, the patient was observed to lose some of the information learned (recall = 9/15 words). Mr. N.'s ability to learn paragraph details on the WMS–Logical Memory subtest also appeared to be disrupted by attention problems (16th percentile). He provided the expected number of paragraph details for his intellectual level when presented with the first paragraph, but his performance dramatically declined on presentation of a second, more difficult paragraph. However, when the second paragraph was reread to the patient, his performance dramatically improved, and his second attempt was in fact at the high average range for his age. Following a 45-minute delay, the patient was only able to recall approximately 56% of the information originally learned, a retention rate below the normal range; however, when provided with cues, the patient's performance actually approximated normal recall.

Nonverbal

The patient's immediate recall reproduction of relatively simple geometric figures was within the average range for his age (WMS–Visual Reproductions); however, following a 45-minute delay, the patient was only able to recall approximately 30% of the information originally learned. Again, when provided with cues, the patient's performance dramatically improved to well within normal limits (100% retention). The patient's recall after three minutes of a complex geometric figure was depressed (Rey-Osterrieth = less than 10th percentile). He was able to retain the overall shape of the design but unable to provide accurate details.

Concept Formation and Response Inhibition

The patient performed rapidly and accurately on the Wisconsin Card Sorting Test, a task involving conceptual tracking and categorization skills. He completed four categories using half of the stimulus cards. There was however one notable finding regarding his performance on this test. Specifically, the patient made one "failure to maintain set" error; he provided nine consecutive correct responses and then sorted a stimulus card according to an incorrect strategy, commenting, "I didn't mean to." This observation suggests that the patient had experienced a brief lapse in concentration and momentarily stopped monitoring his actions. His performance on the Stroop color interference task was at the mean for his age, and only one error was observed.

Academic Achievement

WRAT
Reading: 86th percentile; 10.9 grade equivalent
Spelling: 58th percentile; 9.3 grade equivalent
Arithmetic: 37th percentile; 7.2 grade equivalent

Mr. N.'s sight reading and spelling skills are within the average to high average range for his age. Lower performance, although still within the average range, was observed on the Arithmetic subtest; performance on the task appeared to be significantly affected by inability or unwillingness to exert sustained attention. Specifically, the patient was allotted 10 minutes to complete several mathematical computations, but approximately 8 minutes into the task, the patient stated that he was tired and wished to discontinue the subtest.

Summary and Impressions

Neuropsychological test findings, as well as simple observation of the patient's overt behavior, overwhelmingly point to the presence of significant deficits in attention and concentration abilities. Assessment of other cognitive abilities was problematic due to the significant confounding effect of the attention deficits. However, the patient's overall intelligence, language, motor, abstraction, and conceptualization skills appear to be intact. Results of academic testing suggest that sight reading and spelling skills are within normal limits although mathematical abilities are lower than expected at least partially due to attention factors.

Some impaired performances were observed on learning and recall tasks, but these appeared to be the result of a failure to initially attend to and process the material. Once the material was learned, it was generally available for retrieval or at least could be elicited through cueing. This performance pattern is most consistent with the presence of a marked attentional disturbance as opposed to a true disturbance of memory. However, the fact that processed information could not be sufficiently recalled without the aid of cues suggests the possibility of a retrieval and/or storage disorder.

Variable performance was observed across visual perceptual and construction tasks. Mr. N.'s impulsive and disorganized responses and his distractibility appeared to have negatively impacted his performance on these tasks, but at the present time the presence of a mild perceptual organization disorder cannot be ruled out.

While the patient's attentional difficulties clearly date from childhood, it is not known to what extent his substance abuse has contributed to cognitive difficulties.

In conclusion, substantial evidence for the presence of a significant attention and concentration disorder was observed on neuropsychological testing and behavioral observation. We are quite concerned over the severity of this disorder, and we judge the patient to be considerably disabled by this condition in spite of average intellectual ability. We marvel that the patient has been able to successfully complete any college coursework at all, and we anticipate that these deficits will continue to jeopardize his performance in academic and occupational settings. We personally have seen adult patients with residual attention deficits stemming from childhood diagnoses of hyperactivity who have been successfully treated with stimulant medications such as Ritalin. We would recommend that the patient be evaluated for the feasibility of this type of treatment with due consideration to his past history of drug abuse. In addition, behavioral psychotherapeutic treatment may also be beneficial in helping the patient gain control over his impulsivity and develop structured future goals.

NEUROPSYCHOLOGY TEST SCORE SUMMARY SHEET

Patient: M.N. Age: 23 Sex: M Handedness: R

I. Intelligence WAIS-R Age-Corrected Scores

VERBAL			PERFORMANCE		
Information	12	(75 %ile)	Picture Completion	6	(9 %ile)
Digit Span	9	(37 %ile)	Picture Arrangement	17	(99 %ile)
Vocabulary	12	(75 %ile)	Block Design	9	(37 %ile)
Arithmetic	8	(25 %ile)	Object Assembly	8	(25 %ile)
Comprehension	10	(50 %ile)	Digit Symbol	8	(25 %ile)
Similarities	10	(50 %ile)			
VERBAL IQ =	99	(47 %ile)	PERFORMANCE IQ =	96	(39 %ile)

FULL SCALE IQ = 98 (45 %ile)

II. Attention/Concentration
Digit Span: 6 forward + 4 backwards = 10 Total (37 %ile)
Mental Control, WMS: 2 (1 %ile)
Cancellation Test= 2'44"
Trails A: 23" (55 %ile), Trails B: 96" (2 %ile)

III. Language
Controlled Word Association:F(12) + A(7) + S(12) + Age Corr.=35 (40-44 %ile)

IV. Perceptual/Organizational
Rey-Osterrieth Complex Figure Copy: 20/36 (<10 %ile)
Hooper Visual Organization Test: 23.5 /30 Street Test: 8 /13
Embedded Figures: 22/24 Letter Cancellation: intact
Bender-Gestalt: intact

V. Memory

VERBAL		NONVERBAL	
WMS Logical Memory	6.25 (16 %ile)	WMS Visual Repro.:	10 (36%ile)
45 min. delay:	3.5	45 min. delay:	3
Percent retention:	56	Percent retention:	30

WMS Associate Learning	I Easy 6 , 6 , 5	Rey-Osterrieth Fig:	20 (<10%ile)
	I Hard 0 , 0 , 2	3 min. delay:	12 (<10%ile)
	I Score: 10.5 (3 %ile)		
	Delay: 5 easy, 2 hard 100 % ret.		

Rey Auditory Verbal Learning Test (15 items):
T1: 7 T2: 9 T3: 6 T4: 12 T5: 11 Recall after Interference 9

VI. Motor Exam

	Dominant Hand	%ile	Nondom. Hand	%ile
Finger Tapping:	58	93	49	75
Grooved Pegbd.:	69"	37	75"	36

VII. Sensory
R-L Differentiation: intact

VIII. Frontal Systems
Stroop A: 37", Stroop B: 61" , Stroop C: 117"
Wisconsin Card Sort: Categories: 4 , discontinued
Auditory Consonant Trigrams: discontinued

X. Achievement

WRAT-R:	Standard Score	Grade Equiv.	Percentile Rank
Reading	116	10.9	86
Spelling	103	9.3	58
Arithmetic	37	7.2	37

Case 3: Residual Learning Disorder with Compensation

Reason for Referral

Mr. M.Q. is a 57-year-old, right-handed Caucasian male who was referred for neuropsychological testing by his psychologist to evaluate cognitive functioning for the possible presence of dyslexia and to determine whether possible problems in cognitive processing were related to the patient's difficulty maintaining occupational stability.

Presenting Situation and Background Information

Mr. Q. reported long-standing difficulties in mathematics, left-right confusion, and spelling problems, all of which have been present since childhood. He stated that his arithmetic calculations are usually full of errors and that he had great difficulty learning the multiplication tables, but has had no problems with the conceptual aspects of math. He also stated that he reads slowly but comprehends well. Additionally, Mr. Q. reported that he tends to misplace items (e.g., keys) often, although he rated his memory in general as good. The patient voiced concern that he may have dyslexia and described his long-standing difficulties as "personal deficiencies" and "sins." These problems are associated with intense emotional strife; the patient has reportedly been in psychotherapy for the past three years to help him cope with related tension and nervousness.

Mr. Q. has a history of difficulty maintaining occupational stability. He has reportedly been fired from at least four jobs. The patient stated that he was fired on two occasions for reasons connected, in part, with excessive drinking. Mr. Q. stated that he was a very heavy drinker for many years and also used tranquilizers. He recently enrolled in a drug rehabilitation program to help him curb his drinking habit. He currently admits to drinking seven cocktails an evening. He denies current use of tobacco.

The patient has a B.A. degree in business administration and reportedly graduated with honors. He had been married for 26 years. For the past 10 years he has been operating his own small parcel delivery service.

The patient reported having difficulty sleeping, indicating that he wakes up often during the night and subsequently is often fatigued. He denies involvement in any accidents or head injuries. His family history is positive for a brother who is reportedly schizophrenic and a father who has mood fluctuations. Family history is positive for a left-handed mother. Birth and developmental history are reportedly unremarkable. The patient denies using any medications at present.

Behavioral Observations

Mr. Q. has rather long gray hair, glasses, and a bulbous nose, and he appeared quite disheveled. He also appeared to be somewhat anxious and was quite emotional. In fact, he became tearful at one point when describing his experience as a soldier. He related his cognitive difficulties in a tone of great despair and shame. He exhibited low self-esteem and a rather depressed affect. Mr. Q worked diligently and displayed good effort, although difficulties in attention and concentration were observed throughout the evaluation.

TESTS ADMINISTERED

See data summary sheet.

TEST RESULTS

Intellectual Function

Intellectually, Mr. Q. is functioning overall in the very superior range. He obtained a Verbal IQ of 135 (99th percentile), a Performance IQ of 113 (81st percentile), and a Full Scale IQ of 130 (98th percentile). His intelligence test profile indicated intersubtest scatter and a significant difference of 22 IQ points between his Verbal and Performance IQs. He performed most poorly on a subtest of visual tracking ability involving coding nonsense figures for numbers (Digit Symbol). Subtests that best correlate with visuo-spatial ability (Block Design, Object Assembly) were performed in the average to above average range. In contrast, he performed at ceiling levels on tests tapping his fund of general information, vocabulary range, abstract-reasoning abilities, and ability to discriminate details (i.e., Information, Vocabulary, Similarities, and Picture Completion subtests, respectively).

Attention and Concentration Processes

Mr. Q. displayed a mild depression of his attention and concentration ability. He scored within the average range but below expectation for his intellectual level on subtests on the WAIS-R that are sensitive to basic attention processes (Digit Span, Arithmetic). In addition, several errors were committed on the Consonant Trigrams Test, a test of auditory concentration ability. The patient also exhibited relative difficulty on the Stroop Test, and his performance on the interference condition was below the mean for his age. His performance on Trails A was below average levels, and although he performed within the average range on Trails B, this is still below expection for his intellectual level. Written arithmetic problems were solved slowly but correctly.

Language Function

Speech was fluent and articulate, and there were no gross signs of aphasia. No difficulties were found on confrontational naming as tested with the Boston Naming Test, or in generating words belonging to various letter categories as tested with the Controlled Word Association Test (>95th percentile). He displayed no difficulties in writing to dictation or writing a self-generated paragraph.

Sensory/Perceptual

No gross impairments were observed in Mr. Q.'s perceptual organization ability. He performed without error on the Hooper VOT, a test of visual perception. No disturbances in visual-motor integration were found; he was able to copy three-dimensional figures without difficulty and scored within normal limits on the Beery VMI. He was also able to copy a more complex line drawing fairly accurately (Rey-Osterrieth), although he did display some difficulty with the overall organizational structure of the design. Minor difficulties were observed with spatial confusion; his right-left judgments on a road-map test, while generally correct, were performed slowly (Money's Road Map Test), and his right-left discrimination of body parts intra- and extrapersonally were slow and deliberate with one error. There was no evidence of finger agnosia on gross screening.

Motor

Due to time constraints, assessment of motor skill was not performed.

Learning and Memory

Verbal

Mr. Q. performed within normal limits on tests of new verbal learning and memory. In fact, Mr. Q. performed within the superior range on immediate recall of the Logical Memory subtest of the WMS. Moreover, he was able to retain 91% of this material over a 90-minute delay with interference. The patient exhibited more difficulty on learning items in a 15-item word list with repeated presentation (AVLT). Over the five trials, he learned 4, 6, 6, 12, and 14 of the items respectively. His initial slow acquisition of the material is most likely influenced by problems with attention. Although the items were learned more slowly than expected, he eventually learned all but one and performed above average limits on the last trial. After a brief delay with distraction, he demonstrated memory for 12 of the items, suggesting that he was able to effectively hold the items over the delay interval, despite distraction, and retrieve them normally.

Nonverbal

Similarly, above average performance was found on learning of nonverbal information; however, some difficulties were found on recall of the nonverbal information. Mr. Q. was able to reconstruct the Rey-Osterrieth Complex Figure from memory following a three-minute delay at the 90th percentile despite his disorganized strategy in copying this figure previously. His performance on the WMS-VR was also within normal limits for immediate recall. However, a greater than expected loss was experienced following a 90-minute delay (33% retention).

Academic Achievement

Mr. Q. was administered the WRAT and two subtests of the PIAT, and the following scores were obtained:

Subtest	Standard Score	Percentile
WRAT		
Reading	118	88
Spelling	111	77
Arithmetic	105	63
PIAT		
Reading Comprehension	110	74
Spelling	87	19

The WRAT and the PIAT test results indicate that Mr. Q. is currently functioning in the average to above average range in the academic skills measured, with the exception of his ability to recognize correct spelling. Although the patient had no difficulty producing the correct spelling of words (WRAT Spelling), he was impaired in his ability to discriminate correctly spelled words amidst other choices (PIAT Spelling). These results suggest impairment in holistic spelling possibly related to distraction by alternative choices or difficulties related to scanning or impulsivity.

Personality

Test results depict a fairly vulnerable and sensitive individual who appears in considerable emotional strife. There is a strong depressive content evident on the MMPI and interview. The patient also reports a family history of depressive illness: a brother is diagnosed as schizophrenic and a father experienced mood fluctuations.

Mr. Q. appears to be in a great deal of anguish. A possible source of his anxiety may be his failing attempts to meet his personal standards, which he has obviously set at unrealistically high levels.

Summary and Impressions

The present pattern of neuropsychological testing is essentially free of any significant disturbances in higher-level cognitive processing ability. There is some evidence, however, of a residual minor learning handicap that has probably been well compensated for by this very bright individual. Test results show that Mr. Q. has subtle difficulties with right-left discrimination, organization and retention of visual spatial relationships, attention and concentration, and more significantly, a spelling impairment. These minor difficulties are in striking contrast to his very superior verbal skills (Verbal IQ = 135). One might speculate that these types of tasks, visuo-spatial in nature, were a source of a specific learning handicap at an earlier point in his life but that Mr. Q. has developed strategies, probably through verbal mechanisms, to compensate for them. In fact, these subtle visuo-spatial difficulties may reflect a central nervous system that is functionally different in its organization from the typical right-hander, especially as there is a positive history of maternal sinistrality. At any rate, these slight difficulties do not point to the presence of dyslexia and would probably not account for his presenting difficulties.

There were signs of minor difficulties in attention and concentration processes as evidenced by relatively lower scores on subtests of the WAIS-R that are believed to measure attention mechanisms (Digit Span, Arithmetic). An attention disturbance was also suggested by the patient's performance on the Trail Making Test, the Stroop Test and the Consonant Trigrams Test. The patient's self-report also corroborates these findings. Mr. Q. stated that he often loses his keys and other objects. The present pattern of test results fail to provide significant evidence of verbal memory dysfunction. Rather, these difficulties are believed to be influenced by his current psychological profile, which may interfere with his ability to concentrate or maintain sustained thought processes without intrusion of thoughts. Poor performance on several of these tasks (i.e., Stroop, Consonant Trigrams) may also signal the presence of frontal lobe dysfunction, which may be a factor in his attention problems. History of alcohol abuse may be a contributing factor to these problems in attention.

The most significant findings were gleaned from interview and personality assessment. Mr. Q. is a fairly vulnerable and sensitive man who is currently showing signs of an affective disorder. His symptoms include agitation, decreased energy, feelings of despair and inadequacy, difficulty concentrating, brooding, tearfulness, and a sleep disturbance. Genetic factors may be contributing—the patient reports a family history of depressive illness. Mr. Q. appears to be in considerable emotional strife. This may, in part, stem from his high personal standards. He appears to punish himself for not meeting these standards, which are obviously unrealistic for him. His feelings of self-depreciation and inner turmoil may explain why this highly intelligent individual has had difficulties in the past maintaining employment. Also, his impulsive behavior, which could well be tied to his drinking habit, may have contributed in part to these problems. He related several examples reflecting his impulsive nature, including one tied to his war experiences.

In sum, Mr. Q. is a bright, sensitive, caring, and vulnerable individual with many special strengths and some long-standing weaknesses. Mr. Q. is currently functioning intellectually overall within the very superior range. At the same time, there is some evidence of a subtle residual learning handicap involving visuo-spatial skills that is probably well compensated for. In any case, these minor difficulties are not a significant part of the present profile. Most significant is the affective disturbance that Mr. Q. is currently displaying. We strongly encourage continued psychological intervention.

NEUROPSYCHOLOGY TEST SCORE SUMMARY SHEET

Patient: M.Q. Age: 57 Sex: M Handedness: R

I. Intelligence WAIS-R Age-Corrected Scores

VERBAL			PERFORMANCE		
Information	17	(99 %ile)	Picture Completion	17	(99 %ile)
Digit Span	11	(63 %ile)	Picture Arrangement	14	(91 %ile)
Vocabulary	19	(99.9%ile)	Block Design	12	(75 %ile)
Arithmetic	12	(75 %ile)	Object Assembly	10	(50 %ile)
Comprehension	14	(91 %ile)	Digit Symbol	7	(16 %ile)
Similarities	19	(99.9%ile)			
VERBAL IQ =	135	(99 %ile)	PERFORMANCE IQ =	113	(81 %ile)

FULL SCALE IQ = 130 (98 %ile)

II. Attention/Concentration
Digit Span: 8 forward + 4 backwards = 12 Total (63 %ile)
Trails A: 40" (12 %ile), Trails B: 85" (38 %ile)

III. Language
Boston Naming Test: 60 /60
Controlled Word Association: F(22) + A(18) + S(24) + Age Corr.= 65 (>95 %ile)

IV. Perceptual/Organizational
Rey-Osterrieth Complex Figure Copy: 33.5/36 (75 %ile)
Beery VMI: 23/24 Copy-A-Cube: intact
Hooper Visual Organization Test: 30/30
Money Road Map Test of Directional Sense= 1 error

V. Memory

VERBAL		NONVERBAL	
WMS Logical Memory	11.5 (92 %ile)	WMS Visual Repro.:	12 (95 %ile)
90 min. delay:	10.5	90 min. delay:	4
Percent retention:	91	Percent retention:	33
		Rey-Osterrieth Fig:	33.5 (75 %le)
		3 min. delay:	28 (90%ile)

Rey Auditory Verbal Learning Test (15 items):
T1:4 T2:6 T3:6 T4:12 T5:14 Recall after Interference 12
Recognition: 14 Hits, 0 False Identifications

VI. Motor Exam	Dominant Hand	%ile	Nondom. Hand	%ile
Finger Tapping	45	58	40	54

VII. Sensory
Finger Gnosis: intact R-L Differentiation: slow

VIII. Frontal Systems
Stroop A: 64", Stroop B: 92", Stroop C: 191"
Auditory Consonant Trigrams: 27/60

IX. Achievement		Standard Score	Grade Equivalent	Percentile Rank
WRAT:	Reading	118	11.1	88
	Spelling	111	9.7	77
	Arithmetic	105	6.2	63
PIAT:	Reading Comp.	110	12	74
	Spelling	87	9.4	19

X. Personality

MMPI: 2459'1738-6/ L"F-K:

Commentary on Learning Disorder Cases

This chapter illustrates many typical case protocols of adults with residual signs of learning disabilities. Many of the key features of a learning disorder in adulthood are found, such as difficulty in academic achievement skills, attention problems, emotional problems, and mild neuropsychologic problems. The fact that all cases presented are males reflects the prevalence of this disorder in males in the general population. These learning-disabled adults with histories of childhood learning disability, and particularly M.N. with a documented diagnosis, are consistent with the literature, which indicates that learning disorders are usually not outgrown.

The case of M.Q. highlights how subject moderator variables such as intellectual level plays an important variable in overcoming or compensating for mild learning disabilities. Individuals with above average intellectual levels generally are more successful in terms of finishing school and/or in attaining satisfying employment. Despite evidence of a subtle residual learning handicap involving visuo-spatial skills, M.Q. appears to have compensated for these problems via his very superior intellect. The case of R.F. highlights the importance of personality traits in overcoming academic and occupation obstacles. In spite of his cognitive handicaps, R.F.'s tenacity in striving for his goals resulted in graduation from a major university. His strong motivation and dedication was the key force that helped him to progress through many obstacles and attain his goal.

Similar to children with learning disorders, the cases are characterized by the salient feature of marked difficulty in academic achievement areas despite at least average intellectual functioning. All of the cases had evidence of attention/concentration processing problems; although common, this is not always found among adults with residual learning disorders. The literature suggests the finding of a lower Verbal IQ compared to Performance IQ; however, none of the cases presented in this chapter displayed this pattern. In fact, all three of the cases exhibited a higher Verbal IQ than Performance IQ, although the small selection of cases does not allow for meaningful interpretation of this finding.

In conclusion, this chapter supports the findings that learning disorders are found in adulthood, that adult learning disorders may be attenuated if the patient has an above average intellectual level and/or a high motivation level, and that the general neuropsychological profile for a learning-disabled adult is similar to that of a learning-disabled child with at least an average intellectual level, significantly lower academic achievement scores relative to IQ and grade expectation, and selected mild cognitive deficits.

8
Conscious or Nonconscious Feigning of Deficits

The issue of conscious (voluntary) or nonconscious (involuntary) exaggeration or feigning of cognitive deficits on neuropsychological testing has not received much formal attention in the literature, despite its importance for clinical practice. The credibility of neuropsychology within the legal arena hinges on the ability to accurately detect the presence of actual brain dysfunction. In addition, appropriate treatment is contingent on accurate discrimination of actual brain compromise versus functional disorder.

The American Psychiatric Association's Diagnostic and Statistical Manual III–Revised (1987) describes two types of psychiatric disorders in which physical symptoms are created involuntarily or nonconsciously due to psychodynamic conflicts frequently centered around desires for attention and care from others. *Somatization disorder* (or Briquet's syndrome) refers to the presence of numerous and recurrent physical symptoms involving several organ systems with onset before age 30. The symptoms are not found to have a physiologic basis upon medical evaluation. These individuals tend to present their medical histories in a vague but melodramatic manner and usually have consulted numerous physicians over the years. Conversely, patients with *conversion disorder* usually present with a single symptom during an episode, and the symptom usually mimics neurologic disease (e.g., paralysis, seizures, parathesias). An apparent lack of concern regarding the severity of the symptoms or "la belle indifference" may be present.

The DSM III-R also describes two syndromes in which conscious generation of symptoms is present. *Factitious disorder* refers to voluntary or deliberate creation of physical symptoms (Munchausen's syndrome) or psychological symptoms (Ganser syndrome), but this behavior cannot be readily controlled by the individual. The "goal" of the behavior is to adopt the patient role, and the presence of the disorder implies severe psychopathology. *Malingering* refers to voluntary, deliberate creation or exaggeration of symptoms, but the goal is opportunistic—monetary gain, to obtain drugs, to avoid military duty, or to evade responsibility or consequences for a crime. Malingering implies an "act" rather than a legal or mental status or lifestyle; malingerers don or "wear" their symptoms for medical and legal evaluations but then discard them when they assume they are not being observed, in contrast to patients with conversion or somatization disorders. Associated features of malingering may include: (1) contradictory and inconsistent history and test results, (2) uncooperative and evasive attitude, (3) symptomatology inconsistent with known neuropsychological syndromes, (4) severe disability following minor injury, (5) delay between injury and onset of symptoms, (6) presence of antisocial personality disorder or drug dependency, and (7) ongoing litigation.

Finally, the DSM III-R also includes a diagnostic category describing the initiation or exacerbation of an actual physical disorder due to psychological factors. *Psychological factors affecting physical condition* usually encompasses such descriptive terms as "psychosomatic," "psychophysiological," and "functional overlay." In addition, "compensation neurosis" or "accident neurosis" are included in this category when a documented physical condition is present but, in the absence of objective physical findings, usually refer to malingering. These latter terms have sprung from the belief that symptomology disappeared with financial compensation for injury (Miller, 1961), but research has failed to support this contention. Mendelson (1985) notes that between 35% and 75% of litigating patients are not symptom-free and have not returned to gainful employment two to three years following conclusion of their claim.

Creation or exaggeration of cognitive symptomatology most frequently occurs in patients reporting head injury, and thus it is critical that the clinician have knowledge of the neuropsychological symptoms that commonly accompany head injury (see Chapter 1). Guthkelch (1980) reports that accident neurosis or compensation neurosis is relatively rare in populations presenting for evaluation with post-head-injury symptoms (6–8%). This condition is most prevalent in semiskilled or unskilled manual workers and in patients with industrial as opposed to nonindustrial injuries. Accident neurosis is uncommon in patients with relatively severe injury (7 or more days of post traumatic amnesia) possibly because the actual brain damage sustained may render them unable to formulate and execute a plan to deceive. Of note, in the accident-neurosis patients, Guthkelch found no relationship between severity of symptoms and severity of injury, and many of the complaints were bizarre and inconsistent. In addition, improvement in symptoms over time was denied, in contrast with patients with an actual post-concussional syndrome. Rutherford, Merrett, and McDonald (1979) suggest that development of new symptomology after the six weeks following injury is most likely to be associated with psychogenic factors.

Neuropsychological Literature on Feigning of Cognitive Deficits

Neuropsychological Batteries

Heaton, Smith, Lehman, and Vogt (1978) compared WAIS, Halstead-Reitan Battery (HRB), and MMPI scores of 16 nonlitigating head trauma patients with those of 16 volunteers paid to successfully feign impairment on the tests. The malingerers demonstrated a different pattern of deficits than those shown by the true head injury patients. Specifically, the malingerers scored more poorly on motor and sensory tests (Speech Sounds Perception Test, finger agnosia, hand dynamometer, sensory suppression) but scored relatively well on tests particularly sensitive to brain dysfunction (Category Test, Trails B, Tactual Performance Test). In addition, the malingerers exhibited more extensive personality disturbance on the MMPI (high F scale and marked elevations on scales 1, 3, 6, 7, 8, and 0). Mean IQ scores were within the average range for both groups, but the malingerers tended to score relatively poorly on the Digit Symbol and Digit Span subtests. The authors conclude that the clinician should be suspicious if the obtained neuropsychological test scores resemble this "malingering profile," if they are atypical from a neurologic point of view, and if the MMPI protocol is of questionable validity.

Goebel (1983) was able to achieve a 94% hit rate in classifying 52 brain-damaged patients, 61 controls, and 141 nonimpaired volunteers instructed to fake brain damage on the WAIS, HRB, WMS–Logical Memory, and Milner Facial Recognition. The volunteers were divided into four subgroups and instructed to feign left or right hemisphere damage, bilateral damage, or simply to fake "brain damage" in general. No significant difference in test performance was noted across these groups. However, the nondominant scores on grip strength and finger tapping and the Performance IQ were most helpful in discriminating the control and faking groups. The "fakers" were queried as to the strategies used in feigning symptoms. Ten percent indicated that they had made no attempt to fake, 36% faked on every test, and the majority faked on selected tests. Thirty percent provided wrong answers, 36% performed slowly or attempted to appear confused or dull, 14% demonstrated motor incoordination, and 2% attempted to feign memory impairment. Forty percent reported having some knowledge of brain-behavior relationships, such as contralateral motor control (66%) and left hemisphere language dominance (12%). With regard to patterns of behavior associated with brain damage, 10% were aware that motor incoordination might be present, 7% knew that performance might be slowed, and only 5% were aware of the common presence of memory impairment. Goebel concludes:

> . . . nonimpaired individuals of at least average IQ cannot sufficiently alter their performance on neuropsychological assessment to appear brain-impaired with any significant degree of success. While the faking individuals of this study were able to lower their level of performance somewhat, the degree was generally insufficient to trigger a diagnosis of cerebral damage. In addition, pathognomonic errors (Aphasia, Apraxia) as well as patterns of lateralized impairment across different types of higher adaptive functions (e.g., language, motor function, sensory perception, memory, IQ, etc.) are apparently beyond their abilities to produce voluntarily. (p. 740)

In summary, these findings suggest that malingerers are most apt to show depressed performance on motor and sensory tasks, and may also show lowered scores on timed and attention tests.

Memory

Brandt, Rubinsky, and Lassen's (1985) comparison of 10 actual malingerers feigning amnesia with controls and patients with head trauma or Huntington's disease revealed that the malingerers performed as poorly as patient groups on free recall, but performed more poorly on recognition memory tasks. Scores were frequently below chance on recognition tasks, suggesting censoring of correct answers.

Benton and Spreen (1961; Spreen & Benton, 1963) recruited subjects without cerebral damage to simulate performance on the Visual Retention Test comparable to that of mentally deficient individuals (n = 75) or head injured patients with headaches, fatigue, decreased memory, and mental inefficiency (n = 70). Their performance was compared to that of 48 actual brain damaged patients and 68 mentally retarded individuals. Simulators overestimated the degree of deficit exhibited by the criterion patients and committed more errors. Performance of simulators also differed qualitatively from brain-dysfunctional patients, with brain injured patients showing omission errors, and simulators creating bizarre and distorted responses. Thirty-three to 55% of the simulators provided at least two "peculiar" responses, whereas 17% of the brain injured and 3% of the mentally retarded individuals exhibited two or more such responses. (Peculiar responses included gross distortion of height or width of a design, straight lines reproduced as a jagged "saw-tooth" series of lines, etc.)

Thus, on memory testing malingerers may be identified by a high frequency of bizarre responses and recognition performances below chance, as well as depressed free recall scores.

Constructional Ability

Bruhn and Reed (1975) reported 100% correct discrimination of malingering individuals from brain-damaged patients on the Bender Gestalt Test. Formal scoring systems did not discriminate the two groups, but qualitative feature analysis was effective in correct detection and could be readily taught to novice examiners. Bender (1938) has also provided criteria for identifying malingering on the Bender Gestalt: (1) small drawings, (2) uneven performance, (3) distortion of position or direction of details but with the gestalt of individual items maintained (e.g., squares do not become loops), (4) simplification (continuous line for series of dots but overall shape maintained), and (5) more complex drawing elements added.

Language

Sevash and Brooks (1983) indicate that organic versus functional language impairment can be discriminated by the presence of paraphasias, perseverations, and anomia in the former.

Test Procedures Designed to Detect Malingering

Lezak (1983; cf., Spreen & Benton, 1963) suggests that the "hallmark of malingering" is inconsistency between neuropsychological test scores and/or between test scores and level of daily functioning. McKinlay, Brooks, and Bond (1983) cite the importance of serial testing in the detection of malingering. Lezak (1983) provides instructions for several tests that can be used to assess motivation and cooperation in the testing procedures (e.g., memorization of 15 items, dot counting, word recognition, Symptom Validity Test). In memorization of 15 items, the patient is shown a page with 15 items and instructed to memorize them. The number "15" is stressed to make the test appear difficult, although the items are highly associated and can be readily grouped into 5 series to assist learning (e.g., 1, 2, 3; A, B, C). Failure to recall at least three series of stimuli (nine items) is considered suspicious for feigning. Goldberg and Miller (1986) have recently documented that psychiatric in-patients perform normally on the measure, whereas mentally retarded individuals frequently fail to recall at least nine of the 15 items. The authors suggest that malingerers make errors of omission, frequently involving more than one row of items, rather than perseverative errors seen in mentally deficient individuals. None of the psychiatric patients omitted more than one row of stimuli.

Pankratz, Fausti, and Peed (1975) developed a forced-choice technique (Symptom Validity Test) to detect feigning of deafness, and Pankratz (1983) and Binder (Binder & Pankratz, 1987) have subsequently utilized the technique to document faked memory deficit. In this procedure, the patient is briefly shown a black pen or yellow pencil, and required to count backward from 20 to 1. The patient is then requested to recall which object was presented. This procedure is repeated for a total of 100 trials. An error rate greater than chance (e.g., greater than 50 errors) is evidence of faking. Binder and Pankratz (1987) informally administered the procedure to three severely head injured patients and none of the patients made any errors in 20 trials.

In grouped and ungrouped dot counting, the individual is instructed to count dots on cards as rapidly as possible. The cards have varying numbers of dots and are presented in a randomized order. Cooperative individuals systematically utilize more seconds to count larger numbers of dots, and grouped dots are counted more quickly than ungrouped dots. Deviations in the pattern are indicators of possible feigning. On the word recognition task, an individual is read a list of 15 words, and then given a page with 30 words and instructed to circle all words recognized from the orally presented list. Later in the testing session, the AVLT is administered. If free recall on trial 1 of the AVLT exceeds recognition on the word recognition test, faking of amnesia is suspected.

Stevens (1986) described the "Ganser Syndrome Test" of approximate answers and the "Pierre Marie Test." The first term refers to a response style in which individuals consciously provide incorrect responses that very nearly approximate correct answers (e.g., $4 + 3 = 8$ and on second trial, $4 + 3 = 6$). In the Pierre Marie Test, individuals who claim hypalgesia are instructed to close their eyes and respond "yes" when they are touched by the examiner and "no" when they are not touched.

Bash and Alpert (1980) have developed experimental procedures employing the concept of approximate answers in discriminating psychotic patients and individuals feigning psychosis; the utility of these procedures in detecting individuals who feign brain damage is unknown.

A Note of Caution

The literature cited above provides optimism regarding detection of symptom feigning, but it should be kept in mind that test procedures designed to measure cooperation and motivation are not foolproof and clinical judgment should be exercised (Binder, 1986). It is frequently highly difficult to discriminate between conscious and nonconscious feigning (McMahon & Satz, 1981), and the assignment of the "malingering" label should be undertaken with extreme care. In addition, it is possible for diagnostic categories to overlap; for example, conscious and nonconscious feigning of symptoms may coexist in the same patient (McMahon & Satz, 1981), and conversion symptoms may accompany actual cerebral disease. For example, Merskey and Trimble (1979) report that in a sample of patients with conversion symptoms, half of them also suffered from various types of cerebral disease. Stern (1977) posits a possible link between conversion symptoms and right hemisphere disease; he documents a frequent finding of left-sided lateralization of conversion reactions, and hypothesizes a connection between conversion phenomenon and anosagnosia. Denker and Perry (1954) demonstrated that nearly half of their sample of post-concussive patients with hysterical hemihypalgesia had abnormal EEGs. Gould, Miller, Goldberg, and Benson (1986) found that purported pathognomonic symptoms of hysteria (la belle indifference, history of hypochondriasis, secondary gain, non-anatomical sensory loss, split of midline by pain or vibratory stimulation, changing boundaries of hypalgesia, giveaway weakness) were frequently present in patients with acute structural brain disease. Finally, Slater and Glithero (1965) and Whitlock (1967) report that approximately 60% of patients diagnosed as hysterics eventually are found to have an organic cause for their symptomatology.

Summary

When evaluating for the presence of conscious or nonconscious creation or exaggeration of cognitive symptoms, the clinician should be alert to:

1. inconsistencies in performance across tests;
2. inconsistencies between test performance and daily functioning;
3. test findings that are atypical from a neurologic perspective;

4. depressed motor and sensory performances though scores on tests especially sensitive to brain dysfunction are normal;
5. recognition memory poorer than free recall;
6. bizarre or distorted responses, particularly on constructions;
7. suspicious performance on tests designed to discretely assess motivation and cooperation; and
8. personality testing that is of questionable validity and/or documents hysterical or other characterological pathology.

These indicators are not infallible and clinical judgment must be exercised.

References

American Psychiatric Association. (1987). *Diagnostic and statistical manual of mental disorders* (3rd ed.-Revised). Washington, DC.

Bash, I.Y., & Alpert, M. (1980). The determination of malingering. *Annals New York Academy of Sciences, 347*, 86–99.

Bender, O. (1938). *A visual motor gestalt test and its clinical use.* New York: The American Orthopsychiatric Association.

Benton, A., & Spreen, O. (1961). Visual memory test: The simulation of mental incompetence. *Archives of General Psychiatry, 4*, 79–83.

Binder, L.M. (1986). Persisting symptoms after mild head injury: A review of the post-concussive syndrome. *Journal of Clinical and Experimental Neuropsychology, 8*, 323–346.

Binder, L.M., & Pankratz, L. (1987). Neuropsychological evidence of a factitious memory complaint. *Journal of Clinical and Experimental Neuropsychology, 9*, 167–171.

Brandt, J., Rubinsky, E., & Lassen, G. (1985). Uncovering malingered amnesia. *Annals New York Academy of Sciences, 444*, 502–503.

Bruhn, A.R., & Reed, M.R. (1975). Simulation of brain damage on the Bender-Gestalt Test by college subjects. *Journal of Personality Assessment, 39*, 244–255.

Denker, P.G., & Perry, G.F. (1954). Postconcussion syndrome in compensation and litigation: Analysis of 95 cases with electroencephalographic correlation. *Neurology, 4*, 912–918.

Goebel, R.A. (1983). Detection of faking on the Halstead-Reitan neuropsychological test battery. *Journal of Clinical Psychology, 39*, 731–742.

Goldberg, J.O., & Miller, H.R. (1986). Performance of psychiatric inpatients and intellectually deficient individuals on a task that assesses the validity of memory complaints. *Journal of Clinical Psychology, 42*, 792–795.

Gould, R., Miller, B.L., Goldberg, M.A., & Benson, D.F. (1986). The validity of hysterical signs and symptoms. *Journal of Nervous and Mental Disease, 174*, 593–597.

Guthkelch, A.N. (1980). Posttraumatic amnesia, post-concussional symptoms and accident neurosis. *European Neurology, 19*, 91–102.

Heaton, R.K., Smith, H.H., Lehman, R.A., & Vogt, A.T. (1978). Prospects for faking believable deficits on neuropsychological testing. *Journal of Consulting and Clinical Psychology, 46*, 892–900.

Lezak, M. (1983). *Neuropsychological assessment (2nd ed.).* New York: Oxford University Press.

Mendelson, G. (1985). "Compensation neurosis": An invalid diagnosis. *Medical Journal of Australia, 142*, 561-564.
Merskey, H., & Trimble, M. (1979). Personality, sexual adjustment, and brain lesions in patients with conversion symptoms. *American Journal of Psychiatry, 136*, 179-182.
McKinlay, W.W., Brooks, D.N., & Bond, M.R. (1983). Post-concussional symptoms, financial compensation, and outcome of severe blunt head injury. *Journal of Neurology, Neurosurgery, and Psychiatry, 46*, 1084-1091.
McMahon, E.A., & Satz, P. (1981). Clinical neuropsychology: Some forensic applications. In S. Filskov & R. Boll (Eds.), *Handbook of clinical neuropsychology* (pp. 686-701). New York: John Wiley.
Miller, H. (1961). Accident neurosis. *British Medical Journal, 1*, 992-998.
Pankratz, L. (1983). A new technique for the assessment and modification of feigned memory deficit. *Perceptual and Motor Skills, 57*, 367-372.
Pankratz, L., Fausti, S.A., & Peed, S. (1975). A forced-choice technique to evaluate deafness in the hysterical or malingering patient. *Journal of Consulting and Clinical Psychology, 43*, 421-422.
Rutherford, W.H., Merrett, J.D., & McDonald, J.R. (1979). Symptoms at one year following concussion from minor head injuries. *Injury, 10*, 225-230.
Sevash, S., & Brooks, J. (1983). Aphasia versus functional disorder: Factors in differential diagnosis. *Psychosomatics, 24*, 847-848.
Slater, E.T.O., & Glithero, E. (1965). A follow-up of patients diagnosed as suffering from "hysteria." *Journal of Psychosomatic Research, 9*, 9-13.
Spreen, O., & Benton, A. (1963). Simulation of mental deficiency on a visual memory test. *American Journal of Mental Deficiency, 67*, 909-913.
Stern, D.B. (1977). Handedness and the lateral distribution of conversion reactions. *Journal of Nervous and Mental Disease, 164*, 122-128.
Stevens, H. (1986). Is it organic or is it functional? Is it hysteria or malingering? *Psychiatric Clinics of North America, 9*, 241-254.
Whitlock, F.A. (1967). The aetiology of hysteria. *Acta Psychiatrica Scandinavia, 43*, 144-162.

Case 1: Malingering

Reason for Referral

Mr. H.I. is a 47-year-old, right-handed male referred for neuropsychological testing by the psychiatrist for his employer's workers compensation insurance carrier for evaluation of possible cognitive sequelae of a motor vehicle accident that occurred two-and-one-half years ago.

Presenting Situation and Background Information

Because the patient was a poor historian, most of the history was obtained from the referring physician. Mr. I. reportedly has filed a workers compensation claim involving a motor vehicle accident that occurred two-and-one-half years ago, while the patient was employed as a truck driver. The patient was apparently on top of his truck checking the level of the crude oil load when an explosion occurred that threw him to the ground. He reportedly sustained a fracture of his lower back with possible subsequent nerve root irritation. There was no documentation of head injury or loss of consciousness associated with the accident. The presence of a hearing loss was explored with the conclusion that the patient was not in need of amplification devices.

Psychiatric evaluation 15 months after the accident indicated that the patient was depressed and exhibiting paranoid feelings, and a diagnosis was made of post traumatic stress disorder. The patient was placed on antipsychotic medication (Haldol) and began psychiatric treatment on a weekly basis. Six months later the psychiatrist concluded that the patient was unlikely to show significant future improvement and judged the patient to have a profound and permanent psychiatric disability. A neurologic evaluation conducted 22 months after the accident led to diagnoses of: (1) "post traumatic head syndrome including post traumatic psychotic situational reaction with elements of possible Ganser's syndrome, and possible intracranial mass lesion"; and (2) "suspected organic mental syndrome." The patient was referred for neuropsychological evaluation at that time and was reportedly found to suffer from severe psychosis and severe cognitive deficits. The neuropsychologist entertained the possibility that the patient exhibited Ganser-syndrome features, but he noted that the Ganser features were not consistently given and seemed to reflect psychotic disorganization of thought processes rather than malingering. A CT scan also obtained at that time revealed slight asymmetry of the temporal horns, right greater than left, and minimal left basal ganglion calcification. The patient has not returned to work since the accident.

A telephone interview was conducted with the patient's mother immediately after the current testing of the patient. She described him as "perfect" before the accident. Of note, she stated that if a stranger now approached her son to ask him a question, the stranger "would think he was normal," but that because of her extended contact with him, she can recognize that he has problems. She indicated that he is very apathetic and that she attempts to "keep him busy" during the day. Specifically, she tries to entice him to watch TV programs, but he shows no interest. She bought a piano because before the injury, he had shown an interest in music. But she stated that he has "run his fingers across the keys once" and shown no further desire to play the instrument. She reports that her brothers will stop by the house to take her son with them while they shop just to get him out of the house. When asked what would happen if she made no attempt to keep him occupied, she stated that he "would just sit in a chair." She indicated that friends rarely visit because "they don't want to be bothered, he doesn't respond."

When asked if her son engaged in any bizarre behaviors, the patient's mother paused and stated that he shows memory problems. Specifically, he will put a cup of tea down and then is unable to find it. When others point out where it is, he comments, "I didn't put it there," and he is "so sincere." In addition, she reports that she has discovered socks in the refrigerator that the patient indicated he could not find, and he denied placing them there. She also reports that he has attempted to put shoes on the wrong foot, and she once found a $20 bill in the trash that she had given him to spend on a shopping trip. He also reportedly has trouble remembering noteworthy events such as family reunions. She indicated that she first noticed the "memory problems" when the patient was still in the hospital following the truck accident and that the condition has progressively worsened. When asked if he appeared to talk to invisible people, she responded that occasionally she sees his lips move, but she is unable to hear what he is saying.

She stated that he exhibits considerable fearfulness and nightmares and "is scared to be alone." She indicated that she is attempting to leave him alone more so that he will learn to be "independent"; this was her reason for not staying after she had brought her son to the testing appointment, even though it had been requested that she accompany him. She stated that this was the "first time I have left him alone." (This comment contradicts the referring physician's report that the patient arrived at other evaluations alone.) The mother reports that the patient's sister visited approximately nine months ago and began crying, commenting, "How could the accident cause this [personality changes]?" The mother states that her son is in constant pain from his back injury; she is aware of this because of his frequent groaning. She also indicated that the patient is sensitive to noise and becomes readily irritable.

The patient's mother reported that the patient had no history of head trauma, birth or developmental abnormalities, chronic illnesses, surgeries, or seizure disorder and she indicated that there is no family history of psychiatric and/or cognitive problems. She stated that he is a high-school graduate and was "not a great bright student." She denied that he ever had difficulties in school or problems with the law. She also denied that he ever engaged in substance abuse. She indicated that he had never married and has no children.

Tests Administered

Bender Gestalt
Mini-Mental State Exam
Trailmaking
Mental Control subtest of the Wechsler Memory Scale
Rorschach Inkblot Test

Behavioral Observations and Test Findings

Because of the patient's lack of cooperation in the testing, the discussion of test findings will be combined with observations of test behavior. It is our distinct impression that the patient was attempting to exaggerate, if not actually feign, both the presence of psychotic symptomatology as well as cognitive deficits. Our conclusion is based on the patient's highly inconsistent and contradictory behavioral presentation, and in the following discussion we will cite numerous examples.

Mr. I. is a 47-year-old, right-handed, obese, black male of tall stature. He was casually attired and carried a TENS unit. His beard was carefully groomed; the

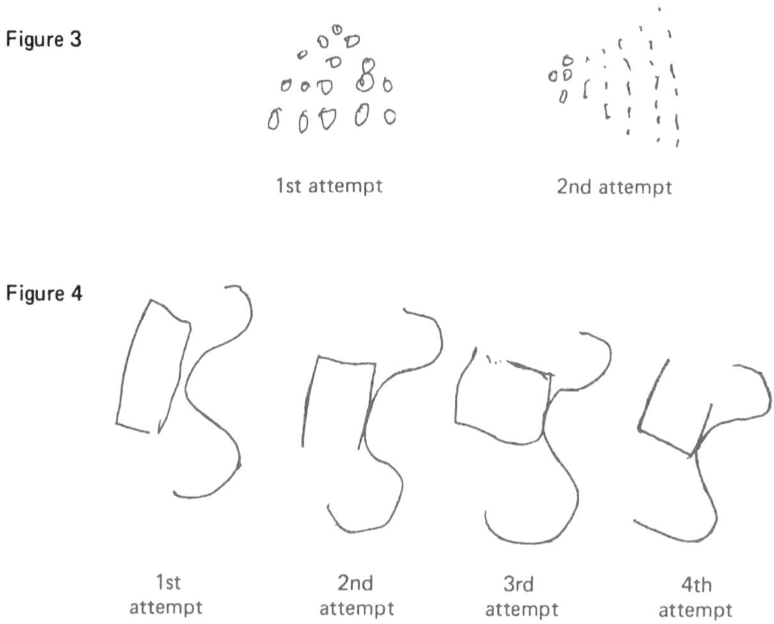

FIGURE 8.1. Case H.I. Bender-Gestalt figures 3 and 4. Reduced by 30%.

growth below the jaw line had been freshly shaven. He carried a grimy cloth pouch and wore an unusual neck ornament that he identified as garlic. The patient was brought to the testing session by his mother, who then left although it had been requested that she accompany him to the session. Late in the session the patient was told that his mother needed to be contacted to transport him home, and it appeared that he did not wish us to speak to her on the phone.

The patient presented a picture of gross impairment. He appeared at times not to comprehend basic questions and would give the examiner a quizzical look and then ask that questions be repeated. He denied knowing how old he was, where he had been born, or how much schooling he had completed. Conversely, the patient demonstrated very good recall of details regarding events surrounding his injury. He reported that he had been at a "bulk station" checking the crude oil level in a truck he was about to drive, "but they [other personnel] didn't hook up the static line and when I went up to check it . . . [explosion] and I landed on my back." It is also possible that Mr. I.'s ability to recount these details is a result of his having been told of them by others, though his detailed account is nevertheless in sharp contrast with his otherwise dramatic inability to recount even simple personal facts, such as the date and place of his birth.

Mr. I. initially provided very defective performances on every cognitive task administered, but when his deficient performance was not accepted and he was pushed to provide correct answers, it is noteworthy that he was able to do so. For example, when he was asked to copy designs from the Bender Gestalt test (Figures 8.1–8.2), his initial renderings were bizarre. When he was told that his

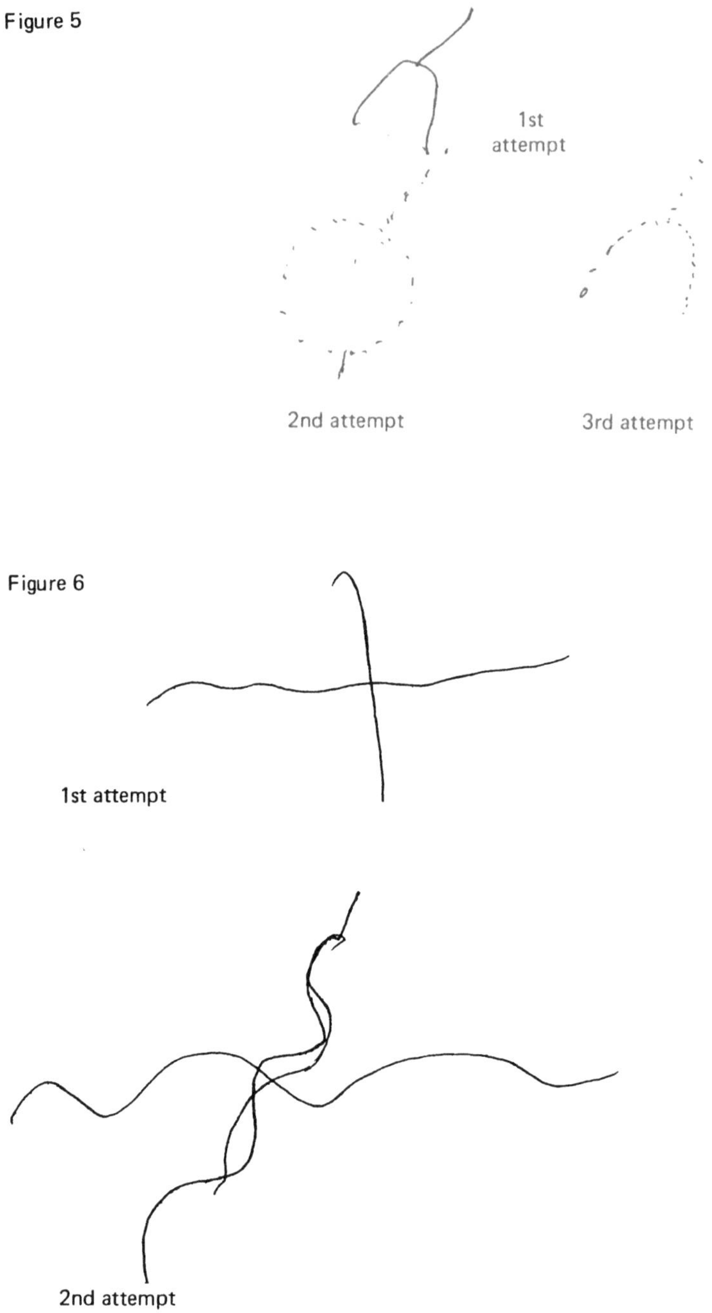

FIGURE 8.2. Case H.I. Bender-Gestalt figures 5 and 6. Reduced by 30%.

copies were incorrect and was asked to draw them correctly (with the implication that we would not move on to another task until he completed the drawings properly), he eventually corrected all of his errors. It also should be noted that when the patient was originally tested 11 months ago, the neuropsychologist noted that the patient's copying ability for simple geometric figures was intact.

When asked to write the day's date on a piece of paper, the patient wrote a date approximately three weeks prior to the actual date; the day and month were incorrect but the year was accurate. However, at a later point when he was asked to report the current year, the patient denied knowing what year it was, and when provided with multiple choice options, he was still "unable" to recognize the correct year.

The patient stated that he could not count to 10 or say the days of the week in order. Such "automatic" tasks are often intact even in severely demented individuals, and again, when the patient was pushed to provide correct responses he eventually did, although he attempted to change the topic (e.g., "Let's talk about something else."). The patient's performance was inconsistent with that observed by the first neuropsychologist who reported that the patient was able to execute simple addition and subtraction operations by counting on his fingers.

Mr. I. claimed that he could not write any words or letters to dictation, yet when asked to write his name on a piece of paper, the letters were well formed and no awkwardness was noted. The patient claimed to be unable to repeat three simple words in sequence (ball, flag, tree) and to say the phrase, "No ifs, ands, or buts"; yet when instructed to take a piece of paper in his right hand, fold it in half, and place it on the floor, the patient spontaneously repeated, "You mean you want me to take it in my hand, fold it in half, and put it on the floor?"

The patient was administered Trails A, a task that involves rapidly connecting numbers in order with a pencil. The patient required extended help to finish the task in 4 minutes, 41 seconds; the normal range is well under 60 seconds. When the patient was initially administered the task during the first neuropsychological evaluation 11 months ago, the patient completed it in 3 minutes, 20 seconds; it is inconsistent that the patient would require 1 minute, 21 seconds longer to complete it during the recent testing.

In regard to the psychiatric symptomatology, it was our distinct impression that Mr. I. was attempting to present himself as psychotic. For example, he spontaneously volunteered the information that he was wearing garlic around his neck, that he could fly without wings, that he wanted to go to the moon except there were "too many people there," that he had an invisible friend named "Ron" downstairs in the waiting room, and that instead of talking about the details of his accident, he wanted to talk about his pet chicken "Frank," a "Rhode Island red." Usually, paranoid individuals are secretive and reluctant to provide personal information, and they also tend to be very frightened and wary of machines. Yet, this patient carries a machine with him to administer "electric shock" to his body (TENS unit).

The Rorschach inkblot test, often sensitive to a thinking disturbance, was administered. The patient's Rorschach responses revealed relatively good form level on some responses in conjunction with inappropriate content responses to other blots (e.g., on the first blot, he saw "Frank," the chicken; on others, he saw "Ron," his imaginary friend). His responses overall did not reveal psychiatric disturbance of the same magnitude as the patient's overt behavioral presentation, though there was some evidence of a post traumatic stress disorder.

Summary and Impressions

It is our conclusion that Mr. I. was deliberately and consciously attempting to present with severe cognitive and psychiatric deficits. Inconsistencies in performance across tasks was noted, as well as inconsistencies between test scores and observed level of adaptive functioning. For example, the patient could not recall basic personal facts but could recall details of events surrounding his injury. Remote personal information is rarely lost except in the most severe organic brain syndrome. On the other hand, the most frequent memory loss seen in head trauma involves loss of recall of events immediately preceding and succeeding the trauma (retrograde and anterograde amnesia). Also of note, the patient showed gross distortion in pencil and paper constructions, but his beard was intricately groomed and shaved. He was able to report the correct year at one point in the testing but later denied knowing the year and guessed incorrectly when provided with multiple choice options. Similar gross inconsistencies were noted in verbal repetition and writing. When his substandard responses were not accepted, he invariably was able to provide correct or improved answers. Interestingly, current test scores were significantly poorer than those reported from a neuropsychological evaluation completed 11 months earlier; cognitive scores typically stabilize or improve following head injury, not decline. Finally, a patient as disoriented and cognitively disabled as the patient presented would not be able to be left alone by family members at doctor appointments or successfully travel by bus (the patient reported that he did indeed travel by bus alone).

The patient may in fact be experiencing more moderate and circumscribed difficulties, but due to his deliberate feigning and uncooperativeness in the testing, no accurate assessment of cognitive and psychological functioning can be obtained at present. It is our belief that at least a moderate level of cognitive functioning and "cleverness" would be required to consciously feign deficits during a three-hour session. This does not rule out the possibility of psychological trauma from his accident, and indeed, some of our findings are consistent with a post traumatic stress reaction to the accident that would not involve the severe cognitive debilitation that the patient attempted to present in our examination.

Again, it should be stressed that Mr. I. may in fact have more subtle deficits, but given his lack of cooperation, these cannot be adequately assessed at this time. It is clear that the patient certainly is not as impaired—cognitively and psychiatrically—as he presents. We recommend that the patient be counseled that it is in his best interest to be truthful during his evaluations so that any actual disability can be appropriately treated and/or recompensed.

Case 2: Psychological Factors Affecting Physical Condition

Reason for Referral

Mr. T.G. was referred for neuropsychological testing by his attorney for his workers compensation claim for evaluation of possible cognitive sequelae of exposure to toxic chemicals. No medical records were available for review, and the findings contained in the following consultation report are based on test findings, observations of the patient's test behavior, and history as provided by the patient.

Presenting Situation and Background Information

Mr. G., a 33-year-old, right-handed male, has been employed as a plant manager for a school district for nine years. Nearly nine years ago he was exposed to a toxic lacquer-like substance (he was unable to name the specific substance) while executing his job duties, and he subsequently became ill and was hospitalized for approximately six days. He reportedly lapsed in and out of consciousness during that time and was placed on oxygen. He reports that he was told that the chemicals contained in the lacquer substance were of such toxicity that they would cause damage to body organs, particularly the brain and liver. He indicated that during his hospitalization he felt like he was "in a dream" and others' voices sounded as if they were "on a slow speed." He experienced visual and tactile hallucinations and had to be physically restrained. He suffered severe pain in his head "like it was being cut apart with a saw." Commencing at the time of the exposure and continuing to the present, the patient has been experiencing headaches that occur on a daily basis and are so severe that the patient has contemplated ending his life. He described them as sharp and throbbing and located on the top and rear of his head. He indicated that they usually begin in the morning and frequently awaken him from his sleep.

Mr. G. reported that approximately one month after the toxic exposure and hospitalization, he began to notice difficulty with his memory. Specifically, he indicated that his remote memories appear to be intact, but that he has difficulty learning and recalling new information, particularly "what people say to me." He also states that his bank contacted him because they had noted that his signature changed since the accident. In particular, the patient indicated that he used to have "good handwriting" but that his handwriting abilities deteriorated following the toxic exposure and that "I was having trouble forming letters." He also reported that since the toxic exposure, he notices that it takes him longer to formulate his thoughts in answer to others' questions and that others have commented on his slowed thinking ability. He indicated that concentration and attention abilities have also been depressed since the accident. Finally, the patient indicated that he has episodes in which he becomes "mean and abusive, like I become another person, I become verbally abusive and afterwards, I can't believe that I did it and my memory of it is kind of vague." The patient reported that these episodes of verbal aggressiveness are not provoked and occur when his headaches are at their worst. Following the outbursts, he lies down and falls asleep. He indicated that during these episodes he is abusive toward his girlfriend but also with other people whom he does not know well. He stated that his friends have commented that they thought he was on drugs because of the change in his personality. He stated that at times, he awakes in the morning with a vague feeling that it might be a "bad day" for him, and he becomes fearful to leave the house.

Four years ago, Mr. G. was also exposed to a toxic asphalt product, which caused pneumonia-like symptoms including breathing difficulties, headaches, and fever. The patient reports that many students and teachers, as well as himself and his work crew, experienced these symptoms and sought medical attention. The patient stated that he was exposed to these toxic chemicals for approximately one year. Since the second toxic exposure, the patient stated that his headaches have worsened.

In addition to the cognitive symptoms, the patient reports prominent psychiatric symptomalogy including nervousness, depression, suicidal ideation, sleep disturbance, weight loss, and reduced sexual interest. The patient was placed on medical leave due to his psychiatric symptoms and has not worked for the past month. He has been receiving psychotherapeutic treatment for the past month.

Mr. G.'s medical history is noteworthy for a head trauma sustained 15 years ago, in which the patient experienced loss of consciousness for approximately three to five minutes. He was treated at a nearby hospital and informed that he had suffered a mild concussion. He reported that he experienced no cognitive sequelae following that accident. The patient denies any chronic illnesses such as diabetes, epilepsy, or high blood pressure. He denies any history of alcohol or drug abuse, birth or developmental abnormalities, surgeries, or psychiatric symptomatology before nine years ago. His current medications include Diltazen, for headaches, and Elavil.

Mr. G. is a high-school graduate and described himself as a "B" student. He denied any history of learning disabilities. He has one brother who obtained a bachelor's degree in English and is currently completing requirements for a teaching credential. He has two sisters: one is currently attending a junior college and the other is employed in the computer industry.

Tests Administered

See data summary sheet.

Behavioral Observations

Mr. G. is a 33-year-old, right-handed, brown-haired Caucasian male of medium height and weight. He arrived on time and unaccompanied for his testing appointment. He was observed to be adequately groomed and casually attired.

Observation of the patient's test behavior strongly suggested that he was not exerting his best effort on the tests, as will be further discussed in the next section. At no time did the patient demonstrate concern or frustration with his substandard performances, despite good awareness. Eye contact was poor. He frequently held his head and sighed in a rather melodramatic manner.

Speech characteristics were unremarkable, and no difficulties were noted in the patient's comprehension of task instructions. Thought content was well organized and relevant. No lengthy response latencies were noted during the interview. No bizarre or peculiar mannerisms were noted, and the patient did not exhibit signs of psychosis such as hallucinations, delusions, or thought disorder.

Test Results

Gross Cognitive Functioning

Performance on a cognitive screening measure was at the cut-off indicating brain dysfunction (MMSE = 23). Mr. G. made errors in subtracting serial 7s. He was only able to recall one of three words following a short delay and, surprisingly, failed to consistently recognize the failed items when they were presented in multiple-choice format, a type of performance found in severely impaired individuals.

Intellectual Scores

The results of intellectual testing revealed scores within the borderline range of general intellectual ability (Full Scale IQ = 75). A mild to moderate discrepancy was noted between overall Verbal and Performance IQs, with the Performance IQ falling 12 points below the Verbal IQ (VIQ = 82; PIQ = 70).

Inconsistencies in performance appeared during the intellectual testing, suggesting that the patient was not fully cooperating in the tasks. For example, he appeared confused by the sample item on the Picture Arrangement subtest and required 17 seconds to arrange the pictures in order. The sample item depicts a worker building a house, and the three pictures included in the sample show the house foundation, the foundation with wood framing, and the finished building being painted. Only severely cognitively impaired individuals show confusion in arranging these simple pictures into a logical order. The patient was unable to correctly arrange any of the remaining Picture Arrangement items. In addition, the obtained forward and backward digit spans were four and two respectively, an extremely poor performance. The patient also showed confusion on the second test item on the Object Assembly subtest, an item that requires assembly of the parts of a face. The patient repeatedly attempted to insert the neck section where the mouth belonged. Interestingly, the patient was able to complete the last and most difficult item in this subtest (assembly of an elephant) in just 19 seconds. An individual who performs well on the last item should have no difficulty in assembling facial features. Dramatic inconsistencies were also observed in the patient's performance on the Block Design subtest. Some of his responses to the Vocabulary subtest suggested a melodramatic presentation; for example, when asked to define the word "ponder," he responded, "darkness," and when asked to define the word "ominous," he said, "suicide."

Attention and Concentration

Performance on rote attention tasks was highly suspicious. The patient made four errors when counting backwards from 20 to 1, and made eight errors when reciting the letters of the alphabet. Specifically, his alphabet recital was as follows: "A, B, C, D, E, F, G, H, K, L, M, P, R, S, T, X, Y, Z." This profound impairment in "automatic" verbal tasks is rare in educated English-speaking individuals.

Language Functioning

The patient's speech was unremarkable, and no difficulties were noted in comprehension of task instructions. However, language screening revealed some grossly deficient performances. The patient spelled "square" as "sqaure," and spelled "triangle" as "trangle." He responded very unusually when asked to repeat "Massachusetts" and "Methodist Episcopal." After he was told to repeat the word "Massachusetts," he paused for a very lengthy period of time and then said, "Mass . . . [long pause] . . . chusetts." When asked to repeat "Methodist Episcopal," he said, "Meth, Meth . . . [long pause] . . . apisabol." This type of grossly impaired verbal repetition was not observed on any other tasks requiring repetition (Digit Span, repeating of an auditorily presented sentence, immediate recall of paragraph details, recall of word lists, etc.). The patient was able to discriminate right and left, read simple material, and gesture appropriately.

Perceptual Organizational Skills

Performance on perceptual organization tasks again showed significant compromise. The patient scored within the impaired range on visual perceptual tasks (Hooper VOT = 18/30; Picture Completion age-corrected score = 3). Paper and pencil constructional skills were also decreased (Beery VMI = 19, 11-6 age equivalent; Rey-Osterrieth Complex Figure = 23/36, <10th percentile–see Figure 8.3) and showed gross distortions and rotations (e.g., detail #11 drawn upside down). Visual sequencing and tracking skills were consistently impaired (Picture Arrangement and Digit Symbol = 2nd percentile; Trails A = 57 seconds; Trails B = patient discontinued at 205 seconds at item #10).

Learning and Memory

The patient performed very poorly in the immediate recall of nonverbal visual material (WMS-VR, see Figure 8.4), and was allowed to directly copy the test stimuli (Figure 8.5). He copied one of the designs partially *upside down* (C-2), and when instructed to draw it correctly, he said that he could not. His 45-minute delayed recall showed marked distortion (e.g., he drew a domino for one of the designs, see Figure 8.6), and he did not correctly recognize any of the stimuli

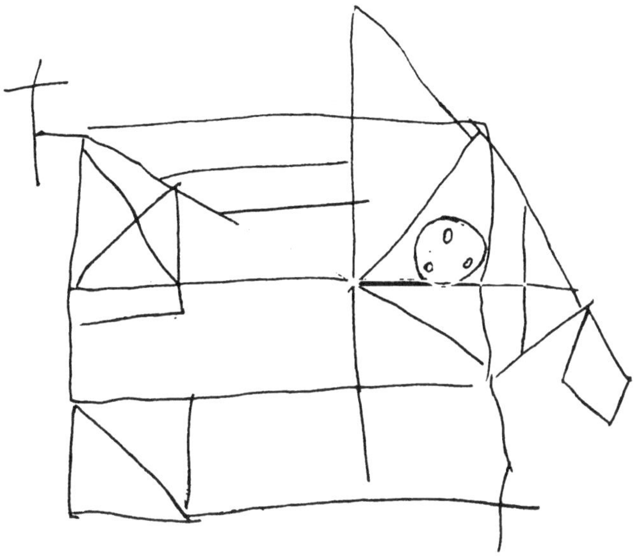

FIGURE 8.3. Case T.G. Rey-Osterrieth Complex Figure: copy. Reduced by 25%.

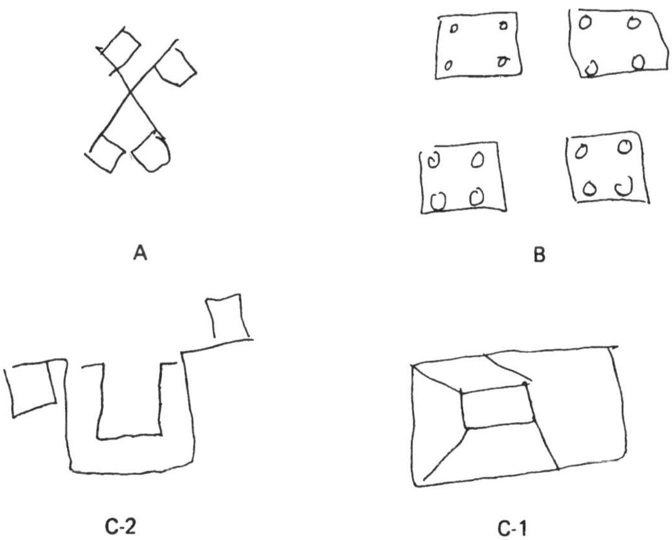

FIGURE 8.4. Case T.G. Wechsler Memory Scale–Visual Reproduction: immediate recall. Reduced by 50%.

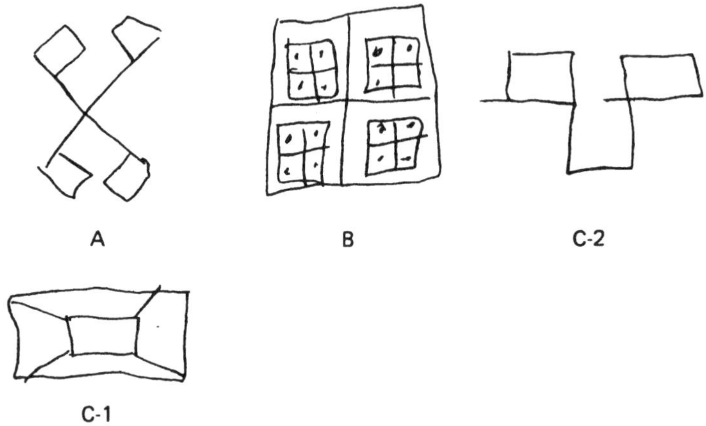

FIGURE 8.5. Case T.G. Wechsler Memory Scale–Visual Reproduction: copy trial. He was requested to attempt figure C-2 a second time, and he refused. Reduced by 45%.

when presented in multiple-choice format. In the learning of word pairs, the patient was only able to learn two of the 10 pairs by the third learning trial (WMS–AL). On a word-list learning task, the patient was only able to learn eight of 15 items by the fifth learning trial (AVLT), and was only able to recall an average of 3.25 paragraph details on immediate recall (WMS–LM). This pattern of test findings is only found in individuals with marked learning and memory impairment.

Motor Examination

Scores on a motor dexterity task were within the average range bilaterally (Tapping: R = 50.8; L = 44.4).

Motivation and Cooperation

Additional tests were administered that are designed to measure motivation level and cooperation, and on these tasks the patient showed performances typical of individuals who are not exerting their best effort and cooperating fully. Specifi-

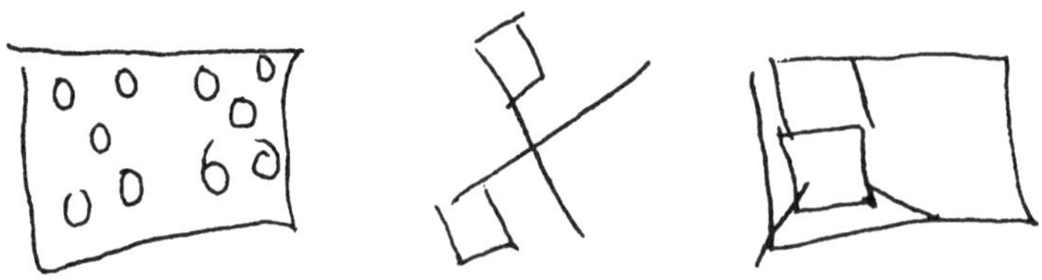

FIGURE 8.6. Case T.G. Wechsler Memory Scale–Visual Reproduction: delayed recall. Reduced by 20%.

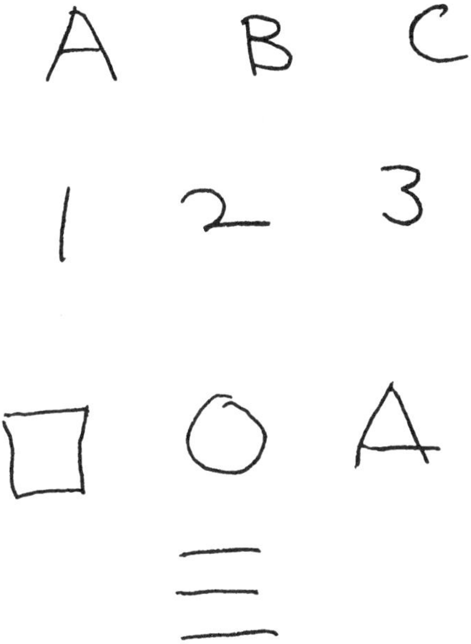

FIGURE 8.7. Case T.G. Memorization of 15 items. Reduced by 10%.

cally, on a word list recognition task, the patient was only able to correctly recognize four words, but on the first trial of the AVLT, the patient was able to recall five words. As recognition is much easier than free recall, the patient's performance suggests that he was not fully cooperative in this learning task. In addition, on a dot counting task, the patient showed a highly suspicious performance. He counted the dots on the test stimuli in a methodical manner, but when he reached the last dot on each card, he paused for several seconds before reporting how many dots were on the cards; his answers were incorrect. Frankly, the patient appeared to be generating an incorrect answer during the several second pause. In the memorization of 15 items, the patient was able to correctly reproduce nine of the items and then gave a final confabulated response (see Figure 8.7).

Personality Functioning

The patient was administered two pencil and paper personality tests, the MMPI and MCMI. The patient's responses on both measures were judged to be valid although the validity scale scores on the MMPI suggested a nonconformist or idiosyncratic response pattern. Significant elevations were noted on all but two MMPI clinical scales, and three scale scores were more than 6 SDs above the mean (1-2-8-7-5-3-6-0). The pattern of scores suggested a pronounced degree of psychiatric disturbance characterized by odd somatic complaints, body preoccupations, worry, and pessimism. The scores suggest a strong likelihood of thought disorder, confusion, and strange thoughts, beliefs, and actions. Individuals with similar elevations may appear unusual, unconventional, and eccentric to others, but they may be able to maintain adequate vocational adjustment. They relate poorly to others and are seen as socially introverted.

Significant elevations (at or above a base rate of 75) were also present on nine of the MCMI scales (2-3-A-1-C-D-8-H-S-C). Patients exhibiting this pattern of scores are described as very withdrawn and aloof, but also dependent and passive-aggressive. They tend to be highly anxious, depressed, and preoccupied with ill health. The patient showed significant elevations on both the Borderline and Schizotypal scales, suggesting the presence of a personality or characterological disorder.

Summary and Impressions

On neuropsychological and intellectual testing, the patient scored at a severely depressed level. Specifically, he scored within the impaired range on tasks measuring memory ability, visual perception and construction skills, attention, and basic language skills. The lowered performance was much more extensive than the mild to moderate disturbances in memory, visual spatial skills, mental processing speed, and eye-hand coordination typically found in patients who are months or years post toxic exposure. Although the low scores could be consistent with the patient's report of dramatically altered consciousness during hospitalization, his report is suspect secondary to psychiatric symptoms.

Additionally, the patient's inconsistent and unusual test responses strongly indicate that he was not fully cooperating in the testing and was not exerting his best effort on the tasks. Also of note, the test findings were not consistent with the patient's current level of functioning in his daily life. For example, patients with the pattern of scores shown by Mr. G. are typically not capable of living on their own, driving themselves to medical appointments, or being employed. Yet, the patient lives on his own and drove himself to the testing appointment, arriving on time. In addition, the patient performed extremely poorly on memory testing, but appeared to have no difficulty recalling and recounting recent events in his life or his numerous symptoms. Thus, although test scores are consistent with dementia, they appear to be the result of an attempt by the patient to appear cognitively impaired. The patient may in fact suffer from subtle cognitive deficits, but these cannot be assessed at the present time because of the psychiatric overlay. Personality testing revealed marked psychiatric disturbance including characterological disorder.

An important question that remains is whether the observed noncompliance in the testing was the result of conscious malingering or was a nonconscious act associated with psychiatric disturbance. This determination is best made by the patient's treating therapist, who has the opportunity to observe the patient over an extended period of time. It is most likely, given the patient's psychiatric disorder, that his noncooperation was a nonconscious, nondeliberate reflection of his psychiatric decompensation, and a desperate attempt to alert others to his psychological pain and distress (i.e., "cry for help" behavior). It is not clear why the patient is exhibiting such psychiatric deterioration at the present time; he denies any recent interpersonal conflict or loss.

It is strongly recommended that the patient not be provided with the results of this report. Disclosure of the contents would not be in the best interest of his psychological functioning and could precipitate more maladaptive behavior. The patient appears to be desperately trying to impress others with the level of his psychiatric dysfunction, and he might view this report as discounting him and his symptoms. He clearly requires psychological treatment at this point in time, and the sooner that he can restructure his life in terms of employment, the sooner his psychological condition will stabilize and improve.

NEUROPSYCHOLOGY TEST SCORE SUMMARY SHEET

Patient: T.G.   Age: 33   Sex: M   Handedness: R

I. Gross Cognitive Functioning
Mini-Mental State Exam: 23 /30

II. Intelligence WAIS-R Age-Corrected Scores

VERBAL			PERFORMANCE		
Information	8	(25 %ile)	Picture Completion	3	(1 %ile)
Digit Span	3	(1 %ile)	Picture Arrangement	4	(2 %ile)
Vocabulary	8	(25 %ile)	Block Design	6	(9 %ile)
Arithmetic	6	(9 %ile)	Object Assembly	10	(50 %ile)
Comprehension	9	(37 %ile)	Digit Symbol	4	(2 %ile)
Similarities	8	(25 %ile)			
VERBAL IQ =	82	(12 %ile)	PERFORMANCE IQ =	70	(2 %ile)

FULL SCALE IQ = 75 (5 %ile)

III. Attention/Concentration
Digit Span: 4 forward + 2 backwards = 6 Total (1 %ile)
Mental Control, WMS: 0 (<1 %ile)
Trails A: 57" (<1 %ile), Trails B: 205" (<1 %ile)

IV. Language
Aphasia Screening Exam: spelling and repetition errors

V. Perceptual/Organizational
Rey-Osterrieth Complex Figure Copy: 23 /36 (<10 %ile)
Hooper Visual Organization Test: 18 /30
Beery VMI: 19/24

VI. Memory

VERBAL		NONVERBAL	
WMS Logical Memory	3.25 (5%ile)	WMS Visual Repro.:	2 (1 %ile)
45 min. delay:	2.75	Direct copy:	9
Percent retention:	42	45 min. delay:	1 (<1 %ile)

WMS Associate Learning
I Easy 2 , 2 , 2
I Hard 0 , 0 , 0
I Score: 3 (<1 %ile)
45 min. delay: 2 easy, 0 hard 100% retention

Rey-Osterrieth Fig: 23/36 (<10 %ile)

Rey Auditory Verbal Learning Test (15 items):
T1:5 T2:6 T3:6 T4:6 T5:8

VII. Motor Exam

	Dominant Hand	%ile	Nondom. Hand	%ile
Finger Tapping:	50.8	64	44.4	48

VII. Personality
MMPI: 12875**3*6"0'4-9/ L:F'K/

VIII. Tests for Malingering
Word Recognition: recog. 4
15-item Memorization: 9 items
Dot Counting:

	Ungrouped		Grouped	
	Time	Answer	Time	Answer
1.	4"	7	1"	8
2.	9"	12	4"	12
3.	9"	17	4"	8
4.	10"	21	5"	20
5.	10"	25	7"	24
6.	13"	29	10"	34

Case 3: Probable Somatization Disorder

Reason for Referral

Ms. D.R. was referred for neuropsychological testing by her attorney for her workers compensation claim to determine whether she is suffering from cognitive impairment related to the work-related head injury she is reported to have sustained three-and-one-half years ago.

Presenting Situation and Background Information

Ms. R. is a 41-year-old, right-handed female who reports that almost three-and-one-half years ago she suffered a head injury while carrying out her duties as a research technician. Specifically, she stated that she was cataloging inventory when a 70-pound instrument fell from a rack approximately 6-feet high, striking her on the head, neck, and right shoulder as she was attempting to rise from a kneeling position. She indicates that she was not knocked unconscious but did suffer a laceration on her scalp that required suturing at an emergency room. The patient attempted to return to work two months after the injury but became dizzy and nauseous, and she has not attempted any work activities since that time. She was rear-ended in a car accident approximately one year ago but denies hitting her head at that time. She reported that three months ago she underwent vocational testing but has not entered into any rehabilitation program.

The patient reports continuing physical, cognitive, and emotional difficulties that began following her injury three-and-one-half years ago. Specifically, she describes the presence of severe headaches, which she describes as "migraine," that usually last three to four days but have continued for as long as 10 days. She indicates that the frequency of the headaches is decreasing, and she now experiences them approximately every two weeks. When the headaches are present the patient states that she "wish[es] I would die. . . I don't function, I don't drive, I don't leave the house." She stated that pain medication does not provide her with any relief. Ms. R. perceives that heat seems to trigger the headaches. Nausea, dizziness, and sensitivity to noise and light accompany the headaches; "I go to the darkest room in the house to get relief. . . I also bought a blindfold." The patient reports that approximately one month after the injury she experienced "terrible head pain and I thought I would die." The pain has not recurred.

Ms. R. also indicates that she periodically experiences numbness in her hands, particularly in the index and middle fingers, while lying down. She states that following her injury she did experience some drooling, but this problem has subsided.

Ms. R. is reporting some symptoms of depression including dysphoric mood, weight gain, and sleep disturbance. She naps during the day and states that she is sleeping more than usual but does not "sleep well." She denied any current suicidal ideation.

The patient states that she is experiencing memory loss for events following the injury and indicates that others have commented on her memory impairment. She reports that she has difficulty remembering people's names and cannot remember how to use surgical instruments she used regularly in her employment—"Things I could do in my sleep before." She indicates that she has difficulty remembering what she has read in books, "like I have never read it at all . . . before the injury I used to pride myself on my memory." She states that when she attempts to cook she frequently burns herself because "I forget to use utensils and attempt to turn things over with my hands." The patient states also that she has forgotten about food she has left cooking on the stove.

Ms. R. also reports that after the injury she has had difficulty concentrating while driving (e.g., missing freeway exits). She indicates that at times she is distracted by such things as windshield wipers and has difficulty diverting her gaze back to the highway. When entering parking structures "I get fixated on the overhead beams." The patient states that she has difficulty tracking while reading and often loses her place on the page. In addition, Ms. R. finds it difficult to look through plastic. She indicates that she frequently knocks objects over.

The patient reports that she has "worked hard to regain my skills" and is currently enrolled in a remedial algebra program. She is a member of a head trauma support group and has received pain-management training for her headaches. When asked to rate the severity of her disabilities, Ms. R. indicated that she believes she is functioning as poorly as the "veggies" (severely impaired individuals) in her head trauma support group. Specifically, she judged her premorbid memory abilities to be "10," whereas present memory capabilities are perceived as "1." Other abilities such as writing, naming, judgment, patience, self-control, computational ability, and planning ability were judged as "10" prior to the injury, and between "2" and "6" following the accident.

The patient denied any prior history of head injury, alcohol or drug abuse, seizure disorder, hospitalizations or surgeries aside from childbirth, or birth or developmental abnormalities. She indicated that she has been diagnosed with borderline hypertension since the head injury. She received a bachelor's degree and denied any history of learning disability. She denied any significant psychiatric history prior to the head injury or prior history of headaches or hypertension, although the review of medical records revealed contradictory information. She currently takes no medications aside from nonprescription pain medication.

Review of Medical Records

The patient was seen in an emergency room at the time of the injury and was observed to have a scalp laceration of the posterior parietal region. No neurologic deficits were noted, however, a post-concussion syndrome was suspected. A skull series was judged to be normal. Paracervical muscle tenderness was observed. The patient was seen again 10 days later for suture removal and was complaining of head pain that did "not fit any anatomical localization," and the physician suggested the possibility of "psychiatric overlay."

Three days after the suture removal, the patient was evaluated by a neurosurgeon. The patient's symptoms of headaches, neck pain, vertigo, and nausea were judged to be "due to the cervical sprain and soft tissue injury, and that any element of concussion is relatively mild." Sensory examination and CT scan were entirely within normal limits. The neurosurgeon reported that he was "convinced that she does not have any neurological problem, and her symptoms continue to be due to her neck sprain." In a report dated two months after the initial evaluation, the neurosurgeon indicated "I am certain that the patient has no neurological problem related to her industrial injury, but I am at a loss to explain her continued, variable, intermittent symptoms."

Ten days later Ms. R. was evaluated by a neurologist. An EEG obtained at that time was read as normal. The neurologist diagnosed the patient as suffering from post traumatic head syndrome and cerebral concussion, cervical sprain, thoracolumbosacral strain, and post traumatic anxiety. The diagnosis of post traumatic head syndrome was made on the basis of "altered consciousness during the original time of injury with subsequent episodes of dizziness, nausea, vomitus, and protracted headaches."

Two months later the patient was evaluated by a psychiatrist who reported that six months before her injury the patient filed a grievance against her employer for sexual discrimination. Hearings were held two months before the head injury, but the grievance was not upheld. The psychiatrist reported that the patient indicated that she had experienced further harassment within her department following the filing of the grievance. He also stated that Ms. R. attempted to return to work following her head injury but had to stop working because "moving her hands caused intense nausea." She attempted to work again two months later, but her headaches and dizziness became worse after only an hour on the job, and the patient has not worked since. The psychiatrist diagnosed the patient as suffering from post-concussion syndrome.

Ms. R. was examined by a second psychiatrist seven months after the industrial injury. He reported that at the time of his evaluation the patient was being seen at a pain clinic four times per week, by a chiropractor two to three times per week, and by a psychotherapist one to two times per week. The psychiatrist indicated that during his examination the patient was able to subtract serial 7s rapidly and accurately and that her memory for recent and remote events was good. He diagnosed the patient as having a mixed personality disorder with histrionic, dependent, passive-aggressive, and paranoid features, and psychological factors affecting physical condition (vascular headaches). He reported a strong tendency for the patient to dramatize and exaggerate her symptomology. He indicated that he felt the personality disorder "existed long before she went to work for her current employer and was not caused by, exaggerated by, nor lit up by her employment." He suggested that "she consciously or unconsciously wishes to remain in the sick role as a way of punishing her employer for what she feels has been harassment." In a supplemental report dated one month later, the psychiatrist compared the history given to him by the patient with that provided by medical reports and concluded that the patient exerted "a deliberate effort to distort the information supplied."

Ms. R. was examined by a second neurologist nine months after her injury. He reports that the patient denied experiencing any industrial injuries prior to the accident in question. He commented on the patient's "rather dramatic histrionic fashion with more importantly, purposeful misgiving of information and distortion of her past medical history." He suggests that her present symptoms are "no different than the ones she had been complaining about prior to the head injury. She still complains of lightheadedness, earaches, headaches, neck pain, low-back pain, left leg pain and borderline hypertension. All of these features were noted prior to her industrial injury on many occasions. She currently appears fixated on her symptoms as she did prior to her industrial injury."

The patient was enrolled in psychotherapy with the first evaluating psychiatrist who provided periodic progress reports. He documented little improvement in her symptoms. Of note, he reports that he had attempted to schedule neuropsychological testing for Ms. R. to determine the presence of subtle organic brain dysfunction complicating the patient's overall recovery. The patient refused this evaluation.

Progress notes from counseling sessions the patient attended eight years before her injury were useful in illuminating her premorbid psychological functioning. Her therapist described her at that time as exhibiting "whining, manipulative, 'victim-playing' behavior. . . . Since childhood, D.R. has consulted physicians . . . with a number of complaints other than accidental injuries. . . . Her life continued to be an almost endless string of problems, including financial problems, parental dissatisfaction, health problems, etc. . . . she complains that she is losing her resiliency, her ability to cope with stresses in her life. The stresses she mentions are so numerous that it appears that she plays the role of 'victim.'"

Behavioral Observations

The patient's test behavior was very unusual, and consequently the test findings must be interpreted very carefully. Specifically, it was the examiner's distinct impression that the patient was not exerting her best effort during the testing. In addition, the patient's behavior was observed to be highly histrionic, manipulative, and passive-aggressive in an obvious, self-defeating manner.

Ms. R. is a 41-year-old, brown-haired, obese Caucasian woman. She wore her hair pulled back in a ponytail and wore plain, unflattering clothing. On arriving at the session, the patient refused to answer questions at the registration office and was emotionally labile. During the interview she spoke rapidly and at length in a whining voice about her numerous symptoms; however, once the testing began she became very withdrawn and sat in silence for long periods of time before providing sparse answers. She refused to guess on answers she indicated that she did not know. Her failures on test items were not accompanied by frustration or irritation but with indifference and unconcern. Most patients will readily provide answers that they think might be correct but are unsure of; however, Ms. R. had to be prodded continually to provide answers that often were correct. For example when asked to define the word "plagiarize," the following interaction occurred:

Patient: "To steal."
Examiner: "Steal what?"
Patient: "Words."
Examiner: "What do you mean 'to steal words'?"
Patient: "To write a story and say it's yours, but you didn't write it."

When the patient was asked to circle words incorporated in a paragraph that she had heard in a word list, she circled approximately half of the target items and indicated that she did not recognize any more. When told to circle more, she circled all the remaining correct words except for one.

Some of the patient's scores appeared to have been lowered because of slowness of responding. For example, on block construction and puzzle-solving tasks, most subjects will work relatively slowly until most of the pieces are in the correct order, and they perceive where the remaining pieces need to be placed. They then proceed quickly because they are aware that the task is timed and they desire to obtain the fastest time possible. Conversely, the patient did not increase the speed of her performance even when the solution to the tasks was obvious.

Following a lunch break, the examiner found a note on the door of the testing office informing her that the patient could be found resting on a sofa in the women's restroom "in case I fall asleep" and was late for the resumption of the testing. The patient refused to complete personality testing on the day of testing, stating that it was "too upsetting." She later phoned the office several days in a row demanding to be allowed to complete one test (MMPI) but "in the morning only because I'm only good in the morning." She explained that she had been reluctant to complete the inventory on the day of testing because "I couldn't take it when we changed [testing] rooms." She reported that the test took an extended amount of time to complete because "I had to ask for a ruler to stay on the lines."

Tests Administered

See data summary sheet.

Test Results

Motivation and Cooperation

Ms. R. was administered two tests designed to evaluate whether a patient is consciously or unconsciously attempting to appear impaired. In the first task, she was informed that she would be required to memorize 15 different items pictured on a piece of paper. The number "15" was stressed to make the test appear diffi-

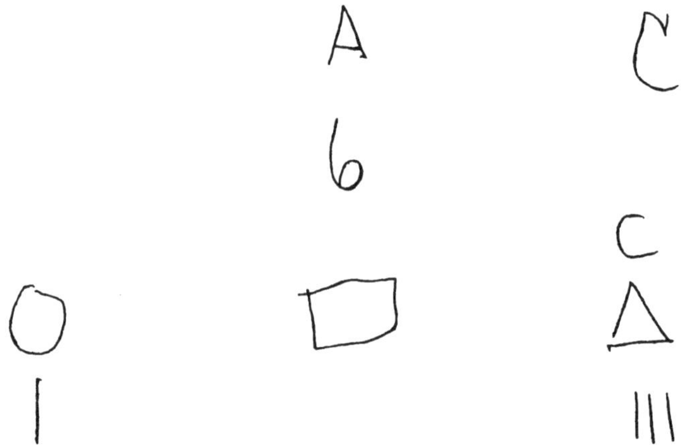

FIGURE 8.8. Case D.R. Memorization of 15 items. Reduced by 30%.

cult. In reality, the patient needed to remember only three or four ideas to recall the items. Anyone not significantly deteriorated can recall at least three of the five series of items (nine items). The patient recalled only one complete series (Figure 8.8).

The patient was also administered a dot-counting task in which she was told to count and report the number of dots on cards as quickly as she could. A cooperative patient's response latency increases gradually with increased number of dots. Although this is a very easy task, the patient generally required considerably more time than the average to count the dots. In addition, her performance was inconsistent; she required only three seconds to count 11 dots but spent 4.5 seconds to count seven dots.

Ms. R.'s performance on these tests would appear to indicate that she was not exerting her best effort on the testing and was attempting to represent herself as impaired. In spite of this lack of cooperation, her test scores generally did not show much deficit, however. Interestingly, when asked at the conclusion of the testing how she thought she had done, she stated, "I didn't feel it went well." The test scores will be presented briefly, although the validity of the scores is highly questionable.

Intellectual Scores

The patient obtained a Full Scale IQ of 99 on the WAIS-R, which places her well within the normal range of general intellectual ability.

Perceptual Organizational Skills

In spite of the patient's report of some visual perceptual and visual tracking problems, she generally scored in the low average to superior range on tests tapping these abilities (Hooper = 29/30; Trails A = 35 seconds, B = 85 seconds;

Picture Arrangement = 75th percentile; Digit Symbol = 25th percentile). The fact that the patient scored extremely well on a visual perceptual task involving identification of disassembled objects (Hooper) would seem at variance with her attempt to present herself as impaired. However, the test administration was altered to control for this behavior. She was instructed that test items would become more difficult as she progressed through the test and that the first few items would be relatively simple. However, she was administered the test backward, with the very difficult items presented first. Constructional skills were intact (Block Design = 63rd percentile; Object Assembly = 25th percentile; Rey-Osterrieth = 36/36).

Language Functioning

The patient's language skills were normal; there was no evidence of any dysnomia, and the patient was able to read aloud, spell, repeat phrases, follow verbal commands, discriminate right and left, and write to dictation (Aphasia Screening Test).

Attention and Memory

Most striking was the patient's behavior on attention and memory testing; when asked to repeat or recall items, the patient would sit and stare at the table for literally minutes before providing any response, and interestingly, her answers were usually correct. This behavior is inconsistent with the neuropsychology of attention and memory functioning. When presented with a stimulus to repeat, the longer the delay before responding, the more likely the memory trace will be lost. In addition, if the person does not remember the information upon initial questioning, it is highly doubtful it will suddenly reappear minutes later. The patient's verbal memory scores were variable, with depressed scores obtained in the learning of unrelated word lists (AVLT). Her learning of word pairs and details of short stories was within the normal range (WMS–AL and WMS–LM = 39th and 41st percentiles, respectively). Visual memory skills were well above average (WMS-VR = 92nd percentile; Rey-Osterrieth Complex Figure = 90th percentile). When the patient was asked to draw geometric designs on delayed recall, she started to add extra details. The examiner told her to stop and draw the designs correctly, and she complied (Figure 8.9).

Personality Functioning

The patient's MMPI profile showed extreme elevations on scales 2 and 3, which is reflective of symptoms of depression associated with a naive, histrionic personality structure. In persons obtaining similar scores, the typical life role is that of "chronic family invalid." The "invalidism" especially tends to occur following major medical intervention or surgery. Excessive medical workups and elective surgery should be avoided due to the possibility of negative physical pathology and prolonged recovery with extensive problems for the covering physician.

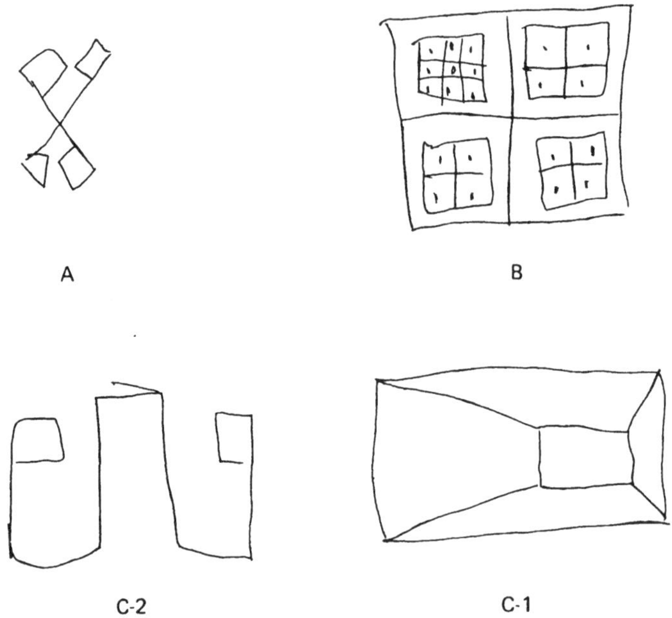

FIGURE 8.9. Case D.R. Wechsler Memory Scale–Visual Reproduction: delayed recall. On figure B, she began to draw the figure incorrectly. She was instructed to draw the remainder of the figure correctly, and she complied. Reduced by 50%.

Impressions and Recommendations

The patient's test behavior and scores on tests designed to evaluate the presence of functional complaints suggest that the patient either consciously or nonconsciously was attempting to present herself as impaired. In spite of this lack of cooperation, minimal evidence of cognitive dysfunction appeared in the test results. The patient's melodramatic manner and refusal to complete the personality testing would argue that she was not consciously malingering; a person deliberately attempting to feign impairment would be expected to comply with all testing but to provide spurious responses. By refusing to take tests one would run the risk of alienating and arousing the suspicions of the examiner and the success of the malingering effort would be placed in jeopardy.

It is our opinion that the patient has long-standing, histrionic, dependent personality features that preceded her injury. Since her accident, Ms. R.'s whole identity seems to have been reorganized around being a head trauma victim; she attends a head trauma support group and clearly identifies with these impaired individuals; "I have the same symptoms they do . . . drooling [etc.]." Her numerous symptoms have elicited much caregiving from others, and she may enjoy this attention and desire to have it continue. For example, following her injury she reports that she moved briefly to her parents' home because she was "starving to death" and they took care of her, and she states that when she is incapacitated by her headaches she has to rely on her son to dispense her medications. As a result of her injury, she is able to see a therapist regularly and receive consultation in pain management. She may in fact be experiencing the physical symptoms she reported, but through her association with head trauma victims, she certainly has been educated as to the symptoms associated with head trauma and either consciously or unconsciously may be simulating them. In addition, review of medical records indicated that the patient was reporting the presence of virtually identical symptoms long before the injury three-and-one-half years ago.

We feel it would be beneficial if Ms. R. stopped receiving attention for "sick" behavior and instead began experiencing attention and reinforcement for productive behavior. For example, she would probably receive more benefit from attending a job-skills development group rather than a head-trauma group. Direct confrontation of the patient regarding the nature of her exaggerated symptomology would not be effective and would only serve to further anger her and result in an escalation of symptoms.

NEUROPSYCHOLOGY TEST SCORE SUMMARY SHEET

Patient: D.R. Age: 41 Sex: F Handedness: R

I. Intelligence WAIS-R Age-Corrected Scores

VERBAL			PERFORMANCE		
Information	15	(95 %ile)	Picture Completion	13	(84 %ile)
Digit Span	7	(16 %ile)	Picture Arrangement	12	(75 %ile)
Vocabulary	10	(50 %ile)	Block Design	11	(63 %ile)
Arithmetic	8	(25 %ile)	Object Assembly	8	(25 %ile)
Comprehension	8	(25 %ile)	Digit Symbol	8	(25 %ile)
Similarities	15	(95 %ile)			
VERBAL IQ =	100	(50 %ile)	PERFORMANCE IQ =	98	(45 %ile)

FULL SCALE IQ = 99 (47 %ile)

II. Attention/Concentration
Digit Span: 5 forward + 3 backwards = 8 Total (16 %ile)
Mental Control, WMS: 6 (37 %ile)
Trails A: 35" (20 %ile), Trails B: 85" (25 %ile)

III. Language
Aphasia Screening Exam: intact

IV. Perceptual/Organizational
Rey-Osterrieth Complex Figure Copy: 36/36 (100 %ile)
Hooper Visual Organization Test: 29 /30

V. Memory

VERBAL	NONVERBAL
WMS Logical Memory 7.5 (41 %ile)	WMS Visual Repro.: 13 (92 %ile)
45 min. delay: 7.25	45 min. delay: 13
Percent retention: 97	Percent retention: 100
WMS Associate Learning I Easy 6 , 6 , 6	Rey-Osterrieth Fig: 36 (100 %ile)
I Hard 0 , 2 , 2	3 min. delay: 29 (90 %ile)
I Score: 13 (39 %ile)	
45 min. delay: 6 easy, 2 hard 100 % retention	

Rey Auditory Verbal Learning Test (15 items):
T1: 5 T2: 9 T3: 8 T4: 10 T5: 9 Recall after Interference 5
Recognition: 14 Hits, 2 False Identifications

VI. Personality
MMPI: 23*681'70-954/ L/F-K:

VII. Tests for Malingering
15 Item Memorization: 9
Dot Counting 1: 3", 2: 13", 3: 8", 4: 16", 5: 23", 6: 45"

Commentary on Feigning of Deficits Cases

As noted in each report, every case was in litigation. Confirmation of creation or exaggeration of symptoms was obtained on the patients through various means. In Case 1, an evaluating psychiatrist had suspected malingering and reported to the examiner several months following the neuropsychological evaluation that the patient had been documented on film changing the carburetor in his car, providing evidence that the patient was not grossly impaired (demented) as portrayed in his test-taking behavior. In the two remaining cases, the treating physicians and therapists had strongly suspected a functional explanation for the symptoms, and EEG and CT scans were negative in all cases except for Case 1. In Case 3, the psychologist associated with the patient's head trauma support group reported that the treatment staff were aware that the patient's behavioral presentation was very different than that seen in the other group members. Only in Case 1 was the examiner informed prior to the testing that a nonorganic etiology for the symptoms was suspected; in Case 3 records were forwarded to the examiner after the testing was completed.

It has been our experience that nonconscious development of cognitive symptoms in association with significant personality disorder is more common than deliberate faking of symptoms, but of course the population characteristics will depend on the clinical setting.

The hallmark characteristic of each test protocol was the illogical inconsistency in performance across similar cognitive tasks, the inconsistency between test performance and level of functioning in activities of daily living, and performance that did not fit with known syndromes from a neuropsychological standpoint. No typical pattern of impaired performance appeared; the first two patients exhibited gross diffuse depression of performance, whereas the third patient showed negligible deficits.

Administration of the tests for functional complaints described by Lezak (1983) was very helpful in detecting questionable motivation and cooperation in testing. In addition, the cases illuminate the importance of obtaining personality testing. In Case 1, involving probable malingering, the patient's responses to projective testing failed to reveal psychiatric disturbance of the same severity as that exhibited in the patient's overt behavior during the testing session. In the latter two cases of probable nonconscious symptom production, significant characterological pathology including hysterical traits was documented.

Observation of patient 3's behavior during the testing revealed a pattern in which she would be quite animated and talkative when describing the accident and subsequent symptomology, but would become very passive and withholding when the actual testing began. Uniformly all patients showed unconcern and indifference regarding their test performances despite intact awareness of cognitive problems. This was in contrast to the common frustration demonstrated by patients with actual brain dysfunction.

Case 1 illustrates the usefulness of sequential testing; part of the evidence that the patient was malingering stemmed from observations that he performed worse on some tasks on retesting than he had during the original neuropsychological evaluation several months previous. This case also demonstrates the importance of obtaining descriptions of the patient's functioning from family members. In this case the patient's mother had described difficulties the patient was experiencing, but her description in no way matched the severity of dysfunction manifested by the patient in person, further bolstering the examiner's perception that the patient was feigning his symptoms.

Case 3 illustrates the often bizarre presenting complaints that can cue the examiner to the presence of a functional as compared to true organic condition (e.g., inability to "look through plastic," forgetting to use utensils when cooking food on the stove and using hands to turn food over in the pan, having her gaze become fixated on windshield wipers and overhead beams of parking structures, drooling).

Appendix

TABLE A. Percentile ranks and IQ equivalents for corresponding Z-scores.

Range	% rank		IQ equivalent	
SD or Z	+SD	−SD	+SD	−SD
2.17–3.00	99	1	133+	67−
1.96–2.16	98	2	130–132	68–70
1.82–1.95	97	3	127–129	71–72
1.70–1.81	96	4	126	73–74
1.60–1.69	95	5	124–125	75–76
1.52–1.59	94	6	123	77
1.44–1.51	93	7	122	78
1.38–1.43	92	8	121	79
1.32–1.37	91	9	120	80
1.26–1.31	90	10	119	81
1.21–1.25	89	11		
1.16–1.20	88	12	118	82
1.11–1.15	87	13	117	83
1.06–1.10	86	14	116	84
1.02–1.05	85	15		
.98–1.01	84	16	115	85
.94– .97	83	17		
.90– .93	82	18	114	86
.86– .89	81	19	113	87
.83– .85	80	20		
.79– .82	79	21	112	88
.76– .78	78	22		
.73– .75	77	23	111	89
.70– .75	76	24		
.64– .69	75	25	110	90
.63– .65	74	26		
.60– .62	73	27	109	91
.57– .59	72	28		
.54– .56	71	29		
.51– .53	70	30	108	92
.49– .50	69	31		
.46– .48	68	32	107	93
.43– .45	67	33		
.40– .42	66	34		94

TABLE A. *Continued.*

Range SD or Z	% rank +SD	% rank −SD	IQ equivalent +SD	IQ equivalent −SD
.38– .39	65	35	106	
.35– .37	64	36		
.32– .34	63	37	105	95
.30– .31	62	38		
.27– .29	61	39	104	96
.25– .26	60	40		
.22– .24	59	41		
.19– .21	58	42	103	97
.17– .18	57	43		
.14– .16	56	44		
.12– .13	55	45	102	98
.09– .11	54	46		
.07– .08	53	47	101	99
.04– .06	52	48		
.02– .03	51	49	100	100

TABLE B. Classification of ability levels.

Classification	Z-score	Percent included	Lower limit of percentile range
Very superior	+2.0 and above	2.2	98
Superior	+1.3 to +2.0	6.7	91
High average	+0.6 to +1.3	16.1	75
Average	±0.6	50.0	25
Low average	−0.6 to −1.3	16.1	9
Borderline	−1.3 to −2.0	6.7	2
Retarded	−2.0 and below	2.2	–

TABLE C. References for nueuropsychological test normative data.

Neuropsychological test	References
Consonant Trigrams Test	Stuss et al. (1982; 1985)
Controlled Word Association Test	Benton (cited in Lezak, 1976)
Finger Tapping Test	Bornstein (1985)
Grip Strength	Bornstein (1985)
Grooved Pegboard	Bornstein (1985)
Mini-Mental State Exam	Folstein, Folstein, & McHugh (1975)
Rey Auditory Verbal Learning Test	Lezak (1983); Butters et al. (1986); Mungas (1983)
Rey-Osterrieth Complex Figure	Osterrieth (cited in Lezak, 1983)
Rey Tangled Lines Test	Lezak (1976)
Shopping List Test	McCarthy et al. (1981)
Stroop Test	Comalli, Wapner, & Werner (1962)
Trail Making Test	Bornstein (1985)
Wechsler Memory Scale	Hulicka (1966); Halland et al. (1983); Delaney et al. (1980); Lezak (1983)

Author Index

Subject Index

MIX
Papier aus verantwortungsvollen Quellen
Paper from responsible sources
FSC® C105338

If you have any concerns about our products,
you can contact us on
ProductSafety@springernature.com

In case Publisher is established outside the EU,
the EU authorized representative is:
Springer Nature Customer Service Center GmbH
Europaplatz 3, 69115 Heidelberg, Germany

Printed by Libri Plureos GmbH
in Hamburg, Germany